Yearbook of
Anesthesiology 13
2024

Indian College of Anaesthesiologists

Office Bearers

Dr B Radhakrishnan
Chief Trustee/Chairman/Vice-Chancellor

Dr Jayashree Sood
President

Dr Baljit Singh
CEO

Dr Kanchi Muralidhar
Dean National

Dr Kumar Belani
Dean International

Dr Kirti N Saxena
Editor-in-Chief, Journal of Indian College of Anaesthesiologists

Dr Mukul Chandra Kapoor
Editor, Yearbook of Anesthesiology

Dr Saneesh PJ
Deputy Dean

Board of Trustees

- Dr Manorama Mittal
- Dr B Radhakrishnan
- Dr Jayashree Sood
- Dr Baljit Singh
- Dr LD Mishra
- Dr Vijay Vohra
- Dr Kanchi Muralidhar
- Dr Roshan Lal Garg
- Dr Surinder Mohan Sharma
- Dr Bimla Sharma
- Dr Pradeep Jain
- Dr Kumar Belani
- Dr Raminder Sehgal
- Dr Naveen Malhotra
- Dr Kamal Fotedar
- Dr Manjula Sarkar
- Dr Mukul Chandra Kapoor

Yearbook of Anesthesiology 13
2024

Editors

Mukul Chandra Kapoor
MBBS MD DNB MNAMS
Chief Consultant, Professor, and Head
Department of Anesthesiology and Critical Care
Amrita Institute of Medical Sciences and Amrita Hospitals
Faridabad, Haryana, India
Chief Editor, Annals of Cardiac Anaesthesia
Director, Scientific Committee
Indian Resuscitation Council Federation (IRCF)
National Adviser, Indian Journal of Anaesthesiology
Former Professor and Senior Adviser
Anesthesiology and Cardiac Anesthesiology, Armed Forces Medical Services
Former President
Indian Association of Cardiovascular Thoracic Anaesthesiologists (IACTA)

Baljit Singh
MD FICA
Professor and Head
Anesthesiology and Intensive Care
SGT University
Gurugram, Haryana, India
CEO, Indian College of Anaesthesiologists
Former Professor (Anesthesiology)
GB Pant Hospital, New Delhi, India

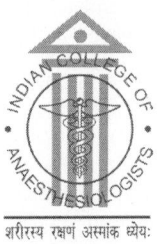

शरीरस्य रक्षणं अस्मांक ध्येय:

Indian College of Anaesthesiologists

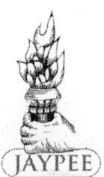

JAYPEE BROTHERS MEDICAL PUBLISHERS
The Health Sciences Publisher
New Delhi | London

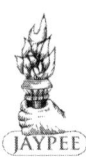 **Jaypee Brothers Medical Publishers (P) Ltd**

Headquarters
Jaypee Brothers Medical Publishers (P) Ltd
EMCA House, 23/23-B
Ansari Road, Daryaganj
New Delhi 110 002, India
Landline: +91-11-23272143, +91-11-23272703
+91-11-23282021, +91-11-23245672
Email: jaypee@jaypeebrothers.com

Corporate Office
Jaypee Brothers Medical Publishers (P) Ltd
4838/24, Ansari Road, Daryaganj
New Delhi 110 002, India
Phone: +91-11-43574357
Fax: +91-11-43574314
Email: jaypee@jaypeebrothers.com

Overseas Office
JP Medical Ltd.
83, Victoria Street, London
SW1H 0HW (UK)
Phone: +44 20 3170 8910
Fax: +44 (0)20 3008 6180
Email: info@jpmedpub.com

Website: www.jaypeebrothers.com
Website: www.jaypeedigital.com

© 2024, Jaypee Brothers Medical Publishers

The views and opinions expressed in this book are solely those of the original contributor(s)/author(s) and do not necessarily represent those of editor(s) or publisher of the book.

All rights reserved. No part of this publication may be reproduced, stored or transmitted in any form or by any means, electronic, mechanical, photo copying, recording or otherwise, without the prior permission in writing of the publishers.

All brand names and product names used in this book are trade names, service marks, trademarks or registered trademarks of their respective owners. The publisher is not associated with any product or vendor mentioned in this book.

Medical knowledge and practice change constantly. This book is designed to provide accurate, authoritative information about the subject matter in question. However, readers are advised to check the most current information available on procedures included and check information from the manufacturer of each product to be administered, to verify the recommended dose, formula, method and duration of administration, adverse effects and contra indications. It is the responsibility of the practitioner to take all appropriate safety precautions. Neither the publisher nor the author(s)/editor(s) assume any liability for any injury and/or damage to persons or property arising from or related to use of material in this book.

This book is sold on the understanding that the publisher is not engaged in providing professional medical services. If such advice or services are required, the services of a competent medical professional should be sought.

Every effort has been made where necessary to contact holders of copyright to obtain permission to reproduce copyright material. If any have been inadvertently overlooked, the publisher will be pleased to make the necessary arrangements at the first opportunity.

Inquiries for bulk sales may be solicited at: jaypee@jaypeebrothers.com

***Yearbook of Anesthesiology 13** 2024*

First Edition: **2024**

ISBN: 978-93-5696-438-9

Printed at: Replika Press Pvt. Ltd.

Dedicated to

Anesthesiology and Critical Care Physicians who toil hard to sustain life. The Anesthesiologists remain behind the screen and seldom get the appreciation they deserve from their patients. Critical Care Physicians are constantly on their toes, see much mortality, and get appreciated often. However, they also face the ire of the patients' relatives and, at times, violence when their patients die!

Contributors

Achal Dhir
MD FRCA FRCPC Diplomate NBE
(Perioperative TEE)
Professor
Department of Anesthesia and
Perioperative Medicine
London Health Sciences Centre
University of Western Ontario
London, Ontario, Canada N6A 5A5

A Kumar MD EDIC FANZCA
Senior Consultant and Anesthetist
Department of Anesthesia
The Queen Elizabeth Hospital
Clinical Senior Lecturer
Discipline of Acute Care Medicine
University of Adelaide
Adelaide, Australia

Amit Prakash MD FRCA EDIC
Consultant
Department of Anesthesia and
Perioperative Medicine
Cambridge University Hospitals
Cambridge, UK

Anavi Prakash
Final Year Medical Student
Faculty of Medicine
Imperial College London
South Kensington Campus, London, UK

Andrea Carsetti MD
Professor
Department of Biomedical Sciences
and Public Health
Università Politecnica delle Marche
Ancona, Italy
Anesthesia and Intensive Care Unit
Azienda Ospedaliero Universitaria
delle Marche, Ancona, Italy

Anisha Nagaria MBBS MD
Assistant Professor
Department of Anesthesiology
and Pain Medicine
Pt JNM Medical College
Raipur, Chhattisgarh, India

Anjali Gera MBBS MD PGDMLE FICA
Senior Consultant
Institute of Anesthesiology, Pain,
and Perioperative Medicine
Sir Ganga Ram Hospital
New Delhi, India

Ashish Sinha MD PhD MBA MSEd FASA
Professor, Loma Linda University
Department of Anesthesiology
Riverside University Health System
Moreno Valley, CA, USA

**Balavenkatasubramanian
Jagannathan** MBBS MD DA
Academic Director and Senior
Consultant, Department of Anesthesia
and Perioperative Medicine
Ganga Medical Centre and Hospital
Coimbatore, Tamil Nadu, India

Baljit Singh MD FICA
Professor and Head
Anesthesiology and Intensive Care
SGT University
Gurugram, Haryana, India
CEO, Indian College of Anaesthesiologists
Former Professor (Anesthesiology)
GB Pant Hospital, New Delhi, India

Bharti Wadhwa MD
Director Professor
Department of Anesthesiology
Maulana Azad Medical College
New Delhi, India

Bimla Sharma
MBBS DGO MD MBA (HCS) FICA
Head
Department of Palliative Medicine
Sir Ganga Ram Hospital
New Delhi, India

Dave Barrett MD MMed BSc
Medical Doctor
Western Australia Country Health
Service, Albany Hospital, University
of Notre Dame, Warrenup, Australia

Contributors

Deepak Pahwa MBBS MD
Senior Consultant (Anesthesiology)
Department of Anesthesiology
Amrita Institute of Medical Sciences
Faridabad, Haryana, India

Eric King BSc MD
Anesthesiologist
Department of Anesthesia
Schulich School of Medicine
Western University
London, Ontario, Canada

Gaurav Kakkar
MBBS (AFMC) FCARCSI CCT (UK) FSNCC
Senior Consultant and Lead
Neuroanesthesia and Neurocritical Care
Amrita Institute of Medical Sciences
Faridabad, Haryana, India

Gian Ignacio BS
Department of Biomedical Engineering
Warren Alpert Medical School
of Brown University
Providence, RI, USA

GS Wander MD DM (Cardiology)
Professor and Head
Department of Cardiology
Hero DMC Heart Institute
Ludhiana, Punjab, India

Haad Arif BS
MD Student
University of California
Riverside School of Medicine
Riverside, CA, USA

Harriette Beard
MBBS BSc (Hons) MRCP FRCA
Anesthetic Registrar
Department of Anesthetics
Cambridge University Hospitals
Cambridge, UK

Harsimran Kaur MBBS MD
Clinical Fellow
Department of Anesthesia and
Pain Medicine
Mount Sinai Hospital
University of Toronto, Toronto, Canada

Hesham Youssef MD FRCPC MBBCh MSc
Assistant Professor
Department of Anesthesia and
Perioperative Medicine
London Health Sciences Centre
University of Western Ontario
London, Ontario, Canada N6A 5A5

Ioana Pasca MD FCCM
Associate Professor
Department of Anesthesiology
Riverside University Health System
Moreno Valley, CA, USA

Kiran Mahendru DM
Assistant Professor
Department of Anesthesiology
Hero DMC Heart Institute
Ludhiana, Punjab, India

Laima M MD
Senior Consultant
Department of Anesthesia and
Intensive Care
South Jutland Hospital
Aabenraa, Denmark

Mukul Chandra Kapoor
MBBS MD DNB MNAMS
Chief Consultant, Professor, and Head
Department of Anesthesiology
and Critical Care
Amrita Institute of Medical Sciences
and Amrita Hospitals
Faridabad, Haryana, India
Chief Editor
Annals of Cardiac Anaesthesia
Director, Scientific Committee
Indian Resuscitation Council Federation
(IRCF)
National Adviser, Indian Journal
of Anaesthesiology
Former Professor and Senior Adviser
Anesthesiology and Cardiac
Anesthesiology
Armed Forces Medical Services
Former President
Indian Association of Cardiovascular
Thoracic Anaesthesiologists (IACTA)

Contributors

Neerja Bhardwaj MD (Anesthesia)
Former Professor and Head
Department of Anesthesia and
Intensive Care
Postgraduate Institute of Medical
Education and Research
Chandigarh, India

Niti Batra MD IDRA
Senior Consultant
Department of Anesthesiology
Amrita Institute of Medical Sciences
Faridabad, Haryana, India
AHA Certified Instructor, ATLS Provider,
Member of ISA, ICA, IAPA, AMF

Pallavi Ahluwalia MD (Anes) PGDHHM
CCEPC MNAMS FIMSA FRCP (Glas)
Professor
Department of Anesthesia
Teerthanker Mahaveer Medical College
Moradabad, Uttar Pradesh, India

Pradeep Bhatia MD
Professor and Head
Department of Anesthesiology
and Critical Care
All India Institute of Medical Sciences
Jodhpur, Rajasthan, India

Prathamesh Milind Patwardhan MBBS DNB (Anesthesia)
Postdoctoral Fellow in Neuroanesthesia (NIMHANS)
Specialty Doctor in Anesthesia
and Intensive Care
The Southport and Ormskirk Hospital
NHS Trust, Liverpool, UK
Former Clinical Fellow in
Neuroanesthesia and Neurocritical Care
The Walton Centre NHS
Foundation Trust, Liverpool, UK

Pratibha Jain Shah MBBS MD FICA FIPM
Professor and Head
Department of Anesthesiology
and Pain Medicine
Pt JNM Medical College
Raipur, Chhattisgarh, India

Puneet Khanna MD
Additional Professor
Department of Anesthesiology, Pain
Medicine, and Critical Care
All India Institute of Medical Sciences
New Delhi, India

Rajesh Bhavsar MD PHD
Senior Consultant
Department of Anesthesia and
Intensive Care
South Jutland Hospital
Aabenraa, Denmark
Post-Doc Scholar
Odense University Hospital, Denmark

Rajiv Chawla MD DNB
Head
Department of Anesthesiology
Rajiv Gandhi Cancer Institute and
Research Centre, New Delhi, India

Ravi P Kanojia
MBBS MS MCh (Pediatric Surgery) MRCS
(Glasgow) MNAMS FIAPS FACS FAIS
Professor
Department of Pediatric Surgery
Postgraduate Institute of Medical
Education and Research
Chandigarh, India

Riccardo Antolini MD
Department of Biomedical Sciences
and Public Health
Università Politecnica delle Marche
Ancona, Italy

Sandeep Lakhani
MBBS MD (Anaes) FRCA FFICM
Consultant in Neuroanesthesia
and Neurocritical Care
Divisional Clinical Director
Neurosurgical Division
The Walton Centre NHS
Foundation Trust, Liverpool, UK
Council Member, Royal College
of Anaesthetists, UK
Chair, Clinical Leaders in Anaesthesia
Network (CLAN)
Royal College of Anaesthetists, UK

Contributors

Sathish Rajaselvam Parameswaran MBBS MD DNB
Junior Consultant
Department of Anesthesia and Perioperative Medicine
Ganga Medical Centre and Hospital
Coimbatore, Tamil Nadu, India

Shagun Bhatia Shah MBBS DA DNB
Senior Consultant
Department of Anesthesiology
Rajiv Gandhi Cancer Institute and Research Centre, New Delhi, India

Shalini Dhir MBBS MD FRCPC MSc (Edin)
Associate Professor and Director
Regional Anesthesia and Acute Pain Services, Department of Anesthesia
Schulich School of Medicine
Western University
London, Ontario, Canada

Shireen Edmends
MBBS DA MMedSci FRCA FANZCA
Consultant Anesthetist
WA Country Health Service Great Southern Warden Avenue
Albany WA 6330

Skule Bakke MD
Senior Consultant
Department of Anesthesia and Intensive Care, South Jutland Hospital
Aabenraa, Denmark

Sophia TH Chew
MBBS MMED (Anaes) FANZCA FAMS
Senior Consultant
Department of Anesthesiology
Singapore General Hospital, Singapore

Stefano Falcetta MD
Medical Director
Anesthesia and Intensive Care Unit
Azienda Ospedaliero Universitaria delle Marche, Ancona, Italy

Swati Chhabra MD DNB
Additional Professor
Department of Anesthesiology and Critical Care
All India Institute of Medical Sciences
Jodhpur, Rajasthan, India

Tejal Desai MBBS DNB FCAI Diplomate NBE (Perioperative TEE)
Assistant Professor
Department of Anesthesia and Perioperative Medicine
London Health Sciences Centre
University of Western Ontario
London, Ontario, Canada N6A 5A5

Thomas Stroem MD PhD
Professor
Department of Anesthesia and Intensive Care
South Jutland Hospital
Aabenraa, Denmark
Senior Consultant
Odense University Hospital, Denmark

Uma Hariharan MBBS
Professor
Department of Critical Care Medicine
Atal Bihari Vajpayee Institute of Medical Sciences and Dr Ram Manohar Lohia Hospital
New Delhi, India

Venkatesan Thiruvenkatarajan MD DA DNB FANZCA
Senior Consultant Anesthetist
Department of Anesthesia
The Queen Elizabeth Hospital
Clinical Associate Professor
Discipline of Acute Care Medicine
University of Adelaide
Adelaide, Australia

Vivekanandan Natarajan MBBS MD
Consultant, Department of Anesthesia and Perioperative Medicine
Ganga Medical Centre and Hospital
Coimbatore, Tamil Nadu, India

Vivek Gupta
DA DNB (Anaesth) FIACTA FICCM
Consultant
Department of Cardiac Anesthesia and Intensive Care
Hero DMC Heart Institute
Ludhiana, Punjab, India

Foreword

Writing a foreword for the *Yearbook of Anesthesiology 13* gives me great pleasure.

The topics are well chosen and include recent advances such as ECMO, Artificial Intelligence, and End-of-Life Care, which will shortly become an essential modality in the armamentarium of the Anesthesiologist.

The chapters are written in simple language that the younger anesthesiologists can easily comprehend.

The authors are all masters in their fields and have contributed with scientific expertise.

The editors, Dr Mukul Chandra Kapoor and Dr Baljit Singh have chosen the authors for this yearbook.

I congratulate all the contributors and the editors for this edition which I am sure will become a must-read for all the anesthesiologists.

Jayashree Sood
MD FFARCS PGDHHM FICA
President
Indian College of Anaesthesiologists
Chairperson
Institute of Anesthesiology, Pain, and Perioperative Medicine
Honorary Secretary, Board of Management
Sir Ganga Ram Hospital
New Delhi, India

Preface

As for the future, your task is not to foresee it but to enable it.
–**Antoine de Saint Exupery**

Anesthesiology and critical care have witnessed remarkable advances in recent years, revolutionizing patient care and improving outcomes. Technological innovations, drug development, and a deeper understanding of human physiology have driven these advancements. The integration of precision medicine, advanced monitoring technologies, minimally invasive surgical techniques, widespread adoption of telemedicine, and enhanced training have collectively raised the standard of care in these fields. In this 13th edition of the *Yearbook of Anesthesiology*, we explore some of the most significant recent advances in anesthesia and critical care and their impact on patient safety and outcomes.

Anesthesiologists are the backbones of all healthcare establishments. They are masters of acute care and the prime movers for safe surgery. Anesthesiologists tailor anesthetic agents and medications to an individual's physiological and pathological status to enhance comfort, safety, and efficacy. They are crucial in optimizing patient conditions for surgical and interventional procedures and planning the administration of anesthesia, sedation, and analgesia. The specialty is constantly progressing to maximize patient comfort and care.

The specialty of critical care has evolved from Anesthesiology. Most physicians practicing critical care today have their basic training in Anesthesiology, and in many ways, it is considered a subspecialty of Anesthesiology. Critical care made significant progress during the COVID-19 epidemic in managing the deadly multisystemic disease. Extracorporeal membrane oxygenator (ECMO) support is a life-saving procedure that has prospered over the last few years. It is today considered the "Bridge to Lung Transplant." In this book, we describe the management of ECMO support.

The advent of advanced monitoring technologies and data analytics has transformed operating rooms and critical care units. Continuous monitoring of vital signs, organ function, and laboratory values provides healthcare providers' real-time information about a patient's condition. Additionally, artificial intelligence and machine-learning algorithms analyze this data to detect subtle changes that may indicate deterioration or the need for intervention. These technologies have enabled early identification of complications, timely interventions, and improved safety. Anesthesiology is matching up with advancements in technology. We deliberate on objective pain monitoring using artificial intelligence-based monitors in this issue.

Minimally invasive surgeries, such as robotic procedures, have become increasingly common. The use of robots in surgery is expanding at a rapid pace. Robotic surgeries offer several advantages, including smaller incisions, reduced pain, shorter hospital stays, and quicker recovery times. Robotic assistance is increasingly used today in the pediatric population. We inform our readers about how to manage such cases.

Ultrasound-guided regional anesthesia has become a safer and more effective alternative to traditional techniques. This approach allows Anesthesiologists to precisely locate nerves and blood vessels to administer anesthesia directly to the affected area and safely access blood vessels. Its use is reducing the risk of complications and improving postoperative pain management. Ultrasound enables real-time visualization of the spread of anesthesia, ensuring better control and optimizing patient comfort. New unusual blocks are being developed for regional anesthesia. Ultrasound has also entered the arena of airway in a big way. We describe the administration of some not-so-common blocks.

Humankind needs to tackle environmental degeneration emergently. Scientists are working tirelessly to help preserve the environment. Anesthesiologists need to develop protocols to reduce our contribution to environmental pollution. Total Intravenous Anesthesia is a step towards that the anesthesiologists need more awareness of total intravenous anesthesia's conduct, so we have deliberated on the subject too.

New commercial ventures have started in the field of space tourism. Commercial spacecrafts are carrying humans for pleasure trips in space. Anesthesiologists must be prepared to manage surgery and critical care on other planets, space missions, and stations. We delved into a futuristic chapter describing potential issues in anesthesia delivery in zero-gravity situations.

The Indian College of Anesthesiologists (ICP) has promoted education and dissemination of current knowledge and advances by regularly bringing out this book on Recent Advances in Anesthesiology for the last 13 years. We endeavor to ensure that the anesthesiologists of our country benefit from this publication. We want to express our gratitude to this book's esteemed contributors, who have put much effort into sharing their expertise with the readers. Thanks to their invaluable contributions, this book is a resounding success every year.

Recent advances in anesthesiology and critical care have ushered in a new era of patient safety, precision, and improved outcomes. As technology evolves and our understanding of patient physiology deepens, we can expect even more ground-breaking developments to enhance the practice of anesthesia and critical care. Indian College of Anesthesiologists will continue to bring out this yearly book of Recent Advances in Anesthesiology for the benefit of the profession.

Mukul Chandra Kapoor
Baljit Singh

Contents

1. **Ultrasound for Airway Assessment** 1
   Riccardo Antolini, Stefano Falcetta, Andrea Carsetti
   - Use of the Probe *3*
   - Ultrasound Anatomy of the Upper Airway *3*
   - Assessment of Difficult Airways Using Ultrasound *8*
   - Confirmation of Endotracheal Intubation *9*
   - Laryngeal Edema Assessment *10*
   - Evaluation for Percutaneous Tracheostomy *11*
   - Evaluation for Cricothyrotomy *11*
   - Pediatric Patients *12*

2. **Negative Pressure Pulmonary Edema** 16
   Niti Batra
   - Pathophysiology *17*
   - Clinical Features *20*
   - Diagnosis *21*
   - Investigations *24*
   - Management *26*

3. **Uncommonly Performed Regional Anesthesia Techniques** 30
   Deepak Pahwa
   - Sphenopalatine Ganglion Block *31*
   - Superior Trunk Block *33*
   - Selective Trunk Block *36*
   - Clavipectoral Fascial Plane Block *37*
   - Medial Cutaneous Nerve of Forearm Block *39*
   - Lateral Cutaneous Nerve of Forearm Block *41*
   - Transversus Thoracic Plane Block/Parasternal Intercostal Plane Block *42*
   - External Oblique Intercostal Plane Block *45*
   - Genitofemoral Nerve Block *47*
   - Pudendal Nerve Block *49*
   - Sacral Multifidus Plane Block *51*
   - Deep Posterior Gluteal Compartment Block *51*

4. **Continuous Spinal Anesthesia** 57
   Pratibha Jain Shah, Anisha Nagaria
   - Historical Background *59*
   - Advantages *60*

- Indications *61*
- Contraindications *61*
- Equipment (Kit) Required *62*
- Technique of Continuous Spinal Anesthesia *64*
- Drugs to be Used *65*
- Problems/Complications *65*
- Continuous Spinal Anesthesia in Obstetrics *67*

5. **The Impact of Perioperative Variables on Morbidity and Mortality of Elderly Hip Fractures** 71
   Ioana Pasca, Haad Arif, Gian Ignacio, Ashish Sinha

   - Type of Fractures *72*
   - Age and Sex *72*
   - Frailty *73*
   - Comorbidities *75*
   - Kidney Disease *76*
   - Chronic Obstructive Pulmonary Disease *77*
   - Cognitive Impairment *77*
   - Infection *78*
   - Causes of Mortality *78*
   - Postoperative Delirium *87*
   - General versus Regional Anesthesia *88*
   - Hypotension *88*

6. **Anesthesia for Spine Surgeries** 97
   Balavenkatasubramanian Jagannathan, Vivekanandan Natarajan, Sathish Rajaselvam Parameswaran

   - Preanesthetic Considerations and Assessment *98*
   - Physiological Changes of Positioning in Spine Surgeries *101*
   - Positioning—Anesthetic Considerations *101*
   - Anesthetic Drugs *104*
   - Anesthetic Equipment *106*
   - Anesthetic Techniques *109*
   - Anterior Approach for Thoracic Spine Surgeries *110*
   - Complications and their Prevention *111*

7. **Total Intravenous Anesthesia: Basic Principles and Practical Aspects** 117
   Gaurav Kakkar

   - History *118*
   - TIVA or TCI: What is the Difference? Or are They Identical? *119*
   - Benefits of Total Intravenous Anesthesia *119*
   - Disadvantages of Total Intravenous Anesthesia *120*
   - Pharmacokinetics *121*

- Commonly Used Models *123*
- Commonly Used Terminologies *124*
- TIVA in Special Circumstances: Elderly/Pediatrics/Obese *125*
- Practical Aspects: Fifteen Rules for TIVA *125*
- Total Intravenous Anesthesia Outside the Operating Room *127*
- Total Intravenous Anesthesia in India *127*

8. **The Contemporary Perioperative Management of Pheochromocytoma** 130
   A Kumar, Venkatesan Thiruvenkatarajan
   - Etiology and Epidemiology *131*
   - Clinical Features *131*
   - Biochemical Investigations and Imaging *132*
   - Preoperative Evaluation and Preparation *132*
   - Pharmacological Preparation for Blood Pressure Control *133*
   - Assessment and Optimization of Myocardial Function *135*
   - Intravascular Volume Optimization *136*
   - Surgical Approach *136*
   - Anesthesia Management *137*
   - Intraoperative Hemodynamic Response *142*
   - Postoperative Management *144*
   - Specific Scenarios *144*

9. **Sedation for Healthcare Interventions: Should Anesthetists be Worried?** 151
   Harriette Beard, Anavi Prakash, Amit Prakash
   - Sedation Outside the Operating Room *152*
   - Patient Selection *155*
   - Monitoring *155*
   - Pharmacology *157*
   - Recovery and Discharge *158*
   - Training *159*
   - Governance *160*

10. **Space: The New Frontier for Nonoperating Room Anesthesia** 162
    Shagun Bhatia Shah, Rajiv Chawla, Uma Hariharan
    - Stressors in the Space Milieu *164*
    - Pathophysiological Effects on the Human Body *164*
    - Logistic Issues *167*
    - The Damage Control Philosophy *167*
    - Surgical Considerations *168*
    - Anesthetic Considerations *169*

- General Anesthesia *173*
- Cardiopulmonary Resuscitation in Space *176*
- Telemedicine Technology *176*
- Imaging Techniques *177*
- Aerospace Medicine Sieve *177*
- Future Directions *178*

11. Premedication in Pediatric Anesthesia 183
Dave Barrett, Shireen Edmends

- Psychological Factors *184*
- Extrinsic Factors *184*
- Choosing the Ideal Agent *184*
- Discussion of Common Agents *185*

12. Anesthesia for Robotic Surgeries in Children 200
Neerja Bhardwaj, Ravi P Kanojia

- The Robotic System *202*
- Laparoscopic Surgery *204*
- Prerequisites for Robotic Procedures *208*
- Preoperative Assessment and Investigations *209*
- Monitoring *210*
- Anesthesia Management *210*
- Postoperative Management of Pain *212*
- Complications *212*

13. Hepatobiliary Disease and Anesthesia 216
Tejal Desai, Hesham Youssef, Achal Dhir

- Anatomy and Physiology *217*
- Liver Disease *219*
- Other System Involvement in Liver Disease *223*
- Scoring Systems *227*
- Patients with Hepatobiliary Disease Coming for Nonhepatic Surgery: Perioperative Risks *229*
- Patients with Hepatobiliary Disease Presenting for Nonhepatic Surgery: Preoperative Assessment *229*
- Preoperative Investigations *230*
- Anesthetic Management of Patients with Chronic Liver Disease *231*

14. Acute Kidney Disease and Anesthesia 241
Sophia TH Chew

- Definition of Acute Kidney Injury *242*
- Normal Physiology of the Kidneys *244*
- Pathophysiology of Acute Kidney Injury *244*

- Formation of Microvascular Thrombi *245*
- Risk Prediction Models *246*
- Perioperative Patient Management *251*
- Renal Replacement Therapy *254*
- Outcomes of Acute Kidney Injury and Acute Kidney Disease *254*
- Postoperative Monitoring and Management *255*

15. Perioperative Management and Anesthetic Implications of Drug Addiction and Substance Abuse 260
Puneet Khanna

- Screening for Substance Abuse *262*
- Opioid Use Disorders *262*
- Alcohol *263*
- Cannabis *264*
- Nicotine *264*
- Vaping Substances *264*

16. Anticoagulation and Regional Anesthesia 267
Eric King, Harsimran Kaur, Shalini Dhir

- Considerations before Regional Anesthesia for Patients on Anticoagulation *268*
- Complications *269*
- Common Anticoagulants *270*
- Management of Antithrombotic Therapy in Obstetric Patients *274*

17. Clinical Outcome Scoring in Intensive Care 279
Pallavi Ahluwalia

- Validation and Testing Model Performance *281*
- Outcome Prediction Scores Used in Healthcare *281*
- Organ Dysfunction Scores *286*
- Severity Assessment Based on Impact on Nurses' Workload *288*
- Single Organ or Disease-specific Scoring Systems *290*
- Do We have an Ideal Scoring System? *290*
- Why do We Need a Scoring System in ICU? *291*
- Problems of Using Severity of Illness Scores to Compare Outcomes between ICUs *291*

18. Extracorporeal Membrane Oxygenation Support in Intensive Care 296
Vivek Gupta, GS Wander

- What is Extracorporeal Membrane Oxygenation? *297*
- Progress of ECMO *297*
- Physiology *298*

- Indications and Patient Selection *301*
- Contraindications *303*
- Circuit Configuration and Design *304*
- Management Strategy during ECMO *305*
- Issues, Challenges, and Complications during ECMO *309*

19. **Delirium in Intensive Care** 318
    Prathamesh Milind Patwardhan, Sandeep Lakhani
    - Incidence and Prevalence *319*
    - Risk Factors *319*
    - Pathophysiology *320*
    - Clinical Presentation *322*
    - Diagnosis and Evaluation *323*
    - Investigations *324*
    - Prevention *325*
    - Treatment *326*
    - Way Forward *327*

20. **Objective Pain Monitoring: A Gift from Artificial Intelligence** 331
    Rajesh Bhavsar, Laima M, Thomas Stroem
    - Pain: Revisited *332*
    - Objective Pain Monitoring: Overview *333*
    - Artificial Intelligence *339*
    - Nociception Level Index Monitor *342*
    - Clinical Applicability *345*
    - Validity *345*
    - Pitfalls *346*

21. **Methadone for Perioperative Pain** 352
    Skule Bakke, Rajesh Bhavsar, Thomas Stroem
    - Methadone: An Interesting Alternative *354*
    - History and Pharmacology of Methadone *354*
    - Clinical Applicability: Previous Experience *356*
    - Methadone: Major Concerns *357*
    - Dose *359*
    - Methadone Advantages *360*

22. **Return to Intended Oncologic Therapy** 366
    Rajiv Chawla, Shagun Bhatia Shah, Uma Hariharan
    - Cancer Treatment *368*
    - Cancer Therapy Options *368*
    - What is "Intended Therapy?" *369*

- Literature Review in RIOT: Equivocal Role of RIOT in Cancer Cure and Cancer Recurrence *373*
- Prospects *373*
- Limitations of Return to Intended Oncologic Therapy *385*

23. Nontechnical Skills in Anesthesiology 388
Pradeep Bhatia, Swati Chhabra

- History of Nontechnical Skills *389*
- Purpose of Nontechnical Skills *390*
- Application of Nontechnical Skills in Anesthesiology *390*
- Training in Nontechnical Skills *393*
- Measuring the Nontechnical Skills *394*
- Role of Organizations *394*
- Global Status of Training in Nontechnical Skills *396*
- Barriers to Effective Implementation of Nontechnical Skills *397*

24. Advanced Features in the Modern Anesthesia Workstation 400
Bharti Wadhwa, Kiran Mahendru

- New Features in Anesthesia Workstations *401*
- Enhanced Gas Delivery Systems *401*
- Drug Delivery Innovations *404*
- Remote Monitoring and Telemedicine *408*
- Integration of Digital Health Technologies *408*
- Ergonomic Designs and User Interfaces *409*
- Simulation and Training Solutions *410*

25. End of Life: Laws and Policies 413
Anjali Gera, Bimla Sharma

- Need for End-of-life Laws and Policies *414*
- Euthanasia *415*
- End-of-life Laws in Other Countries *416*
- The Legal Framework in India *417*
- Legal Evolution of Laws on End of Life *418*
- Law Commission of India Report *422*
- Recent Judgment *422*

Index *427*

CHAPTER 1

Ultrasound for Airway Assessment

Riccardo Antolini, Stefano Falcetta, Andrea Carsetti

ABSTRACT

Managing difficult airways requires specific skills and expertise as it involves life-saving maneuvers that must be rapidly performed. For this reason, anesthesiologists must have good knowledge and skills to manage difficult intubations. Still, they must also be able to identify patients who are likely to have difficult airways preliminarily. In addition to the traditional clinical evaluation, an airway ultrasound (US) assessment may give important information about the patient's airway anatomy. In the presence of any predisposing condition for difficult intubation, all tools for difficult airway management must be readily available, and the cricothyroid membrane (CTM) should be preventively identified to anticipate the need for an emergency cricothyrotomy. Since US is a noninvasive tool, dedicating a little extra time for this preliminary examination allows for better emergency management preparedness.

Keywords: Airway management; Airway ultrasound; Airway assessment; Difficult intubation; Difficult laryngoscopy

■ KEY POINTS

- Current guidelines recommend several clinical tests to identify patients at risk for difficult airway management; airway ultrasound may be usefully integrated with clinical assessment for more accurate risk stratification.
- For a comprehensive airway examination, five views are required: (1) suprahyoid, (2) thyrohyoid, (3) thyroid, (4) cricothyroid, and (5) suprasternal.
- Distance from skin-to-epiglottis (DSE) >2.54 cm reflects the thickness of the pre-epiglottic space. It is the distance that has the main evidence in literature of being correlated with difficult laryngoscopy.
- Ultrasound can be used to confirm the correct placement of the endotracheal tube. Before extubation, ultrasound can be useful for evaluating edematous airways.
- Prior to performing a percutaneous tracheostomy, ultrasound has a role in better defining neck anatomy.

- In pediatric patients, ultrasound serves multiple purposes, including anatomical assessment, confirmation of proper endotracheal tube placement, and selection of the appropriate endotracheal tube size.

INTRODUCTION

Airway management is essential for ensuring adequate ventilation and oxygenation to patients during elective procedures or emergencies. Difficulty or failure in securing a definitive airway can lead to life-threatening complications with a considerable mortality rate, so it is imperative to adhere to international guidelines using all available resources. Several studies present different definitions and criteria for identifying a difficult airway. Furthermore, there is significant interindividual variability, and not all clinical criteria can be objectively measured. These factors contribute to the wide range of reported incidence rates for difficult airways and intubation, between 5 and 22%.[1-3] In emergency departments, intensive care units (ICUs), and prehospital settings, the estimated incidence of failed intubation is approximately 1 in 50–100 attempts, whereas under elective conditions, it is estimated to be 1 in 1,000–2,000 attempts.[4] Nowadays, airway assessment guidelines recommend various tests to predict patients with a high risk of difficult airway management. However, many patients without significant risk factors may hide unexpected challenges.[5] For these reasons, it is necessary to integrate appropriate tools, such as ultrasound (US), with traditional clinical evaluations, especially in patients with difficult anatomical assessments. For many years, the US has been proven to be a helpful, safe, easily accessible, and noninvasive tool for upper airway evaluation. It allows for a preliminary anatomy analysis and through anthropometric measurements, predicts difficult laryngoscopy and intubation. It can also be used for other clinical applications such as:

- Verify the correct positioning of the endotracheal tube (ETT) in the trachea in conditions where end-tidal carbon dioxide (EtCO$_2$) sampling may be unreliable[6,7]
- Choose the correct size of the ETT in the pediatric population[8,9]
- Diagnosis of upper airway obstruction like subglottic stenosis[10]
- Guidance of percutaneous tracheostomy in ICU[10,11]
- Identification of the cricothyroid membrane (CTM) in case of difficult anatomical landmark identification, enabling prompt and accurate cricothyrotomy in case of "cannot intubate, cannot oxygenate" (CICO) scenario[12,13]
- Performing superior laryngeal nerve block to facilitate awake intubation[14]
- Diagnosis of postextubation stridor since the cuff leak test may not always be reliable[15]
- Evaluation of vocal cord mobility after thyroid surgery as an alternative to video rhino-laryngoscope[10,16]

- Confirmation of proper laryngeal mask airway position[17]
- Preoperative gastric emptying assessment; the US is useful for assessing residual gastric volume to identify patients who require nasogastric tube placement and rapid sequence intubation and be prepared for potential risks of aspiration.[18]

USE OF THE PROBE

Convex and linear probes can be used for the upper airway US, depending on the structure to be visualized. Superficial structures are better explored with a high-frequency (5-14 MHz) linear probe, while deeper structures require lower frequencies (4-10 MHz) and the convex probe. High-frequency probes can provide well-defined superficial structures such as vocal cords, epiglottis, and CTM. In contrast, low-frequency probes provide deeper structures, such as the base of the tongue and hyomental distance (HMD). In the US, bone appears hyperechoic, cartilaginous structures and muscles appear hypoechoic, and glands appear more hyperechoic than adjacent structures. Depending on the anatomical structure to be visualized, the probe can be positioned in a transverse, sagittal, or parasagittal orientation, allowing for upper airway evaluation from the oral cavity to the suprasternal notch. The ideal patient position for an upper airway US examination would be the supine position with the neck hyperextended. However, if there are difficulties in achieving this position, the seated position is also acceptable.[19] It is helpful to utilize color Doppler to visualize neck vessels, ask the patient to speak to observe vocal cords movements, or ask the patient to swallow to visualize the esophagus.

ULTRASOUND ANATOMY OF THE UPPER AIRWAY

Ultrasound upper airway assessment can be done from the mouth to the thorax. The following structures can be visualized: tongue base, hyoid bone, epiglottis, thyroid cartilage, vocal cords, CTM, cricoid cartilage, and esophagus.

Ultrasound imaging of the airways has demonstrated significant inter- and intraindividual reliability.[20]

To achieve a comprehensive visualization of the airway, five views are utilized:
1. *Suprahyoid view:* This window allows assessing the oral cavity by placing the curvilinear probe sagittally.
2. *Thyrohyoid view:* This is used to identify the epiglottis. The linear probe is positioned transversely.
3. *Thyroid view:* This is employed to evaluate vocal cord function; the linear probe is positioned transversely.
4. *Cricothyroid view:* This is used to identify the CTM; the linear probe is positioned transversely or sagittally.

4 Ultrasound for Airway Assessment

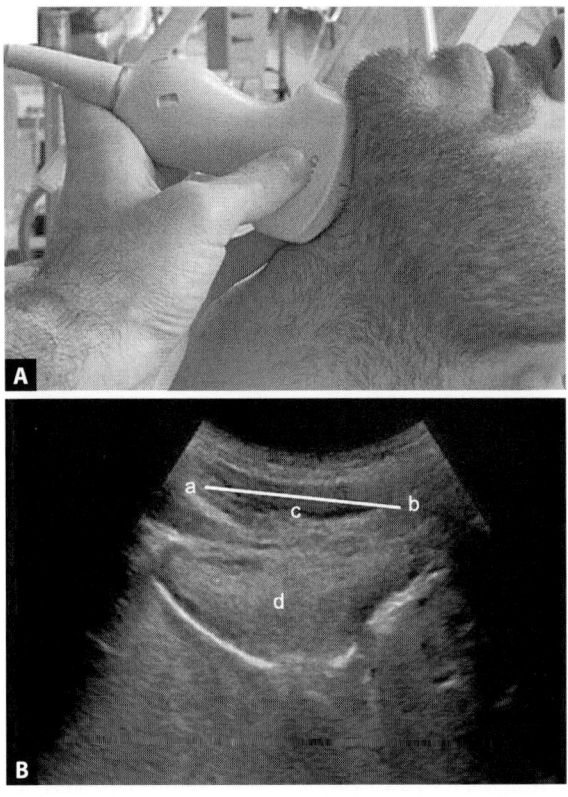

Figs. 1A and B: (A) Probe position for suprahyoid view; (B) a: mentum, b: hyoid bone, c: hyomental distance, d: mylohyoid, and geniohyoid muscle.

5. *Suprasternal view:* This is utilized to confirm the correct placement of an ETT by positioning the linear probe transversely.

Suprahyoid View

The suprahyoid view allows for visualizing the chin, the hyoid bone, the tongue, and the mylohyoid and geniohyoid muscles. The probe should be positioned sagittally with the marker toward the chin **(Fig. 1A)**. Additionally, it is possible to measure the HMD, which is predictive of difficult laryngoscopy, and the thickness of the tongue **(Fig. 1B)**.[21]

Thyrohyoid View

The thyrohyoid view is visualized with the linear probe positioned transversely **(Fig. 2A)**. It allows for the appreciation of the thyrohyoid membrane and the epiglottis. Between these two structures, there is the preepiglottic space, which appears hyperechoic due to its adipose tissue composition. The epiglottis, on the other hand, appears as a thin hypoechoic line. With this window, it is possible to measure the distance from skin-to-epiglottis, which is directly proportionally correlated with Cormack–Lehane grades and predictive for

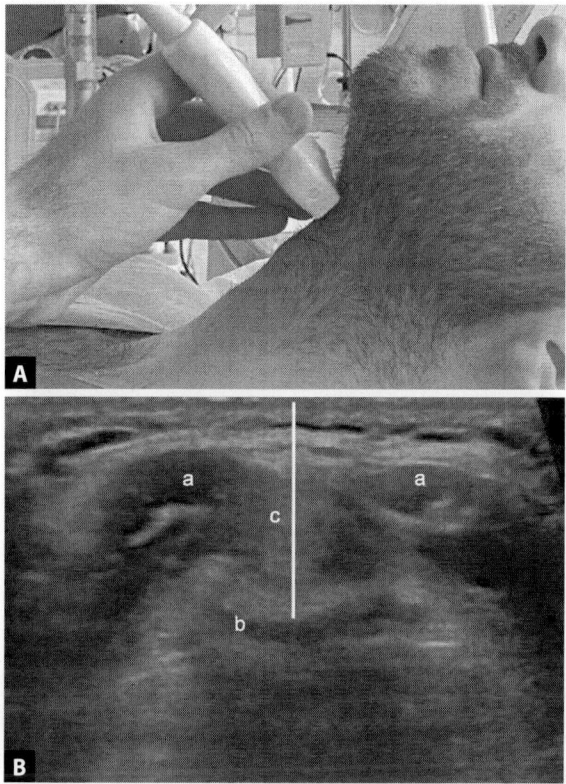

Figs. 2A and B: (A) Probe position for thyroid view; (B) a: strap muscle, b: epiglottis; c: distance from skin-to-epiglottis.

difficult laryngoscopy. A distinctive feature of this window is the "small face sign", where the eyes are represented by the thyrohyoid muscles and the mouth by the epiglottis **(Fig. 2B)**.[22]

Thyroid View

The thyroid view is visualized by placing the linear probe transversely above the thyroid cartilage **(Fig. 3A)**. In this window, the strap muscles, thyroid cartilage, and triangular-shaped vocal cords converge at the anterior commissure, and posteriorly, the arytenoid cartilages are visualized **(Fig. 3B)**. The thyroid cartilage may become calcified in older patients, making visualizing the vocal cords difficult. In such cases, the cricothyroid window can be used to visualize the vocal cords.[19]

Cricothyroid View

The cricothyroid view can be visualized by positioning the linear probe transversely or sagittally **(Figs. 4A to C)**. The thyroid cartilage, CTM, and cricoid cartilage are visualized in this window. It is particularly useful for assessing the localization of the CTM and for the presence of any vessels

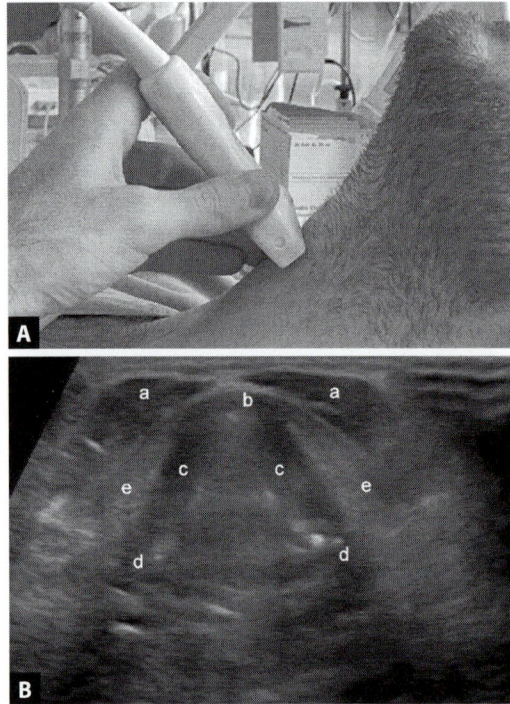

Figs. 3A and B: (A) Probe position for thyroid view; (B) a: strap muscle, b: anterior commissure, c: vocal cord, d: arytenoid cartilages, e: thyroid cartilage.

above it, which could make it challenging to perform a cricothyrotomy. CTM could be visualized in the sagittal position with the "string of pearls" (SOP) technique or in the transverse position with the "thyroid-airline-cricoid-airline" (TACA) technique **(Figs. 4B to D)**.[23] Using the SOP technique, tracheal rings will appear as small hypoechoic oval structures with their posterior border demarcated by a bright hyperechoic linear air-mucosal (A-M) interface. By moving the probe further cranially, the cricoid cartilage and the distal border of the thyroid cartilage can be visualized.[23] For the TACA protocol, the probe should be positioned transversely to identify the thyroid cartilage first and then the cricoid cartilage. The CTM between them will be visualized as a hyperechoic line with parallel hyperechoic lines (reverberation artifacts).[23]

Suprasternal View

The suprasternal view can be visualized by placing the linear probe transversely just above the suprasternal notch **(Fig. 5A)**. In this view, the trachea can be seen in the midline and posteriorly appears the esophagus. Thyroid lobes on either side of the trachea, carotid artery and internal jugular vein, sternocleidomastoid muscles, and vertebrae are also visualized on this site **(Fig. 5B)**. This view can be used to measure the tracheal diameter

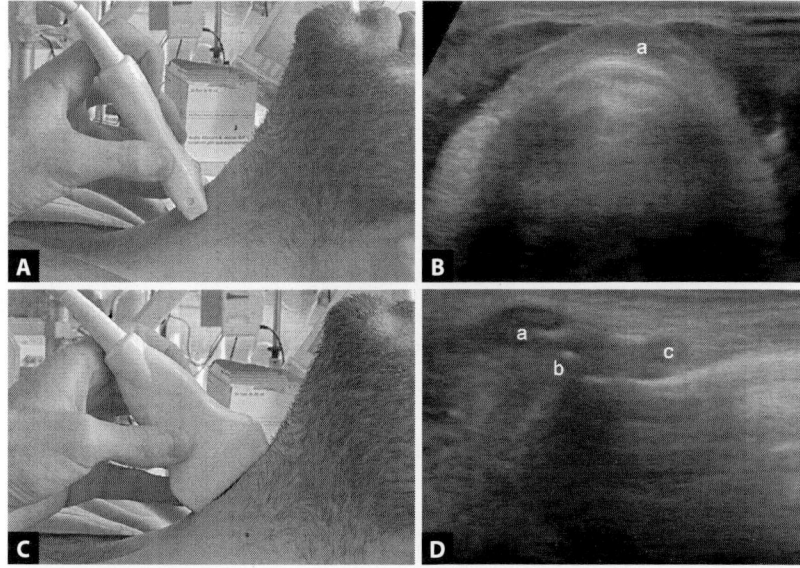

Figs. 4A to D: (A) Probe position for cricothyroid view, transverse orientation; (B) a: cricothyroid membrane with reverberation artifact; (C) probe position for cricothyroid view, sagittal orientation; (D) a: thyroid cartilage, b: cricothyroid membrane, c: cricoid cartilage.

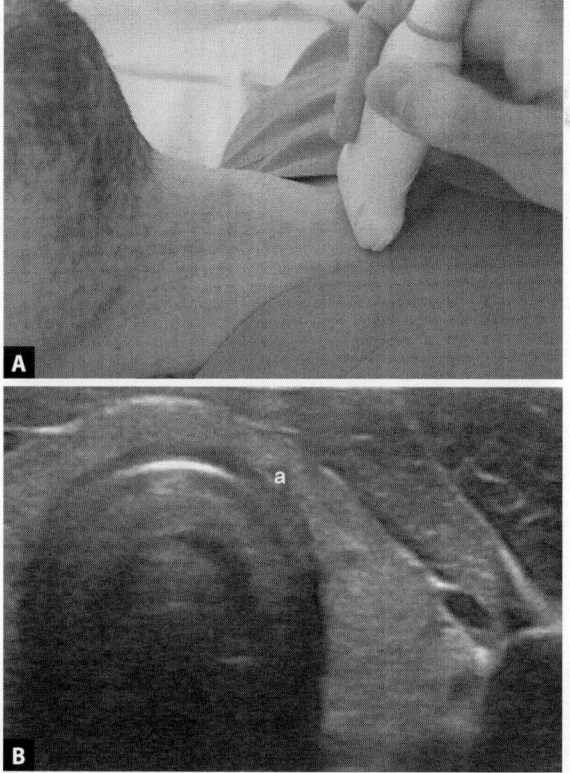

Figs. 5A and B: (A) Probe position for suprasternal view; (B) a: tracheal cartilage.

and confirm the correct placement of the ETT, excluding the intubation of the esophagus, which would reveal a hyperechoic structure adjacent to the trachea, referred to as the "double tract sign" or "double trachea sign."[23]

ASSESSMENT OF DIFFICULT AIRWAYS USING ULTRASOUND

Difficult airways can be predicted based on specific anatomical criteria. However, clinical scores currently used are unreliable in predicting potential difficulties in performing laryngoscopy. Reduced laryngeal view is categorized as Cormack–Lehane grades 2b and 3a, while difficult laryngeal view corresponds to grades 3b and 4. The reported incidence of reduced laryngeal view ranges from 5 to 10%.[22] It is always recommended to evaluate the airways before the induction of anesthesia to plan the management of potential difficulties. Clinical screening tests (such as Mallampati and interincisor distance) have shown low sensitivity and specificity and limited predictive power, primarily when only one test is used.[24,25] There are several reasons for this; e.g., in obese subjects, identifying landmarks is more challenging, and also gender variability is not often taken into account.[26] The El-Ganzouri score combines seven clinical parameters to increase the power of these individual tests.[27] According to American Society of Anesthesiologists guidelines, up to 90% of difficult airways are unpredictable.[28] In emergency departments, airway US evaluation is gaining more prominence due to limitations of traditional clinical scores and the inability to obtain the head and neck sniffing position. It has been demonstrated that US-based anatomical assessment surpasses clinical evaluation and correlates well with measurements obtained from computed tomography (CT) scans.[29] Until now, the Cormack–Lehane scale has been commonly used to identify the difficulty of vocal cord visualization with direct laryngoscopy. A recent meta-analysis identified three domains that correlate with the Cormack–Lehane grade and difficult laryngoscopy:[21,30]

- *Anterior neck soft-tissue thickness domain (TTD):* This is used to evaluate submandibular space and the curvature required for the laryngoscope to overcome the tongue.
  - *DSE:* This reflects the thickness of the preepiglottic space. It is the most supported distance in predicting difficult laryngoscopy.[21]
  - Skin to anterior commissure of the vocal cords
  - Skin to vocal cords
  - Skin to thyroid cartilage
  - Skin to thyrohyoid membrane
- *Anatomical position domain* (APD): A dynamic measure that varies with the patient in the neutral position, ramped position, and hyperextended neck. It reflects the extent to which the tongue can be moved and the neck extended to optimize glottis visualization.

- *HMD:* The distance between the mandible's posterior margin and the hyoid bone's anterior margin measured with a convex probe.
- *HMD ratio (HMDR):* The ratio of HMD measured in the ramped position (HMDR1) or maximal head extension (HMDR2) to the neutral position.
- Condylar translation
- Angle between glottis and epiglottis
- *Oral space domain (OSD):* It evaluates the size of the oral cavity and tongue, which could indicate difficult laryngoscopy.
  - *Tongue thickness (TT):* The most reliable measurement in predicting difficult laryngoscopy within OSD
  - Distance from skin to tongue
  - Tongue volume

The DARES (Difficult Airway Evaluation with Sonography) protocol is a standardized US-based method for assessing the upper airway. It involves sequential measurement of the following:
- DSE ≥2.54 cm
- HMD ≤5.29 cm or TT >6.1 cm
- HMDR2 <1.08
- HMDR1 <1.12

If at least one positive response is present, it could predict difficult airway management.[29]

CONFIRMATION OF ENDOTRACHEAL INTUBATION

Tracheal intubation allows for definitive control of the airways, and the US can be very helpful in verifying the correct placement of the ETT to prevent potentially fatal consequences. The literature reports an esophageal intubation rate in emergency departments of 3.3%.[31] Chest auscultation is commonly used, but it may have restrictions in prehospital settings due to several environmental interferences. $EtCO_2$ is used as the gold standard technique for confirming correct ETT placement. However, it may not be reliable in certain situations, such as low cardiac output, cardiac arrest, and low pulmonary flow. For these reasons, the US is proving to be a promising tool to confirm the ETT's correct placement and appropriate depth. Verification can be done directly in real time during the procedure or after tube placement and indirectly by looking for signs of ventilation, such as pleural sliding or diaphragmatic movements. Combining both techniques increases the sensitivity and specificity of the examination. The probe should be positioned transversely at the suprasternal notch level. ETT is considered in the trachea if only an A-M interface with comet tail artifacts and posterior shadowing are visualized **(Fig. 6)**. In the esophageal tube position, two A-M interfaces with comet tail artifacts and posterior shadowing ("double tract" sign) are seen **(Fig. 7)**.

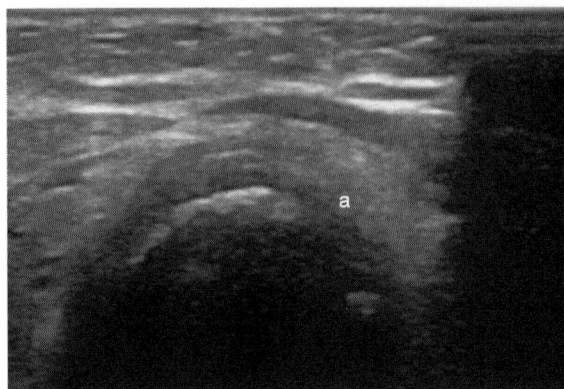

Fig. 6: Suprasternal view with linear probe; a: air–mucosa interface with comet tail artifacts and posterior shadow.

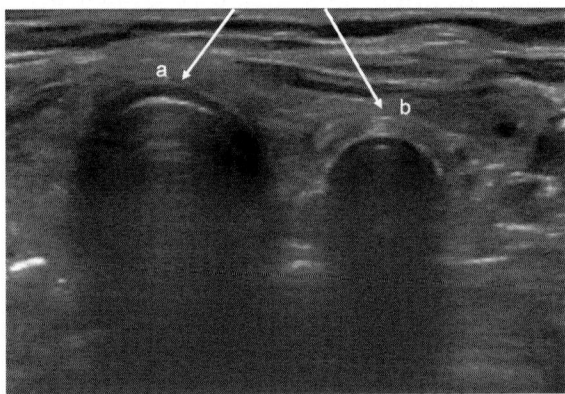

Fig. 7: Suprasternal view with linear probe, "double tract sign"; a: air–mucosa interface in trachea, b: air–mucosa interface in esophagus.

■ LARYNGEAL EDEMA ASSESSMENT

Mucosal edema of the larynx is one of the most common causes of extubation failure, leading to increased mortality, extended hospital stays, and higher costs. The cuff leak test is typically performed before extubation in high-risk patients. It consists in deflating the ETT cuff and assessing for the presence of stridor due to the passage of air between the vocal cords or for volume loss at the ventilator. However, this test is only sometimes reliable. The US is a valuable tool for evaluating laryngeal edema, but there still needs to be a consensus on it predicting postextubation stridor. It has been observed that the width of the trachea correlates with postextubation stridor. A study has demonstrated that a ratio of the transverse diameter of the glottis to the outer diameter of the ETT measured on a CT scan of <1 in females, measured 3 hours before extubation, predicts symptoms of airway obstruction.[32] Furthermore, measurements taken in the US have proven to have the same reliability compared to those taken with CT scans. However, another similar study cautions against using the US in these circumstances due to its low positive predictive value and sensitivity.[33]

EVALUATION FOR PERCUTANEOUS TRACHEOSTOMY

Using US in percutaneous dilatational tracheostomy can improve efficacy and reduce procedure complications. According to a recent study, the mortality rate associated with the procedure is 1 in 600.[34] The most common causes of death are postprocedural bleeding due to altered vascular anatomy, particularly within the 7 days following the procedure, rather than during the procedure itself, and periprocedural airway complications.[34] The US allows for the identification of landmarks, detection of the structures to avoid, selection of the correct size of the tracheostomy cannula, and real-time visualization of the needle during penetration to reduce complications. After identifying the landmarks in the longitudinal plane, an out-of-plane approach is recommended to guide needle insertion, with the probe positioned transversely just above the puncture site.[35] In specific patient populations, such as the obese, it can be difficult to palpate neck anatomy. In these circumstances, the US is a valuable tool for identifying landmarks. Before the procedure, the peritracheal area should be examined to identify the tracheal rings, jugular veins, and their position relative to the midline, the thyroid isthmus, and midline vessels. Any structures crossing the midline should be assessed, ensuring the excessive pressure from the probe does not compress the tissues.[35] An additional advantage of performing US before the procedure is identifying any vascular structures in the neck that should be avoided during the puncture. Periprocedural US allows for the visualization of the tracheal rings, which helps identify the optimal puncture site and ensure proper placement of the tracheostomy tube in the midline. According to sonographic criteria, the tracheal puncture site should be below the first tracheal ring but above the fourth, avoiding vascular structures.[35] The US also provides valuable assistance in selecting the appropriate tracheostomy tube size by measuring the distance from skin to trachea.[36] Currently, the only true advantage of using a bronchoscope over the US for percutaneous dilatational tracheostomy is the ability to identify any damage caused by the needle to the posterior tracheal wall. There are currently no studies analyzing tracheal injuries during US guidance, but it presents an exciting challenge for the future.

EVALUATION FOR CRICOTHYROTOMY

Cricothyrotomy is a life-saving procedure used in CICO situations. The success rate of cricothyrotomy on the first attempt is <36%.[25] Besides operator inexperience, the leading cause of failure is the inability to localize the CTM. This can be challenging, especially in specific categories of patients such as female, obese, and pregnant. US is a valuable tool for identifying

CTM, particularly in individuals where palpation is difficult. To identify the CTM, a linear probe is placed sagittally along the midline looking for the "string of pearls" sign. The cricoid cartilage represents the most prominent "pearl", followed caudally by the thyroid cartilage, and in the middle CTM is visualized. Before the procedure, exploring the area using color Doppler is advisable to check for any vascular structures. For greater precision, the TACA approach can also be used as a "second line" identification of CTM. US enables precise identification of the site and determines the depth at which the CTM is located.

Point-of-care ultrasound (POCUS) approach recommends identifying the membrane before intubating any patient with predictive factors for difficult clinical CTM identification in anticipation of a CICO scenario.[29]

■ PEDIATRIC PATIENTS

Airways US evaluation in pediatric patients is becoming a frontline tool for understanding anatomy. Currently, age is used as the primary criterion for selecting the appropriate ETT size and insertion depth. The US aids in the same objectives as adults: evaluating vocal cords, verifying correct ETT placement, assessing the CTM, visualizing tracheal rings, and choosing the correct ETT size.[8,9] Intubating with a too large tube could lead to edema, increasing the risk during extubation and subglottic stenosis. On the other hand, intubating with a tube that is too small may result in inadequate ventilation, inaccurate $EtCO_2$ monitoring, increased resistance, and a higher risk of aspiration. For these reasons, in addition to choosing the ETT size and position based on age, it is also recommended to select the tube based on the diameter of the subglottic space.[8] US is also useful for verifying the correct placement of the ETT, as incorrect positioning can result in accidental extubation, esophageal intubation, or bronchial intubation. The US is well tolerated in both children and neonates and can be combined with other verification methods such as auscultation and $EtCO_2$ presence.

■ CONCLUSION

The US approach in airway management represents an innovative, practical, and noninvasive tool that can be particularly helpful in critical situations. Clinicians need adequate training in US use, similar to other devices used in difficult intubation scenarios. It is important to emphasize that proficiency in airway US requires appropriate training and expertise in image interpretation. The US examination of the airway represents a reliable and versatile imaging technique gaining popularity in clinical practice. Its role in assessing and managing airway pathologies will continue to evolve, providing new diagnostic and therapeutic opportunities to enhance respiratory patient care.

REFERENCES

1. Frerk C, Mitchell VS, McNarry AF, Mendonca C, Bhagrath R, Patel A, et al. Difficult Airway Society 2015 guidelines for management of unanticipated difficult intubation in adults. Br J Anaesth. 2015;115(6):827-48.
2. Cook TM, Woodall N, Frerk C; Fourth National Audit Project. Major complications of airway management in the UK: results of the Fourth National Audit Project of the Royal College of Anaesthetists and the Difficult Airway Society. Part 1: anaesthesia. Br J Anaesth. 2011;106(5):617-31.
3. Peterson GN, Domino KB, Caplan RA, Posner KL, Lee LA, Cheney FW. Management of the difficult airway: a closed claims analysis. Anesthesiology. 2005;103(1):33-9.
4. Cook TM, MacDougall-Davis SR. Complications and failure of airway management. Br J Anaesth. 2012;109 Suppl 1:i68-i85.
5. De Hert S, Staender S, Fritsch G, Hinkelbein J, Afshari A, Bettelli G, et al. Pre-operative evaluation of adults undergoing elective noncardiac surgery: Updated guideline from the European Society of Anaesthesiology. Eur J Anaesthesiol. 2018;35(6):407-65.
6. Chou EH, Dickman E, Tsou PY, Tessaro M, Tsai YM, Ma MH, et al. Ultrasonography for confirmation of endotracheal tube placement: a systematic review and meta-analysis. Resuscitation. 2015;90:97-103.
7. Sorbello M, Falcetta S, DI Giacinto I, Cortese G, Esposito C, Merli G, et al. Endotracheal intubation confirmation in COVID-19 patients: (ultra)sound is better than silence. Minerva Anestesiol. 2021;87(1):114-6.
8. Daniel SJ, Bertolizio G, McHugh T. Airway ultrasound: Point of care in children-The time is now. Paediatr Anaesth. 2020;30(3):347-52.
9. Adler AC, Siddiqui A, Chandrakantan A, Matava CT. Lung and airway ultrasound in pediatric anesthesia. Paediatr Anaesth. 2022;32(2):202-8.
10. Kundra P, Mishra SK, Ramesh A. Ultrasound of the airway. Indian J Anaesth. 2011;55(5):456-62.
11. Alansari M, Alotair H, Al Aseri Z, Elhoseny MA. Use of ultrasound guidance to improve the safety of percutaneous dilatational tracheostomy: a literature review. Crit Care Lond Engl. 2015;19(1):229.
12. Onrubia X, Frova G, Sorbello M. Front of neck access to the airway: A narrative review. Trends Anaesth Crit Care. 2018;22:45-55.
13. You-Ten KE, Wong DT, Ye XY, Arzola C, Zand A, Siddiqui N. Practice of Ultrasound-Guided Palpation of Neck Landmarks Improves Accuracy of External Palpation of the Cricothyroid Membrane. Anesth Analg. 2018;127(6):1377-82.
14. Lan CH, Cheng WC, Yang YL. A new method for ultrasound-guided superior laryngeal nerve block. Tzu Chi Med J. 2013;25(3):161-3.
15. Ding LW, Wang HC, Wu HD, Chang CJ, Yang PC. Laryngeal ultrasound: a useful method in predicting post-extubation stridor. A pilot study. Eur Respir J. 2006;27(2):384-9.
16. Sorbello M, Corso RM, Falcetta S, Di Giacinto I, Cataldo R. Laryngoscopy, thyroid surgery and recurrent nerve lesions: who is to blame? Minerva Anestesiol. 2020;86(5):576-7.
17. Song K, Yi J, Liu W, Huang S, Huang Y. Confirmation of laryngeal mask airway placement by ultrasound examination: a pilot study. J Clin Anesth. 2016;34:638-46.

18. Ohashi Y, Walker JC, Zhang F, Prindiville FE, Hanrahan JP, Mendelson R, et al. Preoperative gastric residual volumes in fasted patients measured by bedside ultrasound: a prospective observational study. Anaesth Intensive Care. 2018;46(6):608-13.
19. Beale T, Twigg VM, Horta M, Morley S. High-Resolution Laryngeal US: Imaging Technique, Normal Anatomy, and Spectrum of Disease. Radiogr Rev Publ Radiol Soc N Am Inc. 2020;40(3):775-90.
20. Lun HM, Zhu SY, Liu RC, Gong JG, Liu YL. Investigation of the Upper Airway Anatomy With Ultrasound. Ultrasound Q. 2016;32(1):86-92.
21. Carsetti A, Sorbello M, Adrario E, Donati A, Falcetta S. Airway Ultrasound as Predictor of Difficult Direct Laryngoscopy: A Systematic Review and Meta-analysis. Anesth Analg. 2022;134(4):740-50.
22. Falcetta S, Cavallo S, Gabbanelli V, Pelaia P, Sorbello M, Zdravkovic I, et al. Evaluation of two neck ultrasound measurements as predictors of difficult direct laryngoscopy: A prospective observational study. Eur J Anaesthesiol. 2018;35(8):605-12.
23. Zhang J, Teoh WH, Kristensen MS. Ultrasound in Airway Management. Curr Anesthesiol Rep. 2020;10(4):317-26.
24. Frova G, Sorbello M. Algorithms for difficult airway management: a review. Minerva Anestesiol. 2009;75(4):201-9.
25. Gottlieb M, Holladay D, Burns KM, Nakitende D, Bailitz J. Ultrasound for airway management: An evidence-based review for the emergency clinician. Am J Emerg Med. 2020;38(5):1007-13.
26. Fernandez-Vaquero MA, Charco-Mora P, Garcia-Aroca MA, Greif R. Preoperative airway ultrasound assessment in the sniffing position: a prospective observational study. Braz J Anesthesiol. 2022;S0104-0014(22)00088-4.
27. el-Ganzouri AR, McCarthy RJ, Tuman KJ, Tanck EN, Ivankovich AD. Preoperative airway assessment: predictive value of a multivariate risk index. Anesth Analg. 1996;82(6):1197-204.
28. Apfelbaum JL, Hagberg CA, Connis RT, Abdelmalak BB, Agarkar M, Dutton RP, et al. 2022 American Society of Anesthesiologists Practice Guidelines for Management of the Difficult Airway. Anesthesiology. 2022;136(1):31-81.
29. Lin J, Bellinger R, Shedd A, Wolfshohl J, Walker J, Healy J, et al. Point-of-Care Ultrasound in Airway Evaluation and Management: A Comprehensive Review. Diagnostics (Basel). 2023;13(9):1541.
30. Bhargava V, Rockwell NA, Tawfik D, Haileselassie B, Petrisor C, Su E. Prediction of Difficult Laryngoscopy Using Ultrasound: A Systematic Review and Meta-Analysis. Crit Care Med. 2023;51(1):117-26.
31. Brown CA, Bair AE, Pallin DJ, Walls RM, NEAR III Investigators. Techniques, success, and adverse events of emergency department adult intubations. Ann Emerg Med. 2015;65(4):363-70.e1.
32. Shinohara M, Iwashita M, Abe T, Takeuchi I. Association between post-extubation upper airway obstruction symptoms and airway size measured by computed tomography: a single-center observational study. BMC Emerg Med. 2022;22(1):55.
33. Mikaeili H, Yazdchi M, Tarzamni MK, Ansarin K, Ghasemzadeh M. Laryngeal ultrasonography versus cuff leak test in predicting postextubation stridor. J Cardiovasc Thorac Res. 2014;6(1):25-8.

34. Simon M, Metschke M, Braune SA, Püschel K, Kluge S. Death after percutaneous dilatational tracheostomy: a systematic review and analysis of risk factors. Crit Care Lond Engl. 2013;17(5):R258.
35. Rudas M. The role of ultrasound in percutaneous dilatational tracheostomy. Australas J Ultrasound Med. 2012;15(4):143-8.
36. Guinot PG, Zogheib E, Petiot S, Marienne JP, Guerin AM, Monet P, et al. Ultrasound-guided percutaneous tracheostomy in critically ill obese patients. Crit Care Lond Engl. 2012;16(2):R40.

CHAPTER 2

Negative Pressure Pulmonary Edema

Niti Batra

ABSTRACT

Negative pressure pulmonary edema (NPPE) is a noncardiogenic bilateral pulmonary edema that is not so uncommon in anesthesia practice. NPPE represents a pure form of hydrostatic edema. A negative intrathoracic pressure is the primary pathological event in the genesis of NPPE. If prompt treatment is initiated once it is diagnosed, there is complete recovery within 24-48 hours. If overlooked and not understood, it could become fatal. It is more common in young, robust males. Its incidence is always underreported. The negative pressure generated by upper airway obstruction leads to increased hydrostatic pressure in pulmonary capillaries, altering the Starling forces and forming edema. Treatment modalities include oxygen supplementation through a face mask to face mask continuous positive airway pressure (CPAP) application, tracheal intubation, and positive pressure ventilation. Though some cases require minimal supportive care, including maintaining a patent airway and administering supplemental oxygen, most patients require reintubation and ventilation with positive airway pressure. It is essential to apply positive pressure to the airway early to prevent hydrostatic transudation of fluid into the extravascular compartment.

Keywords: Pulmonary edema; Noncardiogenic edema; Upper airway obstruction; Laryngospasm; Obstructive sleep apnea (OSA); Postextubation edema; NPPE

■ KEY POINTS

- Negative pressure pulmonary edema (NPPE) occurs when the patient is breathing against an airway obstruction or a closed glottis.
- The most common cause of NPPE is postextubation laryngospasm.
- It is a noncardiogenic edema due to differential pressure gradients in alveoli caused by upper airway obstruction.
- Prompt and complete recovery is possible if it is diagnosed early.

- Cardiac echocardiography is standard and is needed to differentiate from other causes of pulmonary edema.
- It is more common in young, healthy patients, especially males, smokers, obese, and those undergoing head and neck surgeries.
- Associations between NPPE, obstructive sleep apnea (OSA), and Takotsubo cardiomyopathy have been observed.
- Point-of-care ultrasound (POCUS) has emerged as a rapid diagnostic tool for conclusive diagnosis.

INTRODUCTION

Negative pressure pulmonary edema, sometimes called postobstructive pulmonary edema (POPE), is commonly seen in anesthesia. If identified soon, it can be treated thoroughly, but if left neglected, it can be fatal. In anesthesia, it is commonly seen after laryngospasm due to the forced inspiratory effort against a closed glottis, creating increased hydrostatic pressure in pulmonary capillaries, ultimately leading to edema.

Moore, in 1927, first described NPPE in spontaneously breathing dogs exposed to a resistive load. In 1942, Warren demonstrated the correlation between negative pressure creation and pulmonary edema development. In humans, it was described in 1960 after an autopsy of a postsuicidal hanging case. Capitanio described how children developed edema postcroup and after epiglottitis.[1] Oswalt described the occurrence of pulmonary edema postanesthesia in 1977.[2] Now, it is a known complication after general anesthesia, with the overall incidence being 0.1%.[3] Postextubation pulmonary edema due to laryngospasm accounts for 50% of the cases of NPPE.

There are two types of NPPE: type I and type II.[3,4] Type I is seen after acute obstruction; the incidence is 9.6–12%. Type II is seen in cases of chronic obstruction, with its incidence being 44%.[3] Among pediatric patients, it is seen in acute epiglottitis and croup, leading to upper airway obstruction accounting for 75% of NPPE cases. Type I is seen after acute upper airway obstruction, mainly after surgical manipulation or after laryngospasm, so it is often called laryngospasm-induced pulmonary edema or postextubation edema. Type II NPPE usually results after relief of chronic obstruction caused by enlarged tonsils, hypertrophied adenoids, or redundant uvula.[5,6] Croup is benign but can develop into POPE. The other causes can be hanging, strangulation, upper airway tumors, foreign bodies, choking, and after endotracheal tube obstruction or biting.[7]

PATHOPHYSIOLOGY

According to Starling forces (**Fig. 1**), there are four causes leading to pulmonary edema:
1. Increased hydrostatic pressure
2. Decreased oncotic pressure

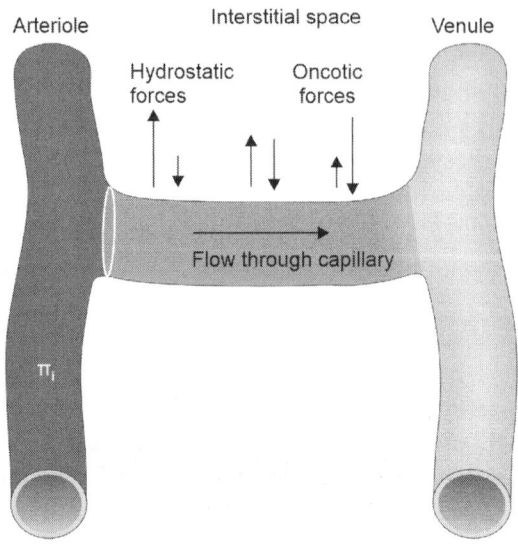

Fig. 1: Starling forces in arteriole and venules.

3. Increased capillary permeability
4. Decreased clearance from lymphatics

The Starling equation says:

$$Q = K[(P_{mv} - P_i) - \sigma(\pi_{mv} - \pi_i)]$$

where Q is the fluid flux outside from capillary lumen to interstitium, K is coefficient of capillary permeability; P_{mv} is the capillary lumen hydrostatic pressure; P_i is the alveolar interstitial hydrostatic pressure; σ is the reflection coefficient (the effectiveness of the vascular barrier in preventing diffusion of protein); π_{mv} is the microvascular protein osmotic pressure; and π_i is the interstitial protein osmotic pressure.

Two mechanisms have been implicated in the pathogenesis of pulmonary edema in cases with upper airway obstruction **(Flowchart 1)**. The first mechanism postulates the development of pulmonary edema due to the fluid shift resulting from changes in the intrathoracic pressure. The increased negative pressure generated by the diaphragm against a closed glottis is called the Muller's maneuver.[8] This creates a negative pressure in the pleural space, which increases the venous return to the right side of the heart resulting in higher hydrostatic pressures in the pulmonary capillaries and a sudden drop of pressures in the alveolar spaces. This creates a huge pressure gradient across the pulmonary capillary wall leading to alveolar flooding and pulmonary edema, exceeding the lymphatics clearance. A young, healthy person can generate as high as 100 mm Hg negative pressure against a closed glottis.[9] This disruption of Starling forces combined with negative intrathoracic pressure results in fluid extravasation leading to pulmonary

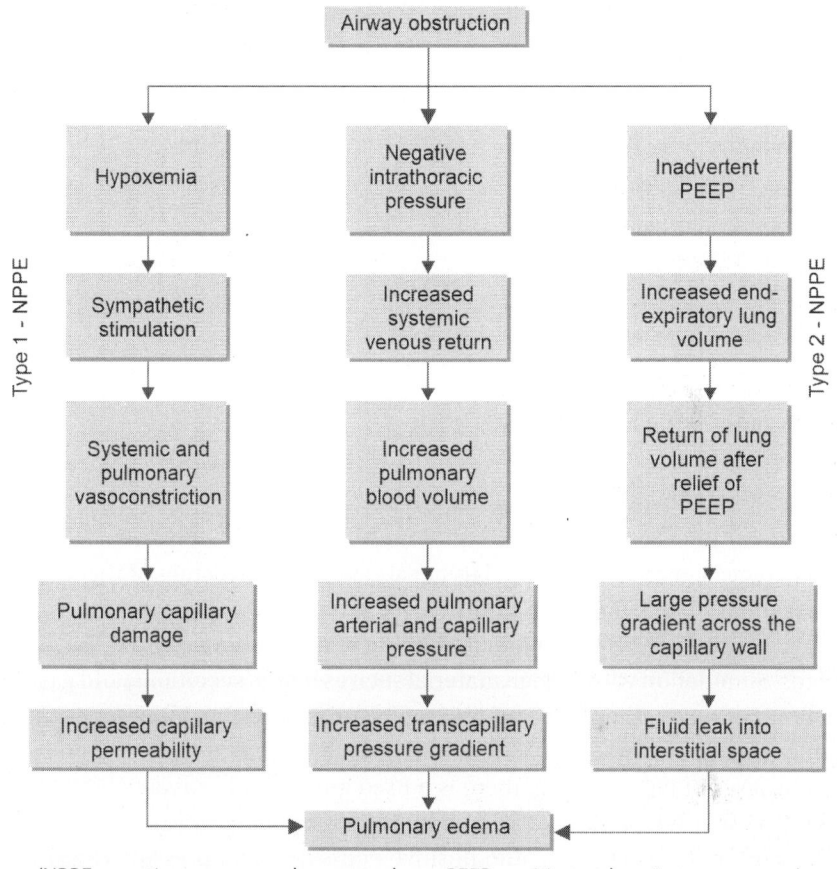

Flowchart 1: Pathophysiology of pulmonary edema.

(NPPE: negative pressure pulmonary edema; PEEP: positive end-expiratory pressure)

edema. The second mechanism involves the break in the alveolar epithelial and pulmonary microvascular membranes, resulting from stress induced due to respiration against closed glottis resulting in increased pulmonary capillary permeability and causing protein-rich pulmonary edema.

Upper airway obstruction creates negative intrathoracic pressure leading to increased venous return, i.e., the preload increases. This causes septal bowing, leading to left ventricular dysfunction. Hypoxia causes peripheral vasoconstriction causing the afterload to increase further. All these changes increase the ventilation–perfusion mismatch. There is a catecholamine surge because of hypoxia and increased hydrostatic pressures. Sometimes along with capillary stress wall failure, a capillary permeability breach occurs, causing exudation of hemorrhagic fluid and alveolar hemorrhage, called negative pressure pulmonary hemorrhage (NPPH). There is almost a 5% chance of NPPE cases developing NPPH.[10]

TABLE 1: Causes of negative pressure pulmonary edema (NPPE).

Type I NPPE	Type II NPPE
Postextubation laryngospasm	Post-tonsillectomy
Epiglottitis	Postadenoidectomy
Choking/foreign body	Choanal stenosis
Strangulation, hanging	Hypertrophic redundant uvula
ETT obstruction, biting, secretions	
Laryngeal tumor, goiter	
Postoperative vocal cord paralysis	
Near drowning	
Intraoperative ETT suctioning	
Migration of balloon of Foley catheter used for epistaxis	
(ETT: endotracheal tube)	

Laryngospasm involves the laryngeal reflex arc consisting of trigeminal, glossopharyngeal, superior, and inferior laryngeal branches of the vagus nerve which innervates the mucosal lining of the nasopharynx till the vocal cords. Stimulation with foreign material such as blood, secretions, and gastric contents causes stimulation of this reflex arc and results in laryngospasm which presents as bradycardia followed by tachycardia.[11]

In cases of type II NPPE, there is a fixed and chronic airway obstruction like OSA in adults and enlarged adenoids, croup, epiglottitis, or tonsils in children. In these patients, auto positive end-expiratory pressure (PEEP) or auto-PEEP is generated due to exhalation against chronic airway obstruction, leading to decreased capillary wall pressure gradient. When this obstruction is relieved, and there is a loss of auto-PEEP, a large pressure gradient across the capillary wall leads to fluid leak into the interstitial space. The effort taken after the relief of obstruction generates an exaggerated negative inspiratory pressure, which aids this further.[12] This mechanism is also thought to explain reexpansion pulmonary edema seen after drainage of large pneumothorax or pleural effusion. The treatment of croup needs to be addressed along with the treatment of edema. Nebulized epinephrine and steroids, along with airway support, are needed.[13] The causes of type I and type II NPPE are listed in **Table 1**.

■ CLINICAL FEATURES

Symptoms of NPPE include breathlessness, air hunger, and pink frothy sputum. On examination, there is tachypnea, tachycardia, fall in oxygen saturation, pulmonary rales, hemoptysis, hypoxemia, and hypercarbia on arterial blood gas analysis.[14,15] The characteristic feature is normal pulmonary pressures on 2D echo. Chest X-ray shows diffuse alveolar and interstitial infiltrates because of the presence of edema in central and nondependent regions of the lungs. With the evidence of Kerley B lines on ultrasound, POCUS has the great advantage of being a bedside noninvasive investigation tool in anesthesia.

Postanesthesia Care Unit Care or Postextubation Emergency

Negative pressure pulmonary edema presents postextubation when the patient takes a breath against closed glottis following laryngospasm.[16,17] It usually presents immediately during extubation but can also present 2-4 hours later. There is a need to observe all patients experiencing respiratory difficulty postextubation in postanesthesia care unit (PACU) for 6-12 hours. A possible explanation for delayed presentation is a positive pressure created by forceful expiration against a closed glottis. As the airway obstruction is relieved, an increased venous return causes blood to shift from peripheral to central circulation, resulting in hydrostatic transudation. Closed postoperative observation thus must be continued for an extended time in patients who experience some respiratory difficulty postoperatively.[9] Respiratory obstruction can result from laryngospasm, breath-holding episodes, or biting on the endotracheal tube[7] inside the operating room. If identified and treated promptly, it shows complete recovery in 12-48 hours.[8]

Spontaneous recovery and resolution of edema is aided by the sodium reuptake into lung interstitial space through sodium channels present in type I and II alveolar epithelial cells. This sodium shift restores the osmotic gradient allowing edematous fluid to be reabsorbed by lung lymphatics.[18,19] This diagnosis must be considered in anesthesia as its manifestations overlap with other pathologies. It can be seen in cases due to postoperative residual neuromuscular blockade in which upper airway dilator muscle strength is impaired, but inspiratory muscle strength is preserved. This has been observed with sugammadex when disproportionate muscle strength leads to high inspiratory pressure culminating in NPPE.[20,21] There is a different degree of sensitivity to muscle relaxants between the upper airway muscle and diaphragm. With a train-of-four ratio (TOF) >0.9, there is still a possibility that upper airway obstruction is there due to increased upper airway collapsibility. The large inspiratory force generated by the diaphragm in a patient with fully recovered muscle relaxation after sugammadex administration can cause increased negative pressure. Rapid recovery of respiratory forces in the presence of upper airway collapsibility results in the development of NPPE.[22,23]

■ DIAGNOSIS

Negative pressure pulmonary edema is defined as the development of acute hypoxemia [pulse oximetry, peripheral oxygen saturation (SpO_2) <92%]

along with signs of upper airway obstruction occurring postextubation or post-laryngeal mask airway (LMA) in the operative room or the PACU. The definite diagnosis is pink frothy sputum and alveolar diffuse infiltrates on chest X-ray.[24]

Differential Diagnosis

Cardiogenic Pulmonary Edema

It is seen due to increased pulmonary hydrostatic pressures due to altered ventricular function, valvular dysfunction, or rhythm disturbances in the heart. The resultant pathology of increased extravascular fluid content in the lung remains common in all forms of pulmonary edema.[25] Pulmonary capillary wedge pressure measurement confirms a cardiogenic edema diagnosis. Cardiac myocytes present in the left ventricle secrete brain-type natriuretic peptide (BNP) as a result of stretching due to increased ventricular blood volume or increased intracardiac pressures. Increased BNP and left ventricular dysfunction point toward a cardiac etiology.[25,26] Treatment, however, remains the same, i.e., with ventilatory support and diuretics.

Anaphylaxis

There is a presence of rash, bronchospasm, hypotension, and a history of allergen exposure that directs toward anaphylaxis-induced edema. On investigation, there are increased tryptase levels. The treatment again is early airway intervention with ventilatory support, but adrenaline is the primary therapy.

Acute Lung Injury

There is a history of an inciting event that gives rise to acute lung injury. This occurs when pulmonary or extrapulmonary insult causes an inflammatory reaction leading to the damaged epithelium, hence pulmonary edema. Also, this entity is commonly seen in intensive care setting with treatment involving ventilatory support and steroids.

Aspiration

This can happen perioperatively and is usually diagnosed by detailed history and examination. Air entry might be unequal. Chest X-ray can be helpful in the diagnosis. The role of steroids is essential along with ventilation.

Neurogenic Pulmonary Edema

There is an associated traumatic brain injury causing catecholamines surge leading to pulmonary edema. There is a need to treat the triggering event in these cases.

COVID Lung

There have been case reports during COVID (coronavirus disease) illness leading to acute inflammatory reactions giving rise to diffuse alveolar infiltrates in the lungs. Treatment involves noninvasive ventilation (NIV) and invasive ventilation.[27]

Sympathetic Crashing Acute Pulmonary Edema

This pathology is seen perioperatively when a catecholamine surge leads to pulmonary edema by increased afterload, decreased contractility, and preload. It can be seen with accelerated hypertension. It is also called flash pulmonary edema. Another example is Takotsubo syndrome (TTS), associated with pulmonary edema. This is again a catecholamine surge mimicking acute coronary syndrome where coronaries are normal, and hence it is a diagnosis of exclusion. Treatment involves supportive care of the heart along with the lungs.

Fluid Overload

This can be seen perioperatively in patients with low ejection fraction (EF) or chronic renal failure who can develop fluid overload. There is hyponatremia and hypoosmolarity that helps in reaching the diagnosis. This is an important differential diagnosis to be considered perioperatively. It needs to be treated with diuretics along with airway support.

An association between TTS cardiomyopathy and NPPE has also been observed. Severe ventricular dysfunction is seen after a catecholamine surge, which leads to increased afterload and pulmonary edema. This embarks an insight to be kept along with NPPE, as TTS is a hyperadrenergic state. TTS is an underdiagnosed condition often named stress-induced acute coronary syndrome. Patients usually do not have any previous cardiac abnormalities. NPPE can get complicated with TTS, but this acute coronary syndrome is typically seen in females above 50 years. The characteristic feature is midventricular or apical left ventricular dysfunction with raised enzymes but a normal coronary angiogram. This gets resolved, and ventricular function gets improved gradually. This catecholamine surge is the link between NPPE and TTS, as attempted inhalation against closed glottis results in negative intrathoracic pressure and catecholamine surge.[28,29] This hyperadrenergic state leads to direct myocyte injury and increases afterload and preload. The increased preload to the right ventricle causes increased pulmonary vasculature volume, hence increased hydrostatic pressures. Due to greater venous return to the right ventricle, septal bowing results in left outflow tract obstruction and decreased EF. Negative intrathoracic pressure increases the left ventricular transmural pressure. Hypoxia further causes peripheral vasoconstriction, increasing peripheral sympathetic activity. This further diminishes the left ventricular function. Though these two identities can coexist, a caveat of research is pending in this field. TTS can coexist, and any hypoxic respiratory failure in the setting of an airway obstruction should prompt search for both cardiogenic and noncardiogenic factors. The population in which NPPE commonly occurs is young males as compared to middle-aged females in TTS.

Negative pressure pulmonary edema is seen in the medical intensive care unit (ICU) in cases associated with OSA. It is often overlooked in medical ICUs because of its low incidence in a medical setting. In a setting where no cardiac or lung etiology is demonstrable, NPPE should be kept as a differential diagnosis. In OSA, intravascular hydrostatic pressure gets increased, favoring excess fluid infiltration. The absence of left ventricular dysfunction makes the diagnosis of acute NPPE likely. Substantial negative intrathoracic pressure is generated against the closed upper airway, increasing the transmural pressure in all intrathoracic structures, including the pulmonary interstitial pressure.[30-32] OSA-related hypoxia contributes to increased pulmonary microvascular hydrostatic pressure due to postcapillary pulmonary venules constriction; these events favor further lung fluid filtration. A portable device used for sleep apnea testing is equipped with technology to estimate intrathoracic pressure. Esophageal pressure can be used as a surrogate for pleural pressure but is challenging to measure it. A device is available that uses pulse wave signals to predict pleural pressure electronically.

In ICUs, NPPE can happen when there is ventilator–patient asynchrony in patients on mechanical ventilation. Adult respiratory distress syndrome (ARDS) patients on low tidal ventilation with increased respiratory drive lead to patient–ventilator asynchrony. This causes increased breathing, leading to negative inspiratory pressures and worsening pulmonary edema. This mimics the cardiothoracic relationships of NPPE and contributes to extubation failure in patients.

INVESTIGATIONS

Imaging

Point-of-care Ultrasound of the Lung

Point-of-care ultrasound is a bedside, noninvasive, and rapid investigation that helps diagnose NPPE using a phased array probe. It is a rapid goal-oriented tool that plays a vital role in perioperative diagnosis and management of hypoxia. It also assesses the cardiac contractility, vena cava compressibility, and pulmonary capillary wedge pressure measurement, thus leading to a conclusive diagnosis.[33,34] Presence of B lines on ultrasound of the lung indicates interlobular septa obliteration with fluid. Extracellular lung water accumulates in loose connective tissue (the continuous space without interruptions with the interlobular septa and subpleural tissues).

This creates an osmotic gradient from the periphery toward the center and allows peripheral clearance, hence an interlobular septum thickening stage before alveolar flooding. In contrast is ARDS, where a damaged membrane leads to random patchy edema and alveolar flooding without the interlobar septa thickening stage. More than three B lines in the same intercostal space suggests fluid filled in alveolar interstitial space. A rapid cardiac exam can also provide information about cardiogenic pulmonary edema by knowing the biventricular size, wall motion, inferior vena cava size, and collapsibility. It helps detect extravascular lung water (EVLW) accumulation before the clinical manifestations present.

Chest X-ray

Central and nondependent alveolar infiltrates point toward NPPE **(Fig. 2)**, with presence of Kerley B lines.

Computerized Tomography Scan

Computerized tomography (CT) scan of chest shows ground glass opacification and typical batwing pattern showing pulmonary opacities from center to periphery. The interlobular septa thickening and dorsocaudal appearance of edema along with normal pulmonary veins helps in differentiating it from other pathologies.

Echocardiography Findings

Pulmonary capillary wedge pressure helps differentiate between cardiogenic and noncardiogenic edema. Pulmonary capillary wedge pressure <18 mm Hg points toward noncardiogenic pulmonary edema. The ventricular contractility, vena cava dimensions, and compressibility give an idea about fluid overload.

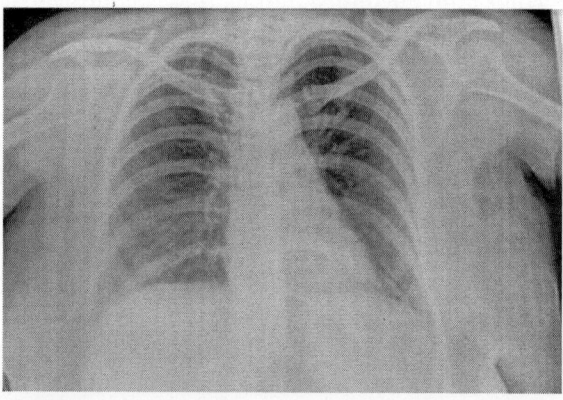

Fig. 2: Chest X-ray showing central and nondependent edema.

Arterial Blood Gas Analysis

Blood gas analyses show hypoxemia along with hypocarbia. Hypercarbia or even normal levels of carbon dioxide indicates ineffective ventilation. This is due to the increased dead space ventilation. There is an increased arterial-alveolar gradient seen in the blood gas picture.

Blood Tests

Cardiac myocytes of the left ventricles secrete BNP in response to stretching caused by increased ventricular blood volume or increased intracardiac pressures. BNP <100 pg/mL points toward noncardiac pathology (NPPE), whereas >500 pg/mL points toward cardiac pathology (cardiogenic edema).[26] Levels between 100 and 500 pg/mL, often seen in critically ill patients, do not help in differentiating it from heart failure. Serum electrolyte levels help in ruling out fluid overload.

■ MANAGEMENT

The management starts with oxygen support and administering positive pressure ventilation, either noninvasive or invasive. Oxygen should be given through a nonrebreathing mask at high flows (15 L/min).[8] In milder cases oxygen might be the only treatment needed.[35] Cases have been observed where delay in diagnosing and starting oxygen have left ventilation as the last option available.[35] Drugs such as furosemide and diuretics can be administered. Loop diuretics reduce sodium and chloride reabsorption to cause diuresis. They help by increasing the lung fluid clearance, but their role remains controversial.[36] Diuretics are helpful in hypervolemia, but one dose gives time to confirm NPPE and it is beneficial. Beta agonists act on the cellular mechanism of clearing lung water; by the cation transport mechanism. β2-agonists promote salt and water transport by increasing intracellular c-AMP (c-adenosine monophosphate) and improving alveolar fluid clearance. But its role is controversial and needs further research. Succinylcholine[8] in low doses of 0.5–1 mg/kg helps break the laryngospasm with low doses of propofol. Larson's maneuver is applied to break the laryngospasm by pressing between the mastoid process and the ramus of the mandible, also called jaw thrust. Dexamethasone is an anti-inflammatory drug, but its role in NPPE is not proven.[37] NIV reduces the work of breathing and helps in alveolar recruitment. Reducing the left ventricular afterload further improves the cardiac output and other hemodynamics. A lung-protective ventilation strategy is the key to establishing a good recovery with low tidal volume ventilation of 6–7 mL/kg and optimum PEEP of 5–10 mm Hg. NIV and mechanical ventilation are the key to recovery. NIV, when started promptly, avoids the use of invasive ventilation.[37]

An extubating strategy should be followed when there is patient–ventilator asynchrony. This highlights the importance of smooth spontaneous breathing before extubating, especially in patients prone to NPPE, like obese, OSA, active smokers, young robust males,[35] ones with recent respiratory infections, or patients for head and neck surgeries. There is a role for pressure support mode, provided in newer anesthesia workstations, as it facilitates assisted breathing while maintaining synchrony with the patient's own breaths. CPAP and pressure support should be preferred during extubation as it helps by applying positive pressure and maintaining the synchrony of respiration. Simultaneously the volatile agent must be removed from the patient system. Before extubation, ensuring that the patient is awake with optimal upper airway muscle tone is prudent.

CONCLUSION

Postextubation pulmonary edema continues to occur and is common in young, healthy males without any significant risk factors. This syndrome can occur in general anesthesia and may develop following lapses in anesthetic technique, especially extubation. Any patient experiencing breath-holding spells or airway obstruction immediately postextubation should be observed closely in postoperative room. There is a significant association between NPPE, OSA, and Takotsubo cardiomyopathy. NPPE is sometimes a diagnosis of exclusion, but it is essential to identify it in patients with certain risk factors, such as obesity with OSA, smokers, and young athletes, for head and neck surgeries.

REFERENCES

1. Capitanio MA, Kirkpatrick JA. Obstructions of the upper airway in children as reflected on the chest radiograph. Radiology. 1973;107:159-61.
2. Oswalt CE, Gates GA, Holmstrom MG. Pulmonary edema as a complication of acute airway obstruction. JAMA. 1977;238:1833-5.
3. Lathan SR, Silverman ME, Thomas BL, Waters WC 4th. Postoperative pulmonary edema. South Med J. 1999;92:313-5.
4. Goli AK, Goli SA, Byrd RP Jr, Roy TM. Spontaneous negative pressure changes: an unusual cause of noncardiogenic pulmonary edema. J Ky Med Assoc. 2003;101:317-20.
5. Chen IC, Chen KH, Tseng CM, Hsu JH, Wu JR, Dai ZK. Croup-induced postobstructive pulmonary edema. Kaohsiung J Med Sci. 2010;26(10):567-70.
6. Guffin TN, Har-el G, Sanders A, Lucente FE, Nash M. Acute postobstructive pulmonary edema. Otolaryngol Head Neck Surg. 1995;112(2):235-7.
7. Dicpinigaitis PV, Mehta DC. Postobstructive pulmonary edema induced by endotracheal tube occlusion. Intensive Care Med. 1995;21(12):1048-50.
8. Bhaskar B, Fraser JF. Negative pressure pulmonary edema revisited: Pathophysiology and review of management. Saudi J Anaesth. 2011;5(3): 308-13.

9. Westreich R, Sampson I, Shaari CM, Lawson W. Negative-pressure pulmonary edema after routine septorhinoplasty: discussion of pathophysiology, treatment, and prevention. Arch Facial Plast Surg. 2006;8(1):8-15.
10. Dolinski SY, MacGregor DA, Scuderi PE. Pulmonary hemorrhage associated with negative-pressure pulmonary edema. Anesthesiology. 2000;93:888-90.
11. Guinard JP. Laryngospasm-induced pulmonary edema. Int J Pediatr Otorhinolaryngol. 1990;20:163-8.
12. Travis KW, Todres ID, Shannon DC. Pulmonary associated edema with croup and epiglottitis. Pediatrics. 1977;59(5):695-8.
13. Sonsuwan N, Pornlert A, Sawanyawisuth K. Risk factors for acute pulmonary edema after adenotonsillectomy in children. Auris Nasus Larynx. 2014;41(4):373-5.
14. Bhattacharya M, Kallet RH, Ware LB, Matthay MA. Negative-pressure pulmonary edema. Chest. 2016;150:927-33.
15. Xiong J, Sun Y. Negative pressure pulmonary edema: a case report. BMC Anesthesiol. 2019;19:63.
16. Arita Y, Yamamoto S, Eda Y, Hasegawa S. Negative pressure pulmonary edema. Intern Med. 2018;57:3673-4.
17. Aay T, Bouti K, Tebay N. Negative pressure pulmonary edema following a cholecystectomy—A case report. Rev Pneumol Clin. 2017;73:267-71.
18. Matthay MA, Folkesson HG, Clerici C. Lung epithelial fluid transport and the resolution of pulmonary edema. Physiol Rev. 2002;82:569-600.
19. Sartori C, Matthay MA. Alveolar epithelial fluid transport in acute lung injury: new insights. Eur Respir J. 2002;20(5):1299-313.
20. Suzuki M, Inagi T, Kikutani T, Mishima T, Dito H. Negative pressure pulmonary edema after reversing rocuronium-induced neuromuscular blockade by sugammadex. Case Rep Anesthesiol. 2014;2014:135032.
21. Sorgenfrei IF, Norrild K, Larsen PB, Stensballe J, Ostergaard D, Prins ME, et al. Reversal of rocuronium-induced neuromuscular block by the selective relaxant binding agent sugammadex: a dose-finding and safety study. Anesthesiology. 2006;104(4):667-4.
22. Osawa T. Different recovery of the train-of-four ratio from rocuronium-induced neuromuscular blockade in the diaphragm and the tibialis anterior muscle in rat. J Anesth. 2008;22(3):236-41.
23. Herbstreit F, Peters J, Eikermann M. Impaired upper airway integrity by residual neuromuscular blockade: increased airway collapsibility and blunted genioglossus muscle activity in response to negative pharyngeal pressure. Anesthesiology. 2009;110(6):1253-60.
24. Ghofaily LA, Simmons C, Chen L, Liu R. Negative pressure pulmonary edema after laryngospasm: a revisit with a case report. J Anesth Clin Res. 2013;3(10):252.
25. Iqbal MA, Gupta M. Cardiogenic Pulmonary Edema. In: StatPearls [Internet]. Treasure Island (FL): StatPearls Publishing; 2023.
26. Rana R, Vlahakis NE, Daniels CE, Jaffe AS, Klee GG, Hubmayr RD, et al. B-type natriuretic peptide in the assessment of acute lung injury and cardiogenic pulmonary edema. Crit Care Med. 2006;34(7):1941-6.
27. Karaman I, Ozkaya S. Differential diagnosis of negative pressure pulmonary edema during COVID-19 pandemic. J Craniofac Surg. 2021;32(5):e421-e423.

28. Lee SH, Chang CH, Park JS, Nam SB. Stress-induced cardiomyopathy after negative pressure pulmonary edema during emergence from anesthesia—A case report. Korean J Anesthesiol. 2012;62(1):79-82.
29. Harmon E, Estrada S, Koene RJ, Mazimba S, Kwon Y. Concurrent Negative-Pressure Pulmonary Edema (NPPE) and Takotsubo Syndrome (TTS) after Upper Airway Obstruction. Case Rep Cardiol. 2019;2019:5746068.
30. Chaudhary BA, Ferguson DS, Speir WA Jr. Pulmonary edema as a presenting feature of sleep apnea syndrome. Chest. 1982;82(1):122-4.
31. Ilyass M, Anass E, Youssef H, Naoufal D, Abderrahmane E, Abdelouahed B, et al. Postoperative acute pulmonary edema: an obstructive sleep apnea syndrome. Ann Med Health Sci Res. 2023;13:404-6.
32. Watanabe Y, Nagata H, Ichige H, Kojima M. Negative pressure pulmonary edema related with severe sleep apnea syndrome: A case report. Respir Med Case Rep. 2020;31:101153.
33. Silva A, Furtado I, Grenho B, Isidoro M. Point of care ultrasound-diagnostic approach of an atypical negative pressure pulmonary oedema. Turk J Anaesthesiol Reanim. 2022;50(4):306-8.
34. Martindale JL, Noble VE, Liteplo A. Diagnosing pulmonary edema: lung ultrasound versus chest radiography. Eur J Emerg Med. 2013;20(5):356-60.
35. Holmes JR, Hensinger RN, Wojtys EW. Postoperative pulmonary edema in young, athletic adults. Am J Sports Med. 1991;19:365-71.
36. Koh MS, Hsu AA, Eng P. Negative pressure pulmonary oedema in the medical intensive care unit. Intensive Care Med. 2003;29:1601-4.
37. Bello G, De Santis P, Antonelli M. Noninvasive ventilation in cardiogenic pulmonary edema. Ann Transl Med. 2018;6(18):355.

…
CHAPTER 3
Uncommonly Performed Regional Anesthesia Techniques

Deepak Pahwa

ABSTRACT

The introduction of ultrasound has brought significant advances in regional anesthesia. Ultrasound has introduced newer nerve and interfascial plane blocks, making them more accurate and reproducible. Anesthesiologists all over the world are using ultrasound to practice regional anesthesia techniques. Regional anesthesia provides better pain relief as compared to opioids and helps in avoiding opioid-related side effects as well as the adverse physiological effects associated with inadequate pain control. This chapter describes, in brief, some of the regional anesthesia techniques that are less commonly used but can still be helpful in several clinical situations.

Keywords: Ultrasound; Regional anesthesia; Analgesia

■ KEY POINTS

- Regional anesthesia provides better analgesia as compared to opioids.
- The use of ultrasound has revolutionized the field of regional anesthesia.
- Ultrasound guidance helps improve the accuracy and the success rate of regional anesthesia techniques.
- Knowledge of less common regional anesthesia techniques can help an anesthesiologist tide over a tricky situation.
- Superior trunk block and selective trunk block can be used for analgesia for surgeries around the shoulder and proximal humerus; and for surgeries involving the whole upper extremity, respectively.
- Clavipectoral fascial plane block along with superficial cervical plexus block can provide anesthesia for surgeries for fracture clavicle.
- The external oblique intercostal plane block is a proper analgesic technique for managing somatic pain arising from the incision of cholecystectomy, hepatic resection, gastrectomy, etc.
- Pudendal nerve block provides analgesia for perineal and vaginal surgeries, hemorrhoids, prostate brachytherapy, and prostate biopsy.
- Sacral multifidus plane block helps relieve pain after perianal surgeries and urogenital procedures.

INTRODUCTION

The last two decades have seen significant advances in surgical techniques. These advances in surgical techniques were only possible with concurrent advances in anesthesia. Adequate perioperative analgesia is essential to any surgery in the enhanced recovery after surgery (ERAS) pathways.[1] Regional anesthesia provides better analgesia as compared to intravenous opioids[2] and helps in avoiding adverse physiological effects due to inadequate pain control.[3]

The adaptation of ultrasound in the mid-1990s for giving peripheral nerve blocks has revolutionized the field of regional anesthesia. Ultrasound has made regional anesthesia safer, more accurate, and easily reproducible. The introduction of ultrasound has led to the developing of newer regional anesthesia techniques. In this chapter, we will be discussing some uncommon but valuable ultrasound-guided regional anesthesia techniques.

SPHENOPALATINE GANGLION BLOCK

The sphenopalatine ganglion (SPG) is the largest parasympathetic ganglion in the body. It is situated in the upper part of the pterygopalatine fossa and is functionally related to the facial nerve.

Indications:[4]
- For treatment of postdural puncture headache (PDPH)
- For perioperative analgesia after cleft palate surgery and functional endoscopic sinus surgery
- Treatment of cluster headache
- For treatment of migraine and other types of headaches
- For treatment of various types of facial pains.

Contraindications:
- Patient refusal
- Patients with coagulopathy
- Patients with facial trauma, which may distort the sonoanatomy
- Allergy to local anesthetics.

Relevant Anatomy

The SPG is situated in the upper part of the pterygopalatine fossa. It is bounded anteriorly by the posterior wall of the maxillary sinus, posteriorly by the lateral pterygoid plate, and medially by the perpendicular plate of the palatine bone; laterally, it continues as the infratemporal fossa while superiorly sphenoid sinus forms its roof **(Fig. 1A)**.

Sensory innervation through the SPG is provided by the fibers arising from the maxillary nerve, and these fibers provide sensations to the nasal membranes, soft palate, and parts of the pharynx. Parasympathetic fibers passing through SPG arise from the superior salivatory nucleus of the pons, pass through nervus intermedius, and form the greater superficial petrosal

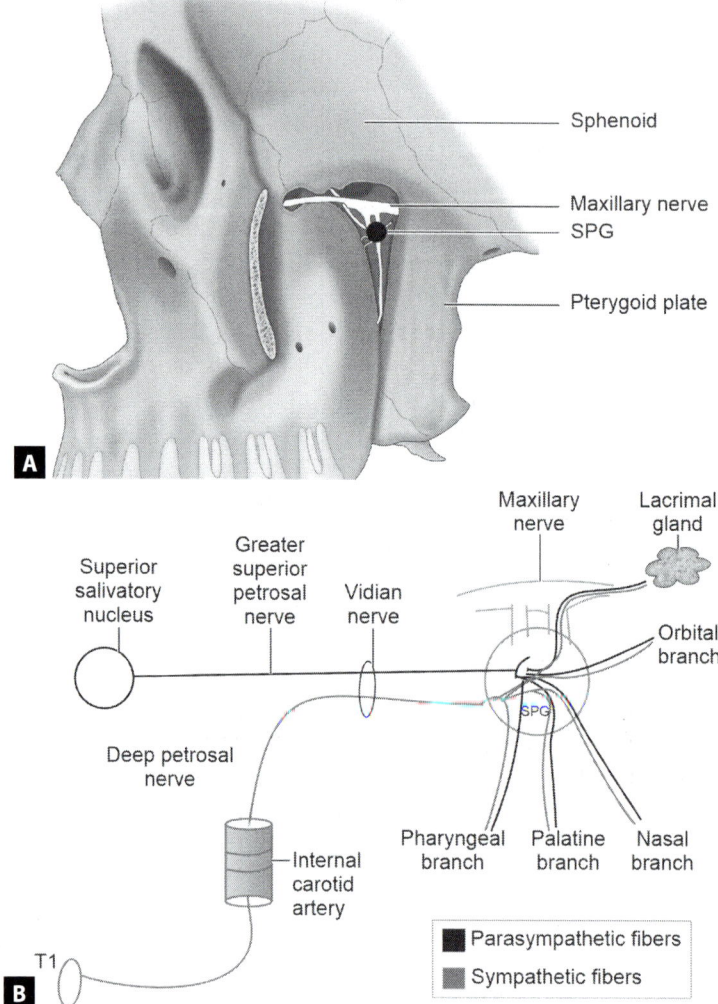

Figs. 1A and B: Sphenopalatine ganglion (SPG) and its relations passage; (B) anatomical illustration showing relay of autonomic fibers in SPG.

nerve. These fibers relay in the SPG. The postganglionic fibers arising from that SPG provide the secretomotor function to the lacrimal glands, the mucus membranes of the nose, the oral cavity, and the pharynx. The sympathetic fibers associated with SPG arise from the upper thoracic spine and synapse with the postganglionic fibers in the superior cervical ganglion. These fibers then pass through the SPG to provide innervation to the lacrimal gland, the nasal, and the palatine mucosa **(Fig. 1B)**.

Block Technique

Various approaches to giving SPG block have been described. These include transnasal, intraoral, suprazygomatic, and infrazygomatic approaches.

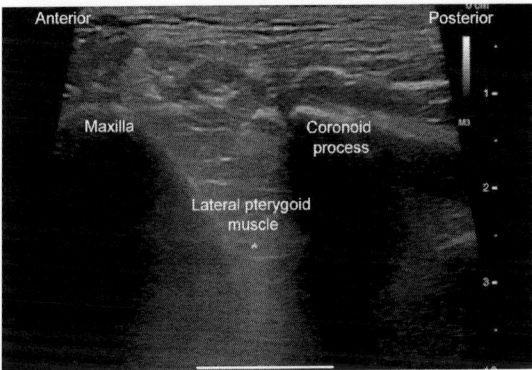

Fig. 2: Sonographic image obtained while giving sphenopalatine ganglion block; the asterisk indicates the needle target.

The transnasal approach has been associated with unpredictable block effects. Serious complications such as needle entry into the orbit, nasal cavity, and serious bleeding episodes have been reported with intraoral and infrazygomatic approaches.[5] Therefore, the author prefers a suprazygomatic approach for giving this block.

For giving the SPG block, the patient is supine with the head turned toward the opposite side. The posterior border of the orbital rim and the zygomatic arch are marked. The area is cleaned and draped. A linear high-frequency transducer is placed just below the inferior margin of the zygomatic arch and directed cranially at an angle of around 45°. The maxilla and the coronoid process are visualized on the ultrasound screen. The infratemporal fossa and the lateral pterygoid plate are between these bony processes. A needle is then introduced from just above the superior margin of the zygomatic arch behind the posterior border of the orbital rim and directed caudally at an angle of around 45°. The tip of the needle is located using the hydrodissection technique. The target for the tip of the needle is the infratemporal fossa just above the lateral pterygoid plate. Once the target is reached, around 5 mL of 0.25% bupivacaine or 0.2% ropivacaine can be injected in an adult patient **(Fig. 2)**.

The side effects of this block include bruising of the skin, and anesthesia in the territory of the maxillary nerve and sometimes in the territory of the whole trigeminal nerve.

Although various observational studies describe the use of SPG block for the treatment of PDPH, the recent guidelines published by the American Society of Regional Anesthesia and Pain Medicine do not support the use of SPG block for the treatment of PDPH.[6]

■ SUPERIOR TRUNK BLOCK

The superior trunk block is used mainly in shoulder surgery as an alternative to the interscalene brachial plexus block. Since the superior trunk is blocked, it provides noninferior analgesia compared to the interscalene brachial plexus block. As the block is given distal in comparison with interscalene brachial plexus block, the chances of phrenic nerve blockade reduce significantly.

Indications:
- Anesthesia for surgeries around the shoulder
- Anesthesia for surgeries around the proximal humerus
- For providing postoperative analgesia after shoulder and proximal humerus surgeries.

Contraindications:
- Patient refusal
- Infection at the needle insertion site
- Contralateral hemidiaphragmatic paralysis
- Bilateral block insertion
- Inability to avoid the overlying vascular structure.

Relevant Anatomy

The shoulder and the proximal humerus receive innervation mainly from the branches of the C5 to C6 nerve roots. The shoulder also receives innervation from the supraclavicular nerves, which arise from C3 to C4 nerve roots. The C5 and C6 nerve roots combine to form the superior trunk. The phrenic nerve lies superficial to the anterior scalene muscle, and as we move distally, it moves away from the brachial plexus. Therefore, a block at the trunk level has a lower chance of causing a phrenic nerve blockade than one at the root level.

Block Technique

For giving this block, the patient is positioned supine with the neck turned toward the opposite side. A linear high-frequency ultrasound probe is placed above the clavicle to identify the subclavian artery and the brachial plexus lying lateral to it. The transducer is slid in a cephalad direction to determine the interscalene groove. The C5 and C6 nerve roots are identified in the groove as the "traffic light sign". The transducer is then slid slightly caudally, and the C5 and C6 nerve roots are seen to merge to form the superior trunk. As we move further in a caudal direction, the suprascapular nerve is seen to leave the trunk. The injection site is the point lying just before where the suprascapular nerve leaves the superior trunk. The color Doppler is switched on to confirm the absence of the transverse cervical and the dorsal scapular arteries. The needle is then introduced in a lateral to medial direction advancing the needle above the middle scalene muscle. The needle tip is targeted to lie just below the superior trunk. Hydrodissection with a small amount of saline confirms the position of the tip of the needle. Once the needle position is confirmed, around 5–10 mL of local anesthetic is deposited below the superior trunk. The needle is then slightly withdrawn and redirected to lie above the superior trunk, and another 5 mL of local anesthetic is deposited at this location. While withdrawing the needle, the supraclavicular nerves (which also supply cutaneous innervation to the shoulder) are blocked as they lie in a plane just superficial to the middle scalene muscle. 5 mL of local anesthetic is sufficient to block the supraclavicular nerves **(Figs. 3A to C)**.

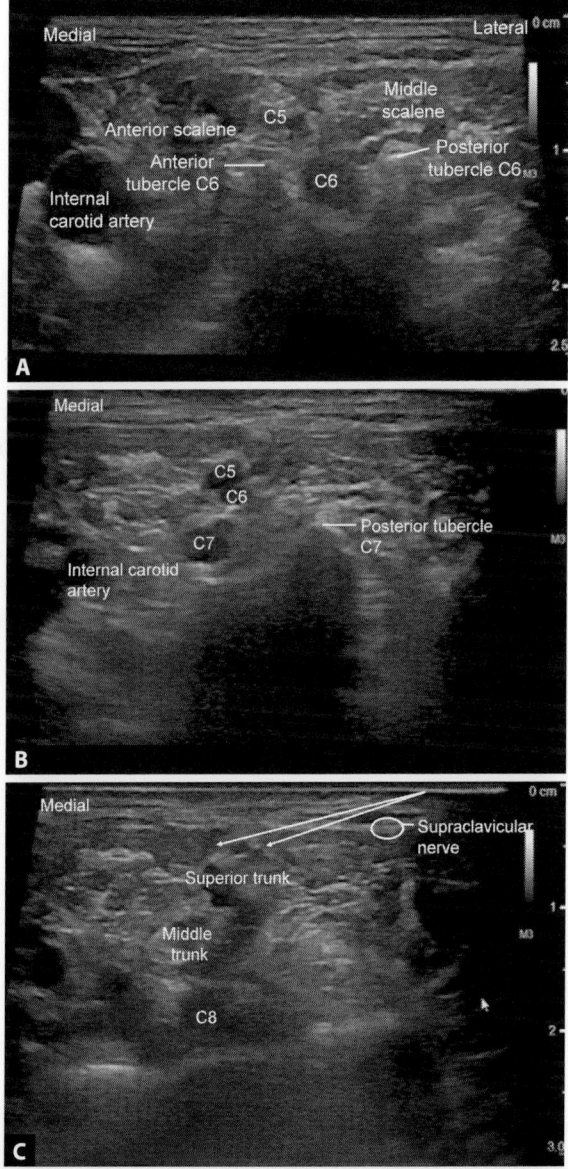

Figs. 3A to C: (A) Ultrasound image of C6 ventral rami coming out of transverse foramen; (B) scanning further caudally—C5 and C6 ventral rami join together to form the superior trunk and C7 ventral rami can be seen coming out of the transverse foramen; (C) needle trajectory for superior trunk block—first lateral and then medial to the superior trunk. Supraclavicular nerves can also be blocked through the same needle insertion point.

The incidence of phrenic nerve blockade with superior trunk block is reported to be around 5% as compared to the interscalene block, where it is seen in around 70% of the patients.[7,8] Horner's syndrome and hoarseness of voice can occur after superior trunk block.

SELECTIVE TRUNK BLOCK

This is a recently described block as an alternative to a combined or hybrid brachial plexus block. The supraclavicular block is considered the "spinal of the upper limb" and is believed to produce anesthesia of the entire upper extremity. However, sparing of the inferior trunk or ulnar nerve can be observed in 2–36% of the cases after the supraclavicular block.[9,10]

Indications:
- Surgery around the proximal humerus
- Surgeries involving the entire upper extremity like combined fractures of the arm and forearm, intramedullary nailing of humerus.

Block Technique

Patient positioning and initial ultrasound scanning are similar to the upper trunk block. A linear high-frequency transducer is placed in the supraclavicular fossa. The transducer is then swiped cranially very slowly to identify the ventral rami of C7, C6, and C5 sequentially. From here, the transducer is slid back in the caudal direction, and the formation of the superior trunk, middle trunk, and C8 ventral rami are identified (*see* **Figs. 3A to C**). The transducer is further moved caudally to identify the fusion of C8 and T1 ventral rami to form the inferior trunk at the level of the corner pocket of the supraclavicular fossa **(Fig. 4)**.

The block is performed through two skin punctures. The first puncture is performed at the level where the superior trunk, the middle trunk, and the

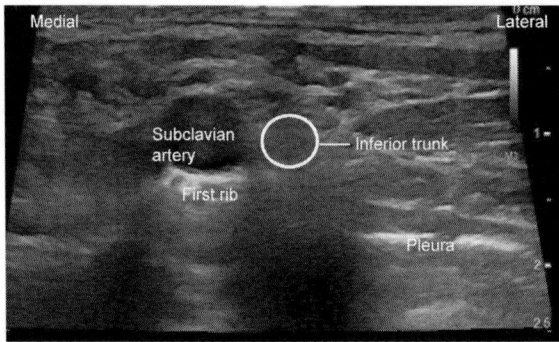

Fig. 4: Ultrasound image obtained by scanning further caudally from the superior and middle trunk to look for the inferior trunk in the supraclavicular fossa in the corner pocket.

C8 ventral rami are identified. A needle is introduced in a plane in a lateral to medial direction, similar to that, giving a superior trunk block. When the needle tip reaches next to the superior trunk, 7 mL of local anesthetic is deposited after negative aspiration of blood. The needle is then slightly withdrawn and redirected caudally to place the tip of the needle close to the middle trunk. Another 8 mL of local anesthetic is deposited at this location. The transducer is then moved caudally into the supraclavicular fossa, and the inferior trunk is identified. The block needle is then inserted from the lateral side of the transducer and advanced so that the tip of the needle lies close to the inferior trunk. 10 mL of local anesthetic is deposited at this site after negative aspiration of blood.[11,12]

There is limited data as of now on the selective trunk block. It offers a few advantages over the hybrid or the supraclavicular nerve block. We can achieve anesthesia over the entire upper limb except the T2 territory using only 25 mL of local anesthetic. It can also be used if there are two surgical sites—one in the proximal part of the upper limb and the other in the distal part of the upper limb.

■ CLAVIPECTORAL FASCIAL PLANE BLOCK

The clavipectoral fascial plane block was described for the first time by Valdes in the year 2017. The significant advantage of this block is that it provides no motor blockade of the upper limb.

Indications:
- Surgeries for fixation of fracture clavicle
- Surgeries for removal of the implant from the clavicle.

Relevant Anatomy

Clavipectoral fascia is a thick fascia that lies deep in the pectoralis major muscle. It extends medially from the costochondral joints, superolateral from the coracoid process, and superiorly from the clavicle. It extends inferiorly from the clavicle and splits and encloses the subclavius muscle. It reunites at the inferior border of the subclavius before splitting again to enclose the pectoralis minor muscle. At the inferior border of the pectoralis minor muscle, the fascia reunites to form the suspensory ligament of the axilla, which in turn attaches to the axillary fascia and forms the floor of the axilla **(Fig. 5)**.

The supraclavicular nerves supply the skin above the clavicle, which arises from the superficial cervical plexus. The sensory innervation of the clavicle, however, remains questionable. It has been proposed that the clavicle receives its innervation from the terminal branches of the suprascapular, the subclavian, the lateral pectoral, and the long thoracic nerves.[13] All these nerves that provide sensory innervation to the clavicle ultimately pass through

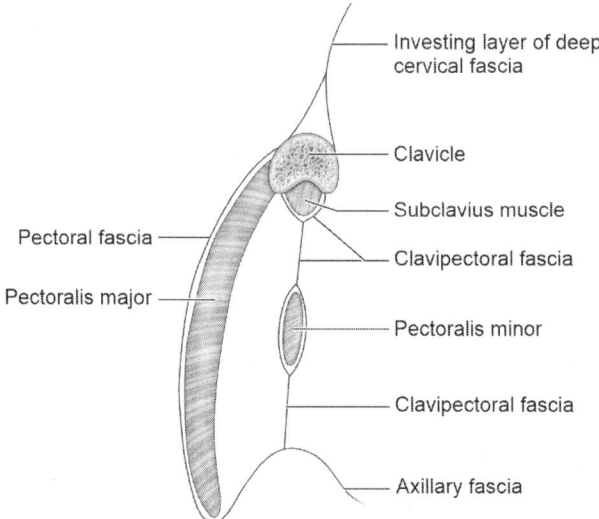

Fig. 5: Clavipectoral fascia and its relations.

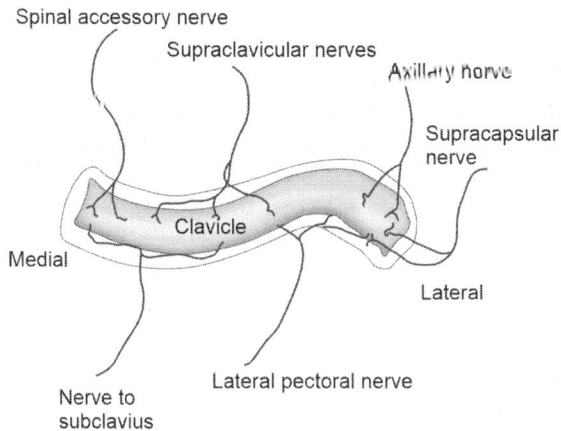

Fig. 6: Nerve supply of clavicle; clavipectoral fascia surrounds the clavicle.

the clavipectoral fascia before supplying the clavicle[14] **(Fig. 6)**. Fracture of the clavicle may cause a break in the continuity of the clavipectoral fascia. Therefore, while performing this nerve block, the drug should be deposited both medial and lateral to the fracture site.

Block Technique

For administering a clavipectoral fascia plane block, the patient is positioned supine with the head slightly turned toward the opposite side **(Fig. 7)**. A linear high-frequency ultrasound probe is then placed in a sagittal orientation first 2–3 cm medial and then 2–3 cm lateral to the fracture site.

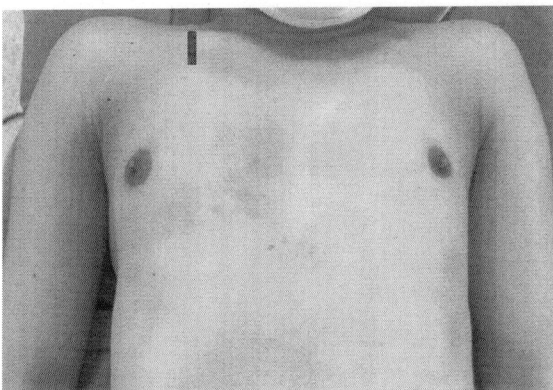

Fig. 7: Probe position for clavipectoral fascial plane block.

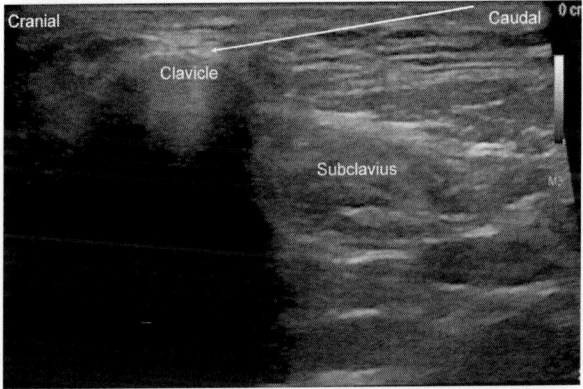

Fig. 8: Needle target for clavipectoral fascial plane block; the line indicates the needle trajectory.

The clavicle, the pectoralis major muscle, the subclavius muscle, and the clavipectoral fascia are then identified. A needle is then advanced in an in-plane technique from inferior to superior direction to place the tip of the needle between the clavipectoral fascia and the periosteum of the clavicle **(Fig. 8)**. About 10-15 mL of local anesthetic is deposited both medial as well as lateral to the fracture site. Clavipectoral fascial plane block and the supraclavicular nerve block or superficial cervical plexus nerve block can provide adequate anesthesia and analgesia for clavicle fracture surgeries.

■ MEDIAL CUTANEOUS NERVE OF FOREARM BLOCK

Indications:
- Superficial surgeries over the medial aspect of the forearm that do not require a tourniquet
- As an adjunct to brachial plexus block when sparing of the medial aspect of the forearm is observed.

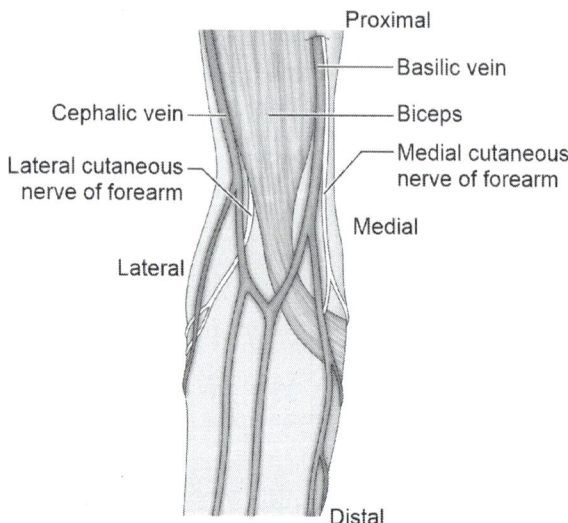

Fig. 9: Diagrammatic representation of the medial and lateral cutaneous nerves of forearm.

Relevant Anatomy

The medial cutaneous nerve of the forearm arises from the medial cord of the brachial plexus. It can be found superficial to the axillary artery and vein in the axillary fossa. It accompanies the basilic vein as it courses distally, enters the brachial fascia overlying the biceps brachii, and runs on the ulnar side of the brachial artery. The nerve travels further distally along the basilic vein lying medial to it. At the elbow level, it divides into anterior and posterior branches, which supply the skin over the anteromedial and posteromedial aspects of the forearm, respectively[15] **(Fig. 9)**.

Block Technique

The ultrasound-guided medial cutaneous nerve of the forearm block is given by positioning the patient supine and asking the patient to abduct his arm at 90° with the elbow in the extended position. A linear high-frequency transducer is kept in the short axis at the midarm level. The brachial artery, median nerve (medial to the brachial artery), ulnar nerve (medially in the subcutaneous plane), and the basilic vein are identified. The medial cutaneous nerve of the forearm can be identified as lying medial to the basilic vein. For blocking the nerve, a needle is introduced in the plane from lateral to medial direction, with the tip of the needle targeting the plane next to the basilic vein. Once the needle has reached its target, 2–3 mL of local anesthetic is deposited close to the nerve after negative aspiration of blood[16] **(Figs. 10A and B)**.

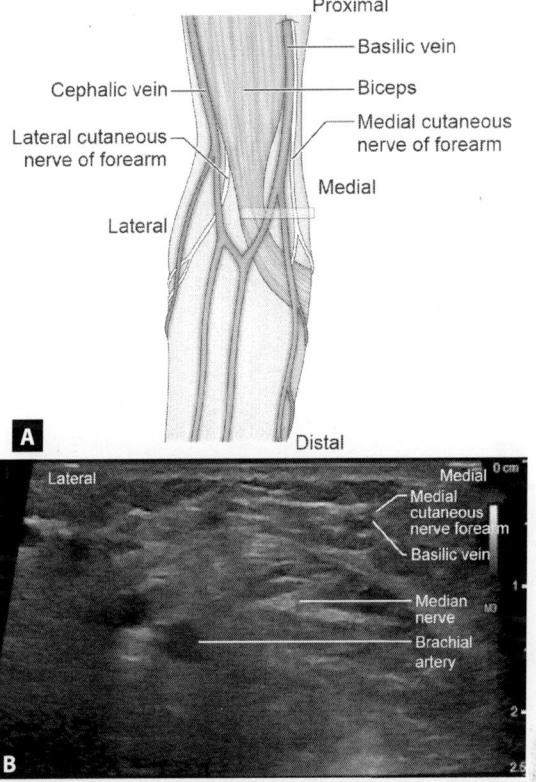

Figs. 10A and B: (A) Probe position for medial cutaneous nerve of forearm block; (B) sonographic image showing medial cutaneous nerve of forearm.

LATERAL CUTANEOUS NERVE OF FOREARM BLOCK

Indications:
- Superficial surgeries over the lateral aspect of the forearm that do not require a tourniquet
- As an adjunct to brachial plexus block when sparing of the lateral aspect of the forearm is observed
- Along with superficial radial nerve block for surgeries of the hand as it provides innovation to the base of the thumb.

Relevant Anatomy

Lateral cutaneous nerve of the forearm arises from the musculocutaneous nerve as its terminal branch. The musculocutaneous nerve travels in a plane between the biceps and brachialis muscle. At the elbow level, it emerges lateral to the tendon of the biceps brachii muscle. Continuing distally, it pierces the deep fascia and continues as the lateral cutaneous nerve of the forearm. At the elbow level, it lies medial or under the cephalic vein, which can be blocked easily (*see* **Fig. 9**).

42 Uncommonly Performed Regional Anesthesia Techniques

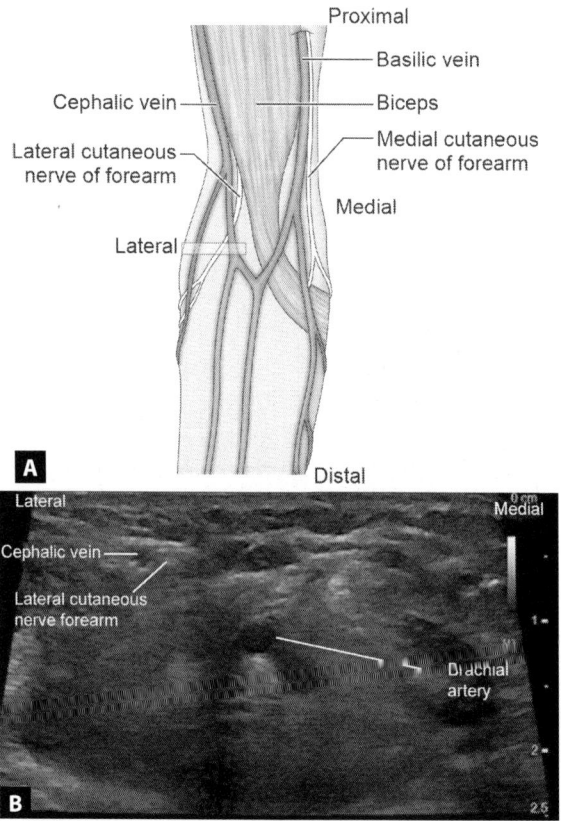

Figs. 11A and B: (A) Probe position for giving lateral cutaneous nerve of forearm block; (B) sonographic image showing lateral cutaneous nerve of forearm.

Block Technique

The patient is positioned supine with the arm abducted at 90° and the elbow extended. A linear high-frequency transducer is then placed at the level of the elbow in the short axis. The cephalic vein is identified as lying in the superficial plane. The lateral cutaneous nerve of the forearm is seen as a hyperechoic structure just medial to the cephalic vein. A needle is then introduced in a lateral to medial direction, with the needle tip targeting the plane next to the cephalic vein **(Figs. 11A and B)**. At this point, 2–3 mL of local anesthetic is deposited next to the nerve after negative aspiration of blood.[16]

TRANSVERSUS THORACIC PLANE BLOCK/PARASTERNAL INTERCOSTAL PLANE BLOCK

Transversus thoracic plane block or the parasternal intercostal plane block is a regional anesthesia technique that is especially useful for providing analgesia to the medial anterior chest wall.

Indications:
- Sternotomy
- Medial rib fractures
- Medial coverage for breast surgery
- Medial coverage for pacemaker/implantable cardioverter-defibrillator placement
- Sternal fractures.

Relevant Anatomy

Sternum is innervated by the anterior cutaneous branches of the second to sixth intercostal nerves and sympathetic plexus around the internal thoracic artery. The nerves pass through the plane between the internal intercostal and transversus thoracic muscles. Local anesthetic deposited between these two muscles at the level of ribs three and four can spread to cover the entire sternum. The internal thoracic artery passes between the internal intercostal and transversus thoracic muscles. The artery should be visualized before placement of the block.

Block Technique

The patient should be positioned supine for placing this block. A high-frequency linear ultrasound probe is placed on the chest in the parasagittal plane in the midclavicular line. Third and fourth ribs, the pectoralis major muscle, intercostal muscle, transversus thoracic muscle, and pleura are identified. The probe is moved medially toward the sternum to identify the transversus thoracic muscle **(Fig. 12)**. Transversus thoracic muscle appears as a hypoechoic layer just above the pleura. The transversus thoracic plane lies between the intercostal and the transversus thoracic muscle. Color flow

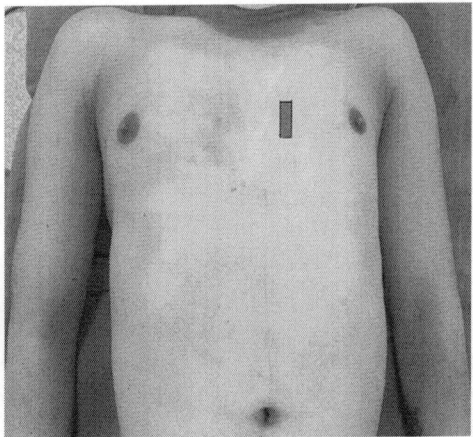

Fig. 12: Position of the transducer for giving parasternal intercostal block.

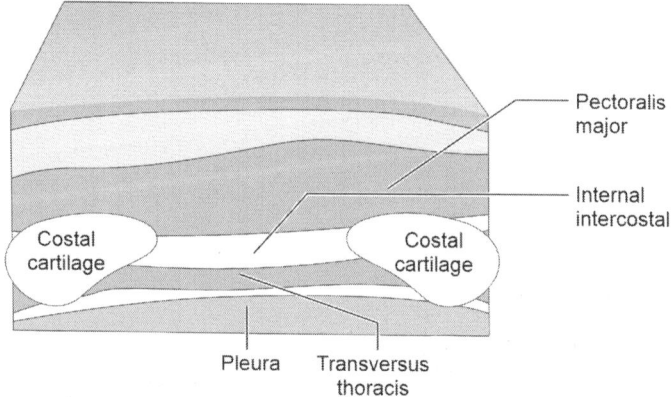

Fig. 13: Schematic view of the structures encountered while giving parasternal intercostal plane block.

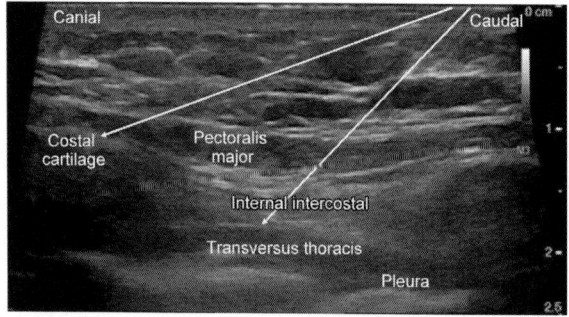

Fig. 14: Sonographic image of the parasternal intercostal block; the lines indicate target points for depositing the drug for the two approaches for the parasternal intercostal block.

Doppler is used before inserting the needle to identify the internal thoracic artery. A needle is then introduced in the plane from the caudal to the cranial direction. Once the needle tip reaches the appropriate plane, 10–20 mL of local anesthetic is deposited after negative aspiration of blood. Care should be taken that the needle tip should not reach the superior rib level **(Figs. 13 and 14)**.

Complications with this block include pneumothorax, hemothorax, and pericardial puncture when giving this block on the left side, leading to pericardial effusion, intravascular injection, and local anesthetic systemic toxicity.[17,18]

Since the placement of the needle tip in this plane can be associated with significant complications, another approach for blocking the anterior cutaneous nerves is targeting the plane between the pectoralis major and the intercostal muscles. The anterior cutaneous nerves pass superficially through the plane between the pectoralis major and the intercostal muscles

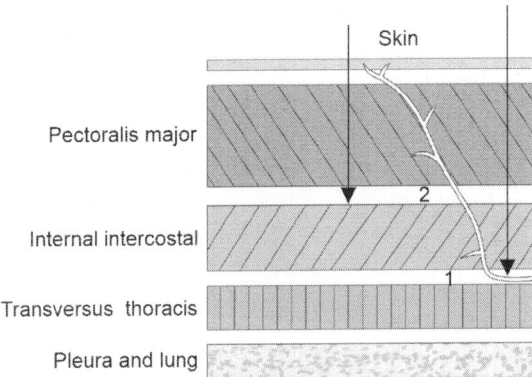

Fig. 15: Two planes of insertion for giving parasternal intercostal block.

before supplying the skin **(Fig. 15)**. A needle is inserted in a caudocranial direction, and the plane between the pectoralis major and the intercostal muscles is targeted. This can be achieved by advancing the needle toward the third costal cartilage and depositing the drug between the pectoralis major and the cartilage. This approach is more straightforward, associated with fewer complications, and equally effective (*see* **Figs. 13 and 14**).

■ EXTERNAL OBLIQUE INTERCOSTAL PLANE BLOCK

The external oblique intercostal plane block was described by Elsharkawy et al. in 2021. They used this block for providing postoperative analgesia in patients undergoing open abdominal surgeries with upper lateral quadrant incisions.

Indications: Upper abdominal surgeries with incision involving the upper lateral quadrant and the midline. For example, hepatic resection, cholecystectomy, gastrectomy, small bowel resection, and fundoplication.

Relevant Anatomy

The upper abdominal wall gets innervation from intercostal nerves T6 to T10. The external oblique muscle is the outermost layer of the abdominal wall. It originates from the lower eight ribs. The muscle fibers then run downward, forward, and medial direction. Around the midclavicular line, the fibers turn into a fibrous aponeurosis, forming the rectus sheath's anterior layer. The plane deep to the external oblique muscle is in continuity with the plane deep to the serratus anterior muscle, the latissimus dorsi muscle laterally, and the plane deep to the rectus abdominis muscle medially. So an injection of local anesthetic deep into the external oblique muscle will spread both laterally as well as medially to block the lateral as well as the anterior cutaneous branches of the intercostal nerves **(Fig. 16)**. It has been observed that the

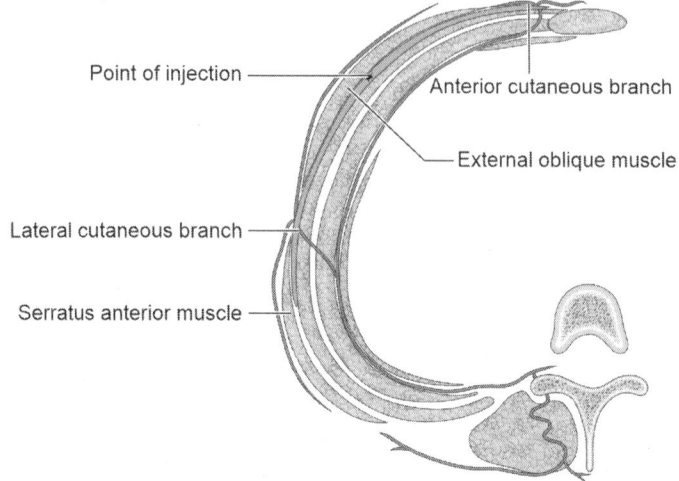

Fig. 16: Spread of drug injected in the external oblique intercostal plane.

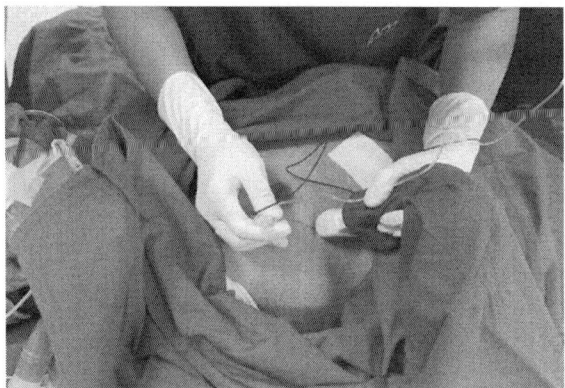

Fig. 17: Probe position for the external oblique intercostal plane block.

drug injected in this plane consistently blocks the lateral and the anterior cutaneous branches of the intercostal nerves T6–T10.[19]

Block Technique

The patient is positioned supine. A linear high-frequency transducer is placed in the sagittal orientation between the midclavicular and the anterior axillary lines at the level of the sixth rib.

The sixth rib is identified by placing the transducer at the level of the lower costal margin, which corresponds to the tenth rib. The transducer is then slid cranially, and the ribs are counted to identify the sixth rib. The transducer is then rotated slightly so that the cranial end of the transducer lies slightly medially while the caudal end of the transducer lies slightly laterally. The transducer now lies in a parasagittal oblique view around 1–2 cm medial to the axillary line **(Fig. 17)**. From superficial to deep subcutaneous tissue,

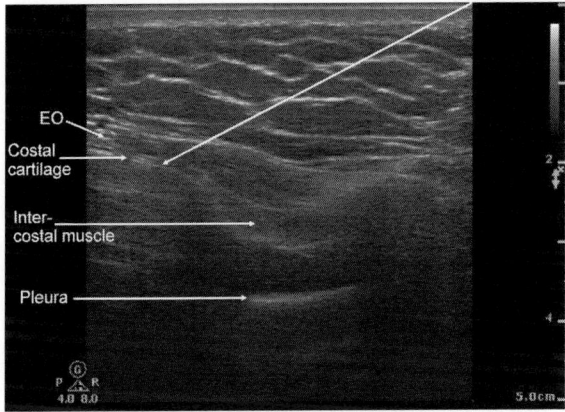

Fig. 18: Sonographic image for external oblique intercostal plane block. (EO: external oblique)

external oblique, and intercostal muscle lying between the two ribs, pleura, and the lung are identified. A needle is then inserted from the cranial end of the transducer and directed so that the needle tip lies between the external oblique and the intercostal muscles **(Fig. 18)**. Around 20–30 mL of the drug is deposited. Although this block provides good somatic analgesia, it does not provide visceral analgesia.

GENITOFEMORAL NERVE BLOCK

The genitofemoral nerve arises from the L1 to L2 nerve roots and, along with the ilioinguinal and iliohypogastric nerves, supplies the area bordering the abdomen and thigh. This nerve and the ilioinguinal and iliohypogastric nerves are commonly blocked for inguinal hernia surgeries.

Indications:
- Open inguinal hernia surgery along with the ilioinguinal and iliohypogastric nerve block
- For surgeries around the scrotum, like hydrocele and pyocele surgery
- For treatment of chronic postsurgical pain because of genitofemoral neuropathy.

Relevant Anatomy

The genitofemoral nerve arises from the ventral rami of the first and second lumbar nerve roots. It runs caudally on the anterior surface of the psoas major muscle and divides into the femoral and the genital branch above the inguinal ligament. The femoral branch of the genitofemoral nerve passes along with the femoral artery beneath the inguinal ligament to enter the femoral sheath. Its terminal branches pierce the femoral sheath to supply the skin over the femoral triangle. The genital branch passes through the transversalis and

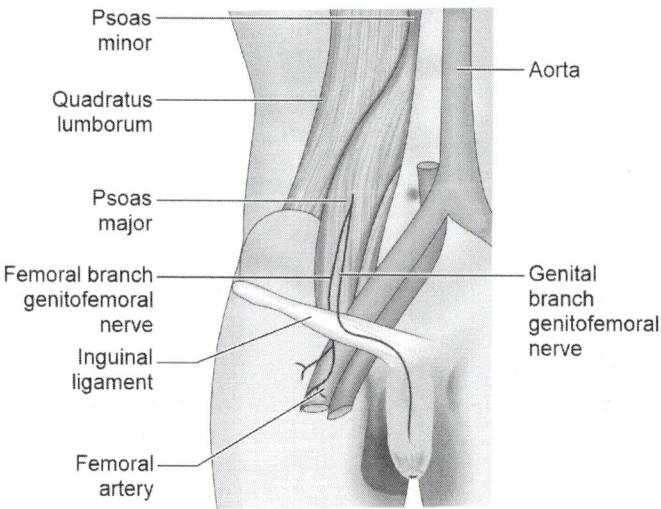

Fig. 19: Course of the genitofemoral nerve and its branches.

spermatic fascia and enters the deep inguinal ring. It runs through the inguinal canal between the cremaster and the internal spermatic fascia, incorporating with the cremasteric fascia, or lying outside the spermatic cord. The terminal branches of this nerve supply the scrotum and the upper, inner, and medial thigh[20] (Fig. 19).

Block Technique

The patient is positioned in the supine position. A linear high-frequency transducer is placed along the inguinal crease, and the femoral artery is seen on the short axis. The transducer is then rotated to visualize the femoral artery in its long axis. The transducer is gradually moved in a cephalad direction along the femoral artery to a point where the femoral artery starts dipping posteriorly. At this point, the femoral artery merges with the external iliac artery. The transducer is again rotated to visualize the external iliac artery in the short axis. The inguinal canal can be located here, lying superficial and medial to the artery as an oval structure. The inguinal canal is then traced medially so that the final position of the transducer is at a distance of around one finger breadth from the pubic tubercle. The inguinal canal contains the spermatic cord in males and the round ligament in females. The testicular arteries may be seen in the spermatic cord with the help of color Doppler. A needle is inserted from the plane to approach the inguinal canal **(Figs. 20A to D)**. In males, 4 mL of local anesthetic is deposited outside the spermatic cord, and 4 mL of local anesthetic is deposited inside the spermatic cord. In females, 5 mL of local anesthetic is deposited around the round ligament.[21]

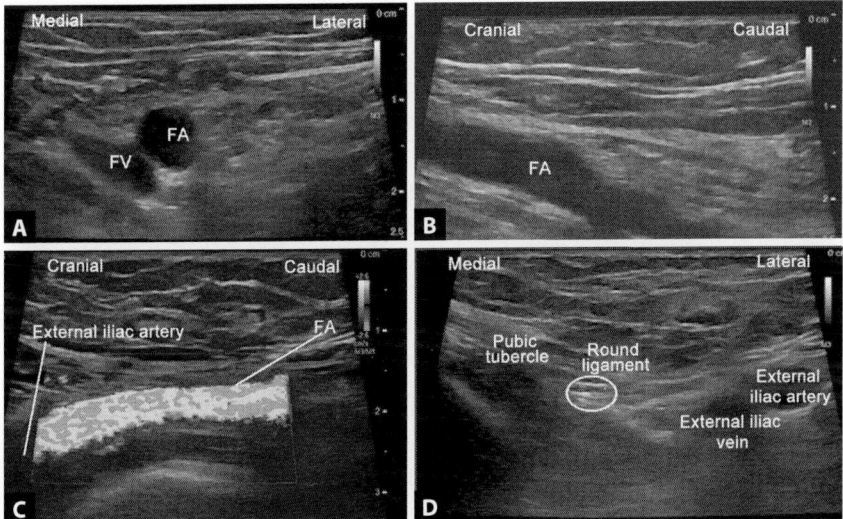

Figs. 20A to D: (A) Transverse scan at the level of inguinal grease; (B) transducer turned 90° to visualize the femoral artery (FA) in a long axis; (C) the FA is traced cranially as it arises from the external iliac artery; (D) the transducer is again rotated 90° to visualize the short axis's external iliac artery and look for a round ligament. (FV: femoral vein)

■ PUDENDAL NERVE BLOCK

The pudendal nerve is one of the primary nerves that supply the area around the perineum, rectum, and posterior part of the scrotum/labia majora. Despite pudendal nerve block being useful for several surgeries, it is not a popular technique, perhaps because of the need for more knowledge of its application.

Indications:
- For postoperative analgesia after hemorrhoids surgery, anorectal surgery, vaginal and perineal surgery, prostate biopsy, prostate brachytherapy, penile surgery, and during labor and episiotomies.
- For diagnosis and treatment of pudendal neuralgia.

Relevant Anatomy

The pudendal nerve arises from the ventral rami of the S2, S3, and S4 spinal nerves. It descends and passes between the piriformis and the ischiococcygeus muscle before leaving the pelvis through the greater sciatic foramen. It then passes dorsal to the sacrospinous ligament and ventral to the sacrotuberous ligament before reentering the pelvis through the lesser sciatic foramen. After entering the pelvis, the nerve passes through the pudendal canal accompanying the internal pudendal vessels. In the pudendal canal, the nerve gives off two branches: the inferior rectal nerve and then the perineal nerve before continuing as the dorsal nerve of the penis or clitoris. During its course through the interligamentous portion and the pudendal canal, it is at risk of compressive neuropathies. The inferior rectal nerve innervates the perianal skin and the lower third of the anal canal. The perineal nerve provides innervation to the skin of the perineum, the posterior part of the scrotum, or the labia majora and minora. The dorsal nerve of the penis or clitoris innervates the skin of the penis or clitoris. It is responsible for the initiation of erection and its maintenance.[22]

Block Technique

The pudendal nerve can be blocked using two approaches: anterior and posterior. The ultrasound-guided anterior or perineal approach was first described by Parras and Blanco in 2013. A linear high-frequency transducer is placed transversely lateral to the vulvar/scrotal junction with the rectum. Slightly medial and deep to the shadow of the ischial tuberosity, one should try to locate the pulsations of the internal pudendal artery. The use of the color Doppler can help identify the internal pudendal artery. The pudendal nerve branches can be identified as hyperechoic structures next to the pudendal artery. A needle is then introduced out of the plane toward the branches of the pudendal nerve. Once the needle reaches its target, 5–7 mL of the local anesthetic is injected close to the nerve after negative aspiration of blood **(Fig. 21)**. The procedure can then be repeated on the opposite side. The complications associated with this block are rare but include vascular injury, muscle weakness in the sciatic nerve territory, urinary or fecal incontinence, numbness in the pudendal nerve area, etc.

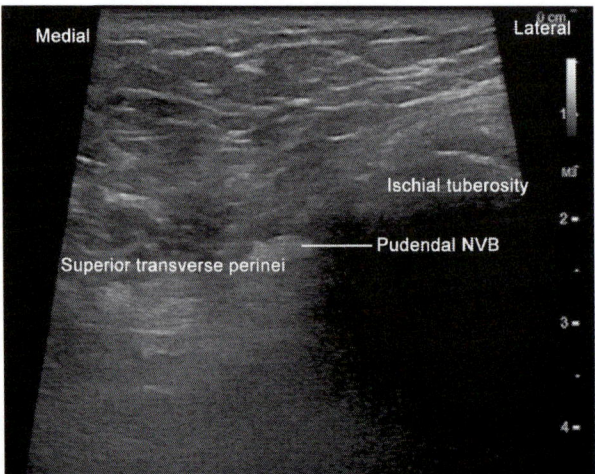

Fig. 21: Ultrasound image of the anterior approach to the pudendal nerve. (NVB: neurovascular bundle)

SACRAL MULTIFIDUS PLANE BLOCK

The sacral multifidus plane block was initially described by Tulgar et al. in 2019.[23] They used this block for analgesia for pilonidal surgery. Since then, it has been used in several surgeries.

Indications:
- Perianal surgeries
- Sacral spine surgery
- Pelvic fracture repair
- Urogenital procedures

Relevant Anatomy

The posterior surface of the sacrum is irregular and has three bony crests: (1) median, (2) intermediate, and (3) lateral. The spinal ganglia are found in the lateral part of the sacral canal. The dorsal rami arising from the spinal ganglia exit the sacral canal through the dorsal sacral foramina. The upper three dorsal rami pass through the multifidus muscle and supply the skin over the posteromedial aspect of the buttocks.

Block Technique

The patient is positioned prone. A curvilinear low-frequency transducer is placed in a paramedian sagittal orientation at the lumbar level. The L5 vertebra is identified, and the transducer is rotated transversely and then moved caudally to identify the first and second median sacral crest. The transducer is slid 3–4 cm laterally to identify the second intermediate sacral crest and the multifidus muscle. A needle is then advanced in an in-plane approach to hit the posterior aspect of the bone. 20 mL of local anesthetic is deposited between the multifidus muscle and the sacral crest in the interfascial plane **(Figs. 22A and B)**. Sacral multifidus plane block possibly blocks the dorsal rami and media cluneal nerves as they pass through the multifidus muscle. Some local anesthetic may also spread anteriorly through the sacral foramina to block the ventral rami. A local anesthetic may also spread anteriorly and cranially to block the pudendal nerve, lumbosacral plexus, and sciatic nerve.[24]

DEEP POSTERIOR GLUTEAL COMPARTMENT BLOCK

Regional anesthesia for surgeries around the hip joint concentrates primarily on the lumbar nerve supply to the hip joint. This is because the highest number of nociceptors are present on the superolateral part of the hip capsule.[25] However, a few patients may have more receptors on the posterior part of the capsule. These patients may experience significant pain despite administering regional anesthesia techniques aimed primarily at the anterior innervation of the hip joint. Deep posterior gluteal compartment block,

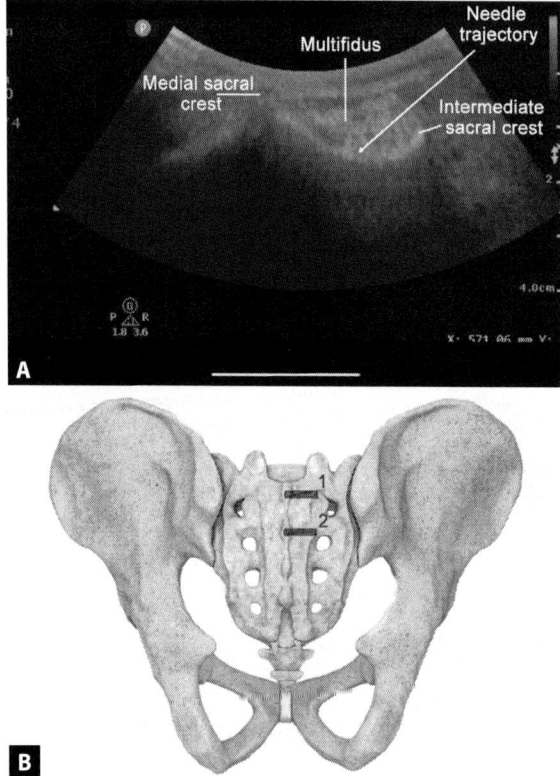

Figs. 22A and B: (A) Sonographic image and needle trajectory for sacral multifidus plane block; (B) stepwise transducer position for sacral multifidus plane block.

which is a recently described nerve block technique, can be especially useful in these patients.[26]

Indications: For postoperative analgesia in patients who underwent hip surgery and complain of pain in the posterior hip after the surgery.

Relevant Anatomy

The posterior part of the hip capsule receives innervation from the sciatic nerve, superior gluteal nerve, and nerve to the quadratus femoris muscle. These nerves arise from spinal nerves L4 to S1.

The superior and inferior gluteal nerves run caudally and emerge just above and below the piriformis muscle, respectively. These nerves then enter the fatty compartment lying superficially and cranially to the triceps coxae, the quadratus femoris muscle, and deep to the gluteus maximus muscle. The superior gluteal nerve travels along with the superior gluteal vessels to reach the plane between the gluteus medius and gluteus minimus muscle. Ultimately, all the nerves supplying the posterior part of the hip pass

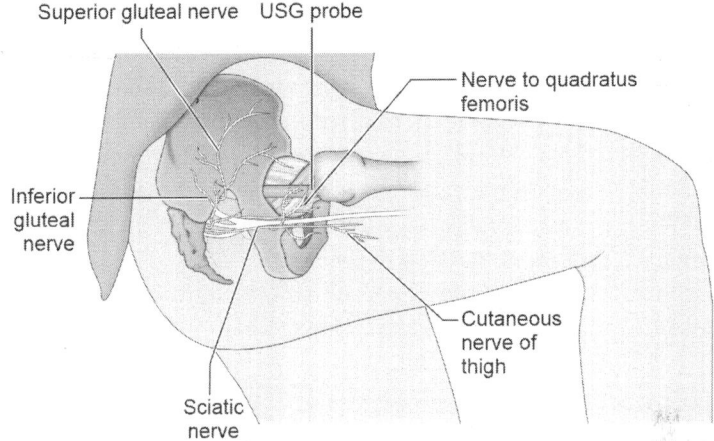

Fig. 23: Various nerves supplying the posterior part of the hip joint and the probe position for giving deep posterior gluteal compartment block. (USG: ultrasonography)

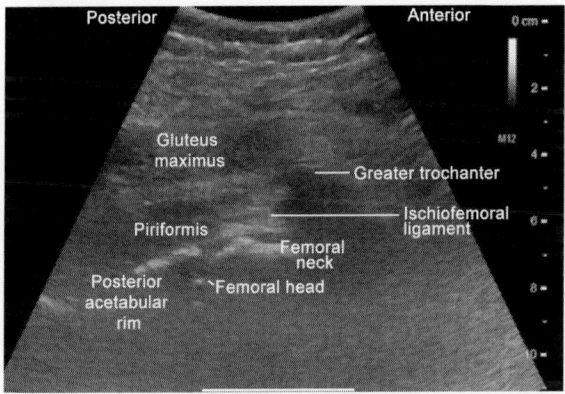

Fig. 24: Sonographic image of the structures encountered during deep posterior gluteal compartment block.

through a fatty compartment that lies cranial to the triceps coxae, caudal to the gluteus medius muscle, anterior to the gluteus maximus muscle, and posterior to the piriformis muscle **(Fig. 23)**.

Block Technique

The patient is positioned in the lateral decubitus position with the side to be blocked, lying non-dependent. The hip and knee of the nondependent side are flexed at a 90° angle. A curved low-frequency transducer is placed at the greater trochanter along the axis of the femur bone. The probe is then moved posteriorly to identify the greater trochanter, the femoral neck and head, and the posterior margin of the acetabulum. The gluteus maximus and piriformis muscles can be identified as lying superficial to deep above these bony landmarks **(Fig. 24)**. A needle is then introduced in a plane in a posterolateral to anterior-medial direction till the tip of the needle contacts the posterior margin of acetabulum near its attachment to the ischiofemoral ligament. 20 mL of local anesthetic is deposited at this point after negative aspiration of blood. The spread of the drug can be seen over the posterior hip capsule, the posterior margin of the acetabulum, and under the piriformis muscle. Since the sacral plexus lies near the injection site, blockade of the posterior femoral cutaneous nerve and the sciatic nerve can be expected. In patients with a fracture of the neck of the femur where 90° flexion of the hip joint is difficult to achieve, the block can still be performed with the bony landmarks identifiable even with lesser degrees of limb flexion.

CONCLUSION

Various less common regional anesthesia techniques have been described in this chapter. These techniques help provide analgesia to the patients, and some can also provide surgical anesthesia. Knowledge and familiarity with these techniques add another tool to the armamentarium of anesthesiologists.

REFERENCES

1. Ripollés-Melchor J, Ramírez-Rodríguez JM, Casans-Francés R, Aldecoa C, Abad-Motos A, Logroño-Egea M, et al.; POWER Study Investigators Group for the Spanish Perioperative Audit and Research Network (REDGERM). Association between use of enhanced recovery after surgery protocol and postoperative complications in colorectal surgery: The Postoperative Outcomes Within Enhanced Recovery After Surgery Protocol (POWER) Study. JAMA Surg. 2019;154:725-36.
2. Schug SA, Palmer GM, Scott DA, Halliwell R, Trinca J; APM: SE Working Group of the Australian and New Zealand College of Anaesthetists and Faculty of Pain Medicine. Acute Pain Management: Scientific Evidence, 4th edition. Melbourne: Australian and New Zealand College of Anaesthetists and Faculty of Pain Medicine; 2015.
3. Hutton M, Brull R, Macfarlane AJR. Regional anaesthesia and outcomes. BJA Educ. 2018;18(2):52-6.
4. Gharaei H, Nabi BN. Sphenopalatine Ganglion Block a Jack of all Trades Block. J Anesth Crit Care Open Access. 2015;3(2):00091.
5. Smith CR, Dickinson KJ, Carrazana G, Beyer A, Spana JC, Teixeira FJP, et al. Ultrasound-guided Suprazygomatic Nerve Blocks to the Pterygopalatine Fossa: A Safe Procedure. Pain Med. 2022;23(8):1366-75.
6. Uppal V, Russell R, Sondekoppam RV, Ansari J, Baber Z, Chen Y, et al. Evidence-based clinical practice guidelines on postdural puncture headache: a consensus report from a multisociety international working group. Reg Anesth Pain Med. 2023;rapm-2023-104817.
7. Kim DH, Lin Y, Beathe JC, Liu J, Oxendine JA, Haskins SC, et al. Superior Trunk Block: A Phrenic-sparing Alternative to the Interscalene Block: A Randomized Controlled Trial. Anesthesiology. 2019;131(3):521-33.

8. Stirling D, Klar G, Cenkowski M. (2023). Ultrasound-guided superior trunk block. [online] Available from: https://resources.wfsahq.org/atotw/ultrasound-guided-superior-trunk-block/ [Last accessed September, 2023].
9. Perlas A, Lobo G, Lo N, Brull R, Chan VW, Karkhanis R. Ultrasound-guided supraclavicular block: outcome of 510 consecutive cases. Reg Anesth Pain Med. 2009;34:171-6.
10. Fredrickson MJ, Patel A, Young S, Chinchanwala S. Speed of onset of 'corner pocket supraclavicular' and infraclavicular ultrasound guided brachial plexus block: a randomised observer-blinded comparison. Anaesthesia. 2009;64(7):738-44.
11. Sivakumar RK, Areeruk P, Karmakar MK. Selective trunk block (SeTB): a simple alternative to hybrid brachial plexus block techniques for proximal humeral fracture surgery during the COVID-19 pandemic. Reg Anesth Pain Med. 2021;46(4):376-8.
12. Songthamwat B, Luangjarmekorn P, Kampitak W, Sivakumar RK, Karmakar MK. Ultrasound-guided selective trunk block (SeTB): a cadaver anatomic study to evaluate the spread of dye after a simulated injection. Reg Anesth Pain Med. 2022;47(7):414-9.
13. Rosales AL, Aypa NS. Clavipectoral plane block as a sole anesthetic technique for clavicle surgery - A case report. Anesth Pain Med (Seoul). 2022;17(1):93-7.
14. Sonawane K, Dixit H, Balavenkatasubramanian J, Gurumoorthi P. Uncovering secrets of the beauty bone: A comprehensive review of anatomy and regional anesthesia techniques of clavicle surgeries. Open J Orthop Rheumatol. 2021;6(1):019-029.
15. Ballard T, Black AC, Smith T. Anatomy, Medial Antebrachial Cutaneous Nerve. In: StatPearls [Internet]. Treasure Island (FL): StatPearls Publishing; 2023.
16. Sehmbi H, Madjdpour C, Shah UJ, Chin KJ. Ultrasound guided distal peripheral nerve block of the upper limb: A technical review. J Anaesthesiol Clin Pharmacol. 2015;31(3):296-307.
17. George R, Dahl K, Blair de Haan J. (2020). How I Do it: Transversus Thoracic Plane Block. [online] Available from: https://www.asra.com/news-publications/asra-newsletter/newsletter-item/asra-news/2020/05/01/how-i-do-it-transversus-thoracic-plane-and-pecto-intercostal-fascial-block [Last accessed September, 2023].
18. Chin KJ, Versyck B, Pawa A. Ultrasound-guided fascial plane blocks of the chest wall: a state-of-the-art review. Anaesthesia. 2021;76 Suppl 1:110-26.
19. Elsharkawy H, Kolli S, Soliman LM, Seif J, Drake RL, Mariano ER, et al. The External Oblique Intercostal Block: Anatomic Evaluation and Case Series. Pain Med. 2021;22(11):2436-42.
20. Mirjalili SA. Anatomy of the lumbar plexus. In: Tubbs RS, Rizk E, Shoja MM, Loukas M, Barbaro N, Spinner RJ (Eds). Nerves and Nerve Injuries. Netherlands: Academic Press; Yeah 2015. pp. 609-17.
21. Peng P, Seib R. (2019). Genitofemoral nerve (inguinal canal) block. [online] Available from: https://www.asra.com/news-publications/asra-updates/blog-landing/legacy-b-blog-posts/2019/08/06/genitofemoral-nerve-(inguinal-canal)-block [Last accessed September, 2023].
22. Rojas Gomez MF, Blanco-Dávila R, Tobar Roa V, Gómez González AM, Ortiz Zableh AM, Azuero AO. Regional anesthesia guided by ultrasound in the pudendal nerve territory. Colombian J Anesthesiol. 2017;45(3):200-9.

23. Tulgar S, Senturk O, Thomas DT, Deveci U, Ozer Z. A new technique for sensory blockage of posterior branches of sacral nerves: Ultrasound guided sacral erector spinae plane block. J Clin Anesth. 2019;57:129-30.
24. Mistry T, Sonawane K, Balasubramanian S, Balavenkatasubramanian J, Goel VK. Ultrasound-guided sacral multifidus plane block for sacral spine surgery: A case report. Saudi J Anaesth. 2022;16(2):236-9.
25. Tomlinson J, Zwirner J, Ondruschka B, Prietzel T, Hammer N. Innervation of the hip joint capsular complex: a systematic review of histological and immunohistochemical studies and their clinical implications for contemporary treatment strategies in total hip arthroplasty. PLoS One. 2020;15:e0229128.
26. Vermeylen K, Van Aken D, Versyck B, Casaer S, Bleys R, Bracke P, et al. Deep posterior gluteal compartment block for regional anaesthesia of the posterior hip: a proof-of-concept pilot study. BJA Open. 2023;5:100127.

CHAPTER 4

Continuous Spinal Anesthesia

Pratibha Jain Shah, Anisha Nagaria

ABSTRACT

Continuous spinal anesthesia (CSA) is a reliable and versatile but underutilized centrineuraxial technique in which a small titrated amount of local anesthetic (LA) is injected into subarachnoid space through an indwelling catheter to achieve the height of block as per the surgical need with stable hemodynamic, to extend block duration for prolonged surgery and to provide post-operative analgesia. Most of the reviewed literature has pointed out the advantages of CSA over general anesthesia (GA), spinal and epidural anesthesia, and combined spinal-epidural, especially in high-risk elderly patients and after an accidental dural puncture in obstetric patients. Most complications associated with CSA, like meningitis, postdural puncture headache (PDPH), and neurological complications, are preventable. As mentioned in the chapter, one must weigh the advantages and disadvantages of CSA in a selected group of patients with specific indications. This technique will be needed more in the coming times because of the increasing age of surgical presentation and associated systemic illness. This chapter also covers the historical background, indications, contraindications, methodology, and precautions to avoid complications.

Keywords: Anesthesia techniques; Continuous spinal anesthesia; Single-shot spinal anesthesia; Intrathecal/spinal catheter; Epidural catheters; Microcatheters; Complications of continuous spinal anesthesia

■ KEY POINTS

- Continuous spinal anesthesia (CSA) is a well-established, reliable centrineuraxial technique in which a small titrated volume of local anesthetics (LAs) is injected intermittently through an intrathecal catheter to produce and maintain a desired level of sensory block to extend the duration of the blockade in case of prolonged surgeries and to provide postoperative analgesia.

- It has an excellent success rate and provides good hemodynamic stability. Hence, safe for lower limb and abdominal surgery in high-risk, trauma, and elderly patients.
- Besides many advantages over single-shot spinal anesthesia (SSSA), epidural anesthesia, combined spinal–epidural anesthesia, and general anesthesia (GA), CSA is not so popular and underutilized by anesthesiologists due to technical reasons and false belief that it is associated with a high risk of postdural puncture headache (PDPH), meningitis, and neurological complications.
- To avoid curling and caudal displacement, the intrathecal catheter should not be advanced beyond 3 cm into subarachnoid space. It should be labeled appropriately to avoid any medication errors.
- Catheter insertion, manipulation, and drug injection should be done under strict asepsis, preferably by a single anesthesiologist or caregiver aware of the intrathecal catheter.
- Despite the high risk of PDPH in the obstetric population, CSA is considered in specific challenging situations such as previous spinal surgery, significant maternal cardiac disease, morbid obesity, difficult epidural catheter placement, difficult airway, and accidental dural puncture.
- With increasing high-risk surgical patients, CSA can be an asset to the anesthesiologist.

INTRODUCTION

Continuous spinal anesthesia is a type of regional anesthesia, where an intrathecally placed catheter allows injection of small titrated doses of LA to produce a well-controlled subarachnoid block. It provides better hemodynamic stability following sympathetic blockade associated with spinal anesthesia, unlike SSSA, where a fixed larger dose can result in an unpredictable block height and hemodynamic instability.[1-6] LA are usually injected intermittently in CSA; intermittent or fractionated spinal anesthesia could be a more appropriate word than CSA.[7] It is one of the most useful, versatile, and reliable centrineuraxial techniques available to provide analgesia and anesthesia in both obstetric and nonobstetric populations.[5,6] For many years, it was considered only for elderly patients with cardiac problems posted for lower abdominal and limb surgeries,[8] but nowadays it is also used in younger population too for various obstetric, gynecological, and urological procedures.[6,9-12] Though the use of CSA in the nonobstetric and obstetric population dates back almost a century and eight decades, respectively, the wider use and acceptance of this technique have been hampered primarily by limitations of the available equipment and associated complications, despite having plenty of inherent advantages.

HISTORICAL BACKGROUND[1,2,4-6,7,9,11]

Continuous spinal anesthesia was first described in 1906 by Henry Percy Dean, a British surgeon, almost 7 years after the introduction of SSSA with cocaine in 1899 by August Bier. It involved intermittent injection of LA through a spinal needle left in the spinal canal throughout the operation. Its popularity and existence remained in a dilemma ever since.

After three decades, in 1940, William T. Lemmon, a Philadelphia surgeon, revived the technique, though it was cumbersome and very tricky. He performed a spinal tap in lateral position in 140 cesarean deliveries using a malleable 17-18G German silver needle (2.5-3.5″ long), which was connected to a flexible, rubber tubing with a stopcock to inject the LA as and when required. Then, the patient was positioned supine on a mattress and table, having a gap to accommodate the indwelling needle and rubber tubing **(Fig. 1)**. The same mattress was used by Hinebaugh and Lang (1944) to administer CSA for labor analgesia in over 50 cases. The usefulness of the CSA approach was constrained by the requirement to anchor needles in the subarachnoid area.

In 1944, Edward Tuohy of Mayo Clinic attempted to overcome this limitation by using a 15G Tuohy spinal needle that allowed easy passage of a 4G lacquered silk urethral catheter, injecting LA intermittently into subarachnoid space. Though continuous access was more manageable, inevitable PDPH secondary to the sizeable dural hole created by the 15G Tuohy needle hindered its widespread use. In 1950, Dripps reported paresthesia and a low success rate following CSA. The inherent drawbacks of CSA, such as technical problems, degree of trauma, and likelihood of cerebrospinal fluid (CSF) loss, put this technique into a long period of quiescence.

The technique of CSA was revisited 20 years later, following the development of 32G microcatheters by Hurley and Lambert in 1987 which

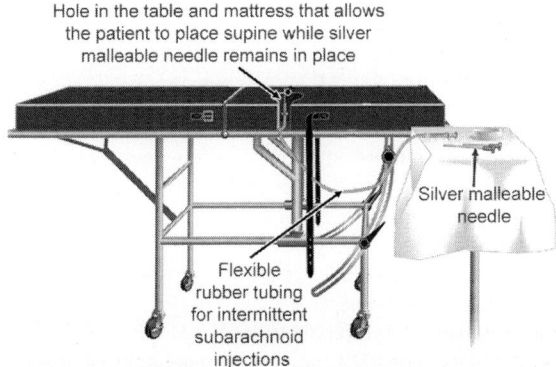

Fig. 1: Special table and mattress used by Lemmon for continuous spinal anesthesia in 1940.

were passed through a 26G spinal needle. Since then, there has been a surge in enthusiasm for using CSA as these microcatheters and the smaller spinal needles required for their placement promised to decrease the incidence of PDPH to certain levels. Unfortunately, these catheters were challenging to manipulate and associated with a high failure rate because of kinking and breakage. A high incidence of cauda equina syndrome was reported with their use by Rigler et al. In 1992, the US Food and Drug Administration (FDA) banned using catheters over 24G size. In 2010, Palmer reported the successful administration of CSA in 300 parturients using a 28G catheter.

There have been many case reports on the successful conduct of anesthesia for abdominal and lower limb surgeries in high-risk elderly populations. However, inhibition of using CSA among anesthesiologists continued because of beliefs of high risk of PDPH, neurological damage, and meningitis.

ADVANTAGES

Continuous spinal anesthesia has definite advantages over single-shot spinal, epidural, continuous epidural, combined spinal epidural, unilateral spinal anesthesia, and sciatic nerve block **(Box 1)**.

- CSA provides reliable and excellent anesthesia because of a definite end point, i.e., free flow of CSF with minimal hemodynamic and respiratory disturbance, and the duration of anesthesia can be extended as per surgical need. Hence, it is helpful for prolonged surgical procedures in high-risk patients.[1,2,7,8,13,14]
- CSA provides better control over the height of the block with low incremental doses, extended duration of anesthesia, postoperative pain relief with better hemodynamic stability, and reduced risk of high or total spinal block compared to SSSA.[3,5,7,8,15-18]
- It avoids the use of multiple anesthetic agents used in GA, autonomic response to intubation and extubation, complications associated with GA,

BOX 1: Advantages of continuous spinal anesthesia.

- Reliable and well-established technique
- High success rate due to definite end point, i.e., free flow of cerebrospinal fluid
- Faster onset
- Better control over the height of the block
- Better cardiovascular and respiratory stability
- Provides extended duration of blockade in case of prolonged surgery
- Provision for postoperative analgesia
- Almost no risk of high and total spinal block
- Avoid the use of multiple anesthetic agents as in general anesthesia
- Relatively easier to perform
- Minimal side effect

and positive pressure ventilation, especially postoperative respiratory and cognitive dysfunction, and provides prolonged postoperative analgesia. Therefore, it is a valuable and excellent alternative anesthesia technique to GA in high-risk patients, such as those with severe aortic stenosis or cardiomyopathy, respiratory diseases posted for noncardiac abdominal and lower limb surgeries.[7,8]

- Compared to epidural anesthesia, CSA is relatively easier to perform, has a faster onset, has a high success rate due to a definite end point (free flow of CSF) and excellent hemodynamic stability, provides adequate level and degree of anesthesia, prolonged duration of sensory blockade with small incremental doses, and dramatically reduces the risk of high spinal anesthesia and LA toxicity. Hence, CSA is a better option for emergency surgeries or patients with limited anesthesia time.[7,18-23]
- Besides lots of advantages of CSA over epidural anesthesia by using smaller anesthetic doses with rapid onset and motor and sensory blockade recovery with better cardiovascular stability, it also provides superior hemodynamic stability during the initial intraoperative period compared to combined spinal–epidural anesthesia.[24]

INDICATIONS

Existing literature suggested that CSA has been successfully used in various types of major high-risk and abdominal surgeries in high-risk patients. There are a number of situations and comorbidities in which CSA becomes an attractive option while weighing the relative risk of treatable side effect against many advantages of CSA, which are as follows:

- Major lower abdominal and lower limb surgeries in patients with severe cardiorespiratory diseases and trauma, where GA is relatively risky.[8,23]
- Labor analgesia and cesarean deliveries, especially in high-risk pregnancy, previous spinal surgery, significant cardiac disease, morbid obesity, difficult airway, and difficult epidural catheter placement.[12,24,25]
- After an accidental dural tap, CSA can provide anesthesia and postoperative analgesia, as it is known to decrease the incidence of PDPH and avoids undue risk of repeat dural punctures.[12,24-26]
- Postoperative pain relief through a patient-controlled analgesic pump. Ansbro et al. (1954) have reported the use of an intrathecal catheter for postoperative analgesia.[27-29]
- Pain relief in cancer patients through an intrathecal pump.[30]

CONTRAINDICATIONS

- *Absolute*: CSA is contraindicated in case of patient refusal, raised intracranial pressure, coagulopathy, blood dyscrasias, sepsis, and marked spinal deformity.

- *Relative*: Mildly impaired coagulation (platelet count $80 \times 10^9/L$) and patients on anticoagulant therapy are relative contraindication due to the risk of spinal hematoma. The risk of spinal hematoma must be weighed against the benefits of avoiding GA in these patients.

EQUIPMENT (KIT) REQUIRED[1,3,7,9]

Continuous spinal anesthesia can be given through a standard epidural macrocatheter or specially designed spinal microcatheter sets. The only catheters available and frequently used to establish CSA are epidural catheters.[1]

- *Standard epidural macrocatheters sets*: These catheters (18G/20G/23G) are inserted into the subarachnoid space after a deliberate dural puncture with an epidural needle (16G/18G/20G), once free flow of CSF is achieved **(Fig. 2)**. These catheters are most commonly used for CSA because of their availability, easy insertion for those familiar with epidural insertion technique, unequivocal confirmation of correct catheter position by CSF aspiration, and better mixing of LAs. However, many experienced anesthesiologists still find deliberate dural punctures challenging to accept. We routinely use a 20G pediatric epidural needle with a 23G catheter for CSA in our tertiary care center.
- *Specially designed microcatheter sets* are available in various sizes as catheter-over-the-needle or catheter-through-needle sets.
  - *Catheter-over-the-needle set*: These sets (marketed as *Spinocath*) consist of a 22G catheter mounted on a 27G Quincke spinal needle or a 24G catheter mounted on a 29G Quincke spinal needle and an 18G epidural needle to access epidural space **(Fig. 3)**. The Quincke spinal needle is connected to a braided wire and has a fluid exit side hole within the catheter. Once the epidural needle is in place, a spinal needle with a mounted catheter is inserted and advanced to puncture

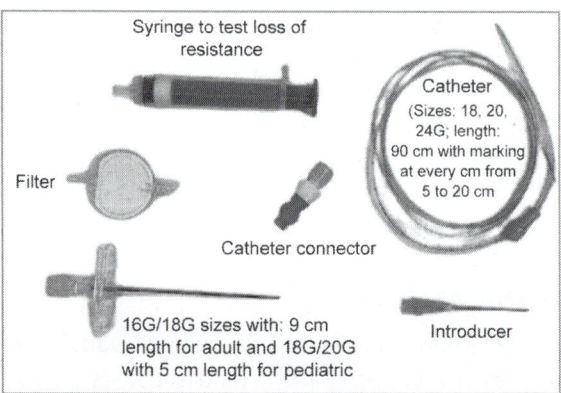

Fig. 2: Standard epidural set.

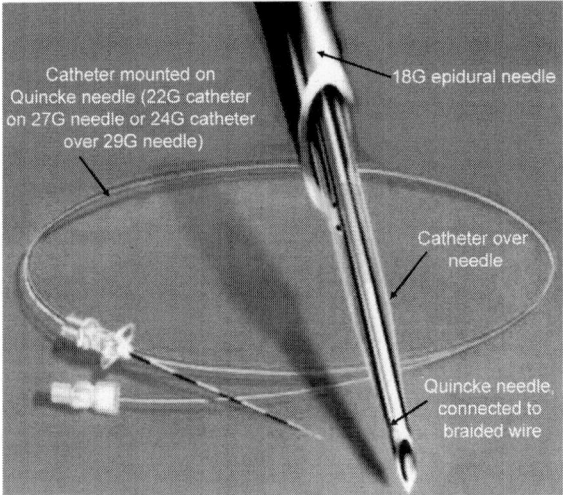

Fig. 3: Catheter over needle (Spinocath).

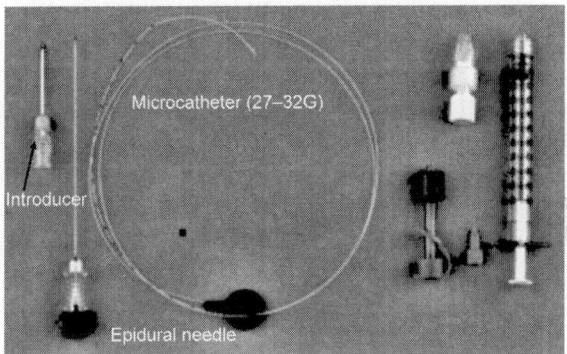

Fig. 4: Microcatheter through needle.

a dura and reach subarachnoid space. This is confirmed by getting CSF into the catheter, which comes through the exit side hole in the spinal needle. Then, braided wire is withdrawn to pull back the spinal needle while leaving the catheter within the subarachnoid space. After that epidural needle is withdrawn carefully, and the catheter is secured on the back using aseptic precautions. The main advantages of these sets are the definite end point of catheter placement and less risk of PDPH as a wide-bore catheter seals the hole made in the dura by the Quincke needle. However, published literature mentions that they are difficult to insert and require a definite skill.

- *Catheter-through-needle set*: These sets consist of microcatheters of varying sizes (25–32G), spinal needle, and introducer **(Fig. 4)**. Different manufacturers produce different types of needles and sizes of microcatheters; e.g., Pajunk IntraLong has 22G Sprotte needles with 25–32G catheters, Smith Medical makes 23G Crawford needles with 28G catheters and Kendell makes 22G Sprotte needles with 28G microcatheters. These catheters get kinked if force is applied during insertion. They may be difficult to insert despite the metal stylet introducer. Once inserted, it is not easy to aspirate CSF. CSF aspiration (an unequivocal end point of spinal catheter placement) is an impractical method for confirming the location of the microcatheter.

■ TECHNIQUE OF CONTINUOUS SPINAL ANESTHESIA

- Before proceeding with CSA, one should do a thorough pre-anesthetic check-up and consider any contraindications for CSA.
- Follow NPO guidelines, insert and secure large-bore cannula, and ensure availability of resuscitative equipment and emergency drugs. No premedication is required.
- Inside the operation room (OR), attach routine monitors. Invasive monitoring may be required in severely compromised surgical patients.
- Standard spinal anesthesia technique is followed for CSA. The lumen volume of the catheter and filter (dead space) should be measured (about 0.8–1.2 mL). This volume of normal saline is used to flush the intrathecal catheter after each aliquot to avoid an overdose of intrathecal LA. Under strict aseptic conditions, an epidural needle (in case of standard epidural macrocatheter set and catheter-over-needle set) and spinal needle (in case of microcatheter through needle set) is inserted, preferably through L3–L4 interspace. Free flow of CSF gives an unequivocal confirmation of correct needle placement.
- The catheter is threaded through the needle. Once it crosses the needle tip, advance it further 2–3 cm in the cephalad direction into the subarachnoid space and confirm the free flow of CSF.[1] Secure it in place and label it clearly to avoid confusion with the epidural catheter. Advancement of the catheter >3 cm increases the risk of malposition (caudally directed catheter) and coiling.[7] Caudally directed catheter lead to pooling of LAs in the sacral sac around cauda equina that has a potential risk of neurotoxic damage. Curled-up catheters can snare nerve roots at removal.
- The patient is positioned supine and small aliquots of preservative-free either mixture of iso- and hyperbaric or plain hyperbaric LAs (<1 mL) are injected through the subarachnoid catheter and flushed in with a small volume of saline (equal to dead space volume) to achieve the desired dermatomal block height as per surgical need.
- If the desired block height is not achieved in 10 minutes after the initial dose, inject the second aliquot of LA. Wait another 10 minutes and give third aliquot if desired block height still needs to be achieved. The procedure should be abandoned if there is no effect after three incremental doses.
- The patient's hemodynamics should be monitored every 5 minutes throughout the procedure.

- To extend the duration of anesthesia, a small volume of LA, followed by a saline flush, can be injected to increase the block height.
- The catheter should preferably be removed at the end of surgery after giving an analgesic concentration of LA or opioid alone unless there is a pressing reason to keep it in place. This is to avoid confusion with the epidural catheter and catastrophe, as staff in the ward may not be familiar with these catheters.
- A strict sterile technique is mandatory during the catheter placement, manipulation, and drug injection to minimize the risk of infection.[6,31]
- Clear labeling of the catheter is essential to alert all caregivers about the location of the catheter to avoid mistaking it for an epidural catheter. The same anesthesiologist should preferably administer the aliquots.[6,31]

DRUGS TO BE USED

Any preservative-free preparation of LA can be injected through spinal catheters for CSA. Bupivacaine 0.5% and 0.25% are the most frequently used.[1] Adjuncts, like opioids, midazolam, and clonidine, can be added to enhance the quality of blockade and prolong the duration of analgesia. Plain isobaric solutions spread by diffusion and produce a block centered around the segment of catheter insertion in both caudad and cephalad directions. Hyperbaric solutions are spread by physical movement of the solution around the floor of the uneven dural sac. The spread is limited by lumbar lordosis and thoracic curve up to T10.[1,6,7] Some researchers have used hyperbaric preparation for the initial bolus and isobaric for top-ups. Others have used a mixture of both hyperbaric and isobaric while some have just used isobaric preparation. Isobaric preparation is preferred for CSA to achieve more controllable anesthesia without posture manipulation and to avoid pooling of 8% dextrose that may exert hyperosmolar pressure on neurons.

PROBLEMS/COMPLICATIONS[1,5,7]

Factors preventing frequent use of CSA are listed in **Box 2**. The issues are:
- *Technical problems*: Difficulty in inserting and manipulating the fine catheters through needle, injecting drugs due to high resistance offered

BOX 2: Problems and complications associated with continuous spinal anesthesia.

- Technical problems
- Breakage, kinking, curling and caudally directed catheter
- Hemodynamic instability with large volume of local anesthetic
- Postdural puncture headache
- Meningitis
- Neurological complications (cauda equina syndrome)
- Intrathecal hematoma/hemorrhage
- Medication errors

by fine catheters and confirmation of correct catheter placement by CSF aspiration. Their incidence is approximately 20%.
- *Breakage/kinking of catheter*: It was more common with microcatheters, but can occur with macrocatheters. This can be minimized by slow removal of catheter with patient's back in flexed position and pulling the catheter as close to its insertion point as possible to avoid overstretching.
- *Hemodynamic instability*: This can cause hypotension and bradycardia, due to high level of block caused if large volume of LAs is given at frequent intervals. If small aliquots (<1 mL) are given at intervals to achieve adequate block height, no or transient hypotension follows CSA.
- *PDPH*: This is the common reason for the underutilization of CSA. The incidence of PDPH is directly proportional to the needle size and inversely proportional to patient age. The reported incidence of PDPH is quite low (<1% in the elderly population in Standl, 5.6% in Kumar and 1.5% in Lux studies). This low incidence of PDPH may be due to microcatheters, small-bore spinal needles, and an inflammatory reaction of the dura around the catheter that seals the hole at catheter removal. The reported incidence is high, around 29–33% in the obstetric population and young ambulatory patients.[2,4,7]
- Neurological complications such as cauda equina syndrome, although rare it is associated with the pooling of a large volume of hyperbaric LAs around the nerve roots secondary to microcatheters and caudally directed position. The high concentration of LAs causes direct LA toxicity and indirect nerve injury due to spinal cord ischemia. Accumulation of LAs may be avoided by threading only 3 cm of a catheter in subarachnoid space to prevent caudal displacement, injecting only <1 mL volume at any time, abandoning the technique if a total 3 mL of LA would not produce an adequate block, and avoiding administration of hyperbaric preparation.[1,7]
- *Infection*: Theoretically, drugs may spread directly via catheter into CSF and cause meningitis, but studies suggest a rare incidence of subclinical infection after 24–72 hours catheter in situ. This problem can be minimized by following strict aseptic precautions while placing and manipulating catheters and injecting drugs, avoiding frequent disconnection and reconnection, maintaining a closed system by continuous infusion, and using a bacterial filter.[7,11,31]
- *Intrathecal hemorrhage/hematoma* is rare with CSA and usually associated with heparin and urokinase use.[7]
- *Medication errors* can occur due to drug administration through incorrect routes or drug administration. Injecting a large epidural dose through catheters can lead to high spinal anesthesia, hypotension, and respiratory arrest. There are reports of intrathecal administration of labetalol and

tranexamic acid instead of intravenous administration. This can be minimized by clearly labeling catheters, syringes, and infusion pumps, providing clear instructions, and educating the staff.[31]
- One article reported intraoperative coughing, discomfort, hypotension, and nausea and vomiting following CSA, but that was possible because of the high spinal blockade required for laparotomy and excessive bowel handling by the surgeon.[9]

■ CONTINUOUS SPINAL ANESTHESIA IN OBSTETRICS

Continuous spinal anesthesia provides excellent, reliable, and rapid neuraxial blockade for labor analgesia and anesthesia for cesarean section. However, it is not frequently used in obstetrics because of the high incidence of PDPH and technical issues compared to single-shot spinal, epidural, and combined spinal–epidural anesthesia. However, in particular circumstances, intentional CSA is preferred over other centrineuraxial techniques, such as previous spinal surgery, significant maternal cardiac disease, morbid obesity, difficult epidural catheter placement, difficult airway, and accidental dural puncture.[7,11,12,26] The risk of PDPH is significantly reduced when the catheter is inserted into the subarachnoid space following an accidental dural puncture and is left in situ for >24 hours. The mechanical barrier prevents CSF leak from the dural hole and promotes early inflammation at the puncture site[29,31] **(Table 1)**. A long study was done on 761 obstetric population by Cohn et al. which reported no severe complications such as meningitis,

TABLE 1: Clinical indications of continuous spinal anesthesia (CSA) in obstetric population with reason.[6]

Clinical indications	Reason
Previous spinal surgery	Difficult epidural placement—about 40% failure rate
Significant maternal cardiac disease	Cannot tolerate slight changes in hemodynamics and additional IV anesthetics. CSA provides excellent anesthesia with minimal hemodynamic changes with slow titration of LA
Morbid obesity	Higher rate of epidural catheter failure and unintentional dural puncture. CSA conveys protection against PDPH
Difficult epidural catheter placement	CSA avoids risk of further dural puncture, provides immediate analgesia, and reduces rate of PDPH for 24 hours
Difficult airway	Though somewhat controversial, CSA provides immediate reliable and flexible route to induce anesthesia safely without worrying about loss of airway

(IV: intravenous; LA: local anesthetic; PDPH: postdural puncture headache)

TABLE 2: Suggested drugs for labor analgesia and anesthesia through continuous spinal catheter.[6,7,31]

Technique		Drugs
Labor analgesia	Intermittent bolus	Preservative-free plain bupivacaine 0.25%, 0.5–1 mL (1.75–2.5 mg) + fentanyl 15–20 µg as needed (roughly each 1–2 hours) or sufentanil 5.0 µg initial bolus, repeated as needed
	Continuous infusion	0.05–0.125% bupivacaine + fentanyl 2–5 µg/mL @ 0.5–3.0 mL/h and titrated to a T8–T11 sensory level Or sufentanil 2.5–5.0 µg/h
	Patient-controlled intrathecal analgesia	0.125% bupivacaine + fentanyl 2 µg/mL @ 1–2 mL/h Bolus 1 mL; lockout 20–30 minutes
	Top-ups	Bupivacaine 0.25%, 0.5–1 mL (1.75–2.5 mg) +/– fentanyl 15–20 µg as needed (roughly each 1–2 hours) Or sufentanil 5.0 µg
Surgical anesthesia		Preservative-free 0.5% bupivacaine 5.0 mg (1 mL) + fentanyl 15 mg for the initial dose followed by 0.5 mL boluses of 0.5% bupivacaine (2.5 mg) every 5 minutes until the desired block height is obtained

arachnoiditis, cauda equina syndrome, spinal and epidural abscess, and hematoma during the 12-year follow-up.[6,32] No clinical trial has compared or studied a particular drug for labor analgesia or anesthesia. However, according to the available case reports and series, opioids alone or a combination of opioids with LA are suggested for labor analgesia and anesthesia **(Table 2)**.

CONCLUSION

Continuous spinal anesthesia is a reliable, flexible, and well-established technique that provides excellent analgesia and surgical anesthesia in nonobstetric and obstetric patients using standard epidural catheters (preferably pediatric epidural catheters 24G). Fear of PDPH, meningitis, and neurological complications are the primary reason for its infrequent use; however, the relative risk of these preventable and treatable side effects should be weighed against many advantages of this technique, especially in specific, challenging populations. With the increasing rate of high-risk surgical patients, CSA can be an asset for an anesthesiologist to conduct abdominal and lower limb surgeries without complications.

REFERENCES

1. Burnell S, Byrne AJ. Continuous spinal anaesthesia. BJA CEPD Rev. 2001;1(5):134-7.
2. Kuczkowski KM. Continuous spinal anesthesia: New pearls from old practice. J Clin Anaesth. 2007;19(1):67-72.
3. Lux EA. Continuous spinal anesthesia for lower limb surgery: A retrospective analysis of 1212 cases. Local Reg Anesth. 2012;5:63-7.
4. Hay R, Gupta A. Continuous spinal anaesthesia. BJA Educ. 2022;22(8):295-7.
5. Moore JM. Continuous spinal anesthesia. Am J Ther. 2009;16:289-94.
6. Palmer CM. Continuous Spinal Anesthesia and Analgesia in Obstetrics. Anesth Analg. 2010;111(6):1476-9.
7. Parthasarathy S, Sheeba AJ. Continuous Spinal Anesthesia: A Need for a Re-emergence? Asian J Pharm Clin Res. 2015;8(6):50-3.
8. Amin SM, Sadek SF. Continuous spinal anesthesia for elderly patients with cardiomyopathy undergoing lower abdominal surgeries. Egypt J Anaesth. 2016;32:535-40.
9. Jaitly VK, Kumar CM. Continuous spinal anaesthesia for laparotomy. Curr Anaesth Crit Care. 2009;20(2):60-4.
10. Minville V, Fourcade O, Grousset D, Chassery C, Nguyen L, Asehnoune K, et al. Spinal anesthesia using single injection small-dose bupivacaine versus continuous catheter injection techniques for surgical repair of hip fracture in elderly patients. Anesth Analg. 2006;102(5):1559-63.
11. Veličković I, Pujic B, Baysinger CW, Baysinger CL. Continuous Spinal Anesthesia for Obstetric Anesthesia and Analgesia. Front Med (Lausanne). 2017;4:133.
12. Tao W, Grant EN, Craig MG, McIntire DD, Leveno KJ. Continuous Spinal Analgesia for Labor and Delivery: An Observational Study with a 23-Gauge Spinal Catheter. Anesth Analg. 2015;121(5):1290-4.
13. Beh ZY, Yong PSA, Lye S, Eapen SE, Yoong CS, Woon KL, et al. Continuous spinal anaesthesia: a retrospective analysis of 318 cases. Indian J Anaesth. 2018;62:765-72.
14. Nasr IAH, Nofal OA, Elsayed KM, Hegab AS. Continuous spinal anesthesia for selective spinal block in lower limb surgery. Zagazig Univ Med J. 2022;28(4):701-10.
15. Jain SP, Rashmi N, Chandrapal B, Kumar GR. Effect of Continuous Spinal Anesthesia and Single Shot Spinal Anesthesia on Hemodynamics for Lower Abdominal and Hip Surgeries in Adults: An Observational Study. HSOA J Anesth Clin Care. 2019;6:39-45.
16. Saber R, Metainy SE. Continuous spinal anesthesia versus single small dose bupivacaine–fentanyl spinal anesthesia in high risk elderly patients: A randomized controlled trial. Egypt J Anaesth. 2015;31:233-8.
17. Moawad HE, El-Gendy HA. Comparison between continuous spinal anesthesia and single shot spinal anesthesia in lower abdominal surgeries. Anesth Essays Res. 2016;10(3):510.
18. Kilinc LT, Sivrikaya GU, Eksioglu B, Hanci A, Dobrucali H. Comparison of unilateral spinal and continuous spinal anesthesia for hip surgery in elderly patients. Saudi J Anaesth. 2013;7:404-10.
19. Akkamahadevi P, Ramadas K, Adarsh E. Comparison of continuous spinal anesthesia and epidural anesthesia for lower limb surgeries. Anesth Essays Res. 2017;11(3):631-4.

20. Shah PJ, Shah K, Vipul N, Agrawal P. Comparison of block characteristics in continuous spinal anesthesia and continuous epidural anesthesia for lower limb orthopedic surgeries: An interventional study. J Indian Coll Anaesth. 2022;1:68-73.
21. Ebied RS, Ali MZ, Khafagy HF. Comparative study between continuous epidural anaesthesia and continuous Spinal anaesthesia in elderly patients undergoing TURP. Egypt J Anaesth. 2016;32:527-33.
22. Elfeky MA, Stohy AM, Sabra MM. Randomized comparison of continuous spinal anesthesia versus continuous epidural anesthesia in high-risk elderly patients undergoing major orthopedic lower limb surgeries. Res Opin Anesth Intensive Care. 2019;6:72-9.
23. Ahmed F. Continuous spinal versus continuous thoracic epidural anesthesia for major abdominal surgery in patients with chronic obstructive pulmonary disease. Res Opin Anesth Intensive Care. 2019;6:362.
24. Ahmed Abd El-Ali S, Soliman Abd El-Magid A, Ahmed Abd El-Sadek Sayed AA. Comparative study between continuous spinal anesthesia and combined spinal epidural anesthesia in knee arthroplasty. AMJ. 2020;49:197-208.
25. Tsen LC. Continuous spinal anesthesia: Back to the future. Int J Obstet Anesth. 2017;30:10-13.
26. Kuczkowski KM, Camann WR. Spinal anesthesia in the obese parturient. Curr Opin Anaesthesiol. 2010;23(3):330-4.
27. Jadon A, Chakraborty S, Sinha N, Agrawal R. Intrathecal catheterization by epidural catheter: Management of accidental dural puncture and prophylaxis of PDPH. Indian J Anesth. 2009;53:30-4.
28. Kakel R, Abdelhaq J, Hammoudeh M. Continuous spinal anesthesia after accidental dural tap: A retrospective study. Local Reg Anesth. 2017;10:7-11.
29. Matturu S, Singam A, Madavi S, Verma N. Continuous spinal anesthesia technique after accidental dural puncture. Cureus. 2022;14(9):e29046.
30. Deer TR, Prager J, Levy R, Rathmell J, Buchser E, Burton A, et al. Polyanalgesic consensus conference–2016: recommendations for the management of pain by intrathecal (intraspinal) drug delivery: report of an interdisciplinary expert panel. Neuromodulation. 2017;20(1):6-19.
31. Moaveni D. Management of intrathecal catheters in the obstetric patient. BJA Educ. 2020;20:216-9.
32. Cohn J, Moaveni D, Sznol J, Ranasinghe J. Complications of 761 short-term intrathecal macrocatheters in obstetric patients: a retrospective review of cases over a 12-year period. Int J Obstet Anesth. 2016;25:30-6.

CHAPTER 5

The Impact of Perioperative Variables on Morbidity and Mortality of Elderly Hip Fractures

Ioana Pasca, Haad Arif, Gian Ignacio, Ashish Sinha

ABSTRACT

With the aging United States population, there is a parallel increase in the number of patients presenting with hip fractures—these fractures in the elderly present unique challenges that arise from age and frailty. Improving perioperative management for these patients can enhance morbidity, mortality, and economic outcomes. Optimizing outcomes in elderly hip fracture repair relies on multidisciplinary collaboration to manage perioperative comorbidities.

Keywords: Hip fracture; Morbidity; Mortality; Postoperative complications; Frailty; Anesthesia management; Geriatrics; Elderly; Fracture repair

KEY POINTS

- Elderly patients presenting for the hip fracture repair are susceptible to postoperative complications of nearly all organ systems that frequently increase mortality risk.
- Preoperative conditions, including age, sex, frailty, comorbidities, American Society of Anesthesiologists (ASA) class, and type of fracture, all factor into postoperative risk of morbidity and mortality.
- Minimizing delays to surgery, a comprehensive preoperative cardiac and renal assessment, and administration of iron, erythropoietin, hemoglobin, albumin, and tranexamic acid (TXA) may all help to decrease postoperative mortality.
- Pre- and postoperative troponin, B-type natriuretic peptide (BNP), and renal resistive index (RRI) monitoring may help with the early detection of postoperative complications.
- Dental hygiene, physical therapy, and incentive spirometry have been shown to decrease the incidence of postoperative pneumonia significantly.
- Intraoperative hypotension should be treated promptly.

INTRODUCTION

Hip fractures are the most common trauma-related injuries and the most common reason for elderly patients to undergo emergency surgery.[1-3]

The incidence of hip fractures is chronologically skewed, with 87–96% occurring in patients over 65 years and up to 75% of hip fractures occurring in women.[4] Globally, about 18% of the women and 6% of the men, over their lifetime, will be impacted by such hip trauma.[5]

There are over 300,000 hip fractures annually in the United States, generating approximately 19 billion dollars in healthcare costs. With life expectancy rising globally, hip fractures are a growing challenge worldwide.[6] In 2017, France, Germany, Italy, Spain, the UK, and Sweden spent €37 billion on hip fracture care.[7] In the USA, hip fractures account for 72% of fracture-related healthcare costs, representing only 14% of all osteoporotic fractures.[8] The expenditure in the first 6 months on medical care is directly related to the hip fracture repair and ranges between \$34,509 and \$54,054.[9] Thus, in a population with a growing proportion of elderly patients where fractures are becoming increasingly prevalent, hip fractures pose an increasing burden functionally and financially.

Hip fractures are associated with significant physical, psychological, and financial burdens, with up to half of the patients unable to return to the same quality of life as before their injury.[5,8] Nearly every organ system is negatively affected, with a considerable decline in cardiovascular, respiratory, renal, and cognitive function.

■ TYPE OF FRACTURES

Hip fractures are classified by their anatomical location. They are generally divided into two categories: (1) intracapsular, which occur in the region of the femoral head and neck within the joint capsule of the hip; and (2) extracapsular, which occurs anywhere outside the joint capsule **(Fig. 1)**.[10]

■ AGE AND SEX

In addition to increased morbidity and substantial economic burdens, hip fractures are significantly linked to increased mortality in the geriatric population. Mortality after hip fracture occurs at a rate three-fold higher than in an equivalent nontraumatized group.[4] Unfortunately, and significantly, one-fifth to one-third of the patients will die within 1 year of their hip fracture.[15] The risk of postoperative mortality is 68% higher in patients over 85 years.[14] Although, females are more likely to suffer from a hip fracture, males have a significantly higher mortality rate following hip fracture repair.[4,16,17] Females are more likely to suffer from a hip fracture at a younger age than males, which may be due to postmenopausal osteoporosis and bone fragility. Thus, female patients, being younger, better handle the stress of fracture, subsequent surgery, and management.[17,18] On the other hand, males tend to fracture their hip at a later age and, therefore, present in a state of greater frailty and have higher mortality from coexisting comorbidities.[4,11,16,17]

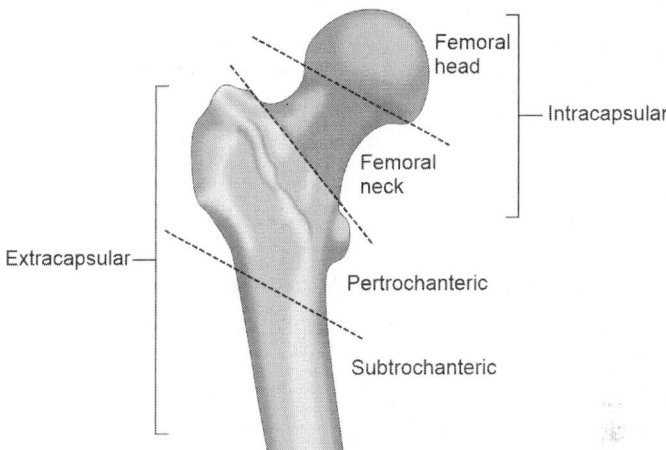

Fig. 1: *Intracapsular fractures* affect the femoral head and neck, while *extracapsular fractures* are those located inferior to the femoral neck and outside the joint capsule.

Note: Intracapsular fractures, particularly femoral neck fractures, are associated with a 77% greater risk of postoperative mortality when compared to the extracapsular fractures,[11-14] most likely due to the critical and vulnerable blood supply to the femoral neck and head resulting in worsened healing and increased susceptibility to necrosis.[10]

■ FRAILTY

Frailty, arguably the most significant determinant of clinical outcomes in older adults, is increased vulnerability to external stressors. The degree of disability due to frailty can be quantified using numerous validated scales. The clinical frailty scale (CFS) is one of the most used scales detailed in **Table 1**.[19,20]

Associated 30-day mortality risks for the individual CFS scores in a retrospective observational study of emergency room patients requiring resuscitation who were subsequently admitted to intermediate care and intensive care units are shown in **Table 2**.[21]

Not only is increased frailty associated with increased 30-day mortality and increased occurrence of one or more complications following hip fracture repair,[13,22,23] but the consequences of higher frailty secondary to comorbidities, polypharmacy, and osteoporosis have been strongly linked as precipitating factors for hip fractures themselves.[23] Frailty scores have also been shown to predict discharge disposition, which may provide insight into the risk of morbidity and mortality following hip fracture repair. Specifically, discharge to skilled nursing facilities (SNFs) or assisted living facilities is associated with more excellent survival rates due to the emphasis on remobilization (defined as mobility in the first 24–48 hours after surgery) and re-enablement defined as resumption of activities of daily living (ADLs) within 3–5 days after surgery.[4,24] Early ambulation within 96 hours of surgery and return to normal ADLs in elderly patients have been shown to improve

TABLE 1: Clinical frailty scale (CFS).[19,20]

CFS	Category	Description
1	Very fit	Robust, active, energetic, and motivated. Exercise regularly. Fittest for their age
2	Well	No severe disease symptoms but are less fit than category 1. Very active but only occasionally
3	Managing well	Well-controlled medical problems but are not regularly active beyond routine walking
4	Living with very mild frailty	While not dependent on others for daily help, symptoms often limit activities
5	Living with mild frailty	Need help in higher-order instrumental activities of daily living such as finance, transportation, heavy housework, and medication management
6	Living with moderate frailty	Need help with all the outside activities and housekeeping. Inside, they often have problems with stairs, need help bathing, and may need minimal assistance with dressing
7	Living with severe frailty	Completely dependent on cognitive and physical personal care. Not at high risk of dying (within 6 months)
8	Living with very severe frailty	Completely dependent on personal care and approaching the end of life. Typically, they could not recover even from minor illnesses
9	Terminally ill	Approaching the end of life. Life expectancy of under 6 months who are not otherwise living with severe frailty

TABLE 2: Mortality rates by clinical frailty score (CFS).[21]

CFS	1–4	5	6	7–9
30-day mortality, n (%)	19 (8.4)	18 (14.2)	21 (21.0)	24 (26.4)
Unadjusted analysis:				
Risk difference (95% CI), %	Reference value	8.0 (−2.1–18.0)	15.9 (4.5–27.3)	21.8 (9.6–34.1)
Risk ratio (95% CI), %	Reference value	1.58 (0.96–2.61)	2.25 (1.42–3.56)	2.81 (1.81–4.35)
Adjusted analysis:				
Risk difference (95% CI), %	Reference value	6.3 (−3.4–15.9)	11.2 (0.4–22.0)	17.7 (5.3–30.1)
Risk ratio (95% CI), %	Reference value	1.45 (0.87–2.41)	1.85 (1.13–3.03)	2.44 (1.50–3.96)

long-term results by helping to decrease the risk of blood clots, pneumonia (PNA), disorientation, and deconditioning.[17,25]

COMORBIDITIES

With increased age comes an increased prevalence of comorbidities, including heart disease, diabetes, chronic obstructive pulmonary disease (COPD), renal dysfunction, and cognitive decline.[26] The use of the ASA class as a proxy for comorbidities is well established, with the assumption that a higher ASA class (class III or more significant) correlates with a greater degree of worsened postoperative outcomes.[27,28] The frequency of a higher ASA class in geriatric hip fractures varies between one-third to more than half of the patients;[25,29] this designation has also been linked to a higher risk for postoperative pulmonary complications.[30] Higher ASA classes have been correlated with increased mortality rates postoperatively, with patients facing a 44% increased mortality risk.[11,14,16,31]

The ASA classification is a systematic risk-stratification method whereby patients receive a class of one through six with examples of comorbidities shown in **Table 3**.[32]

TABLE 3: American Society of Anesthesiologists (ASA) classification system.[32]

ASA class	Definition	Example
ASA I	A typical, healthy patient	Average adult, nonsmoker, and minimal alcohol use
ASA II	A patient with mild systemic disease	Mild disease without functional impairment, current smoker, obese, and well-controlled DM/HTN
ASA III	A patient with a severe systemic disease that is not life-threatening	Substantial function impairment, morbid obesity, poorly-controlled DM/HTN, alcohol dependence, ESRD on dialysis, and mildly reduced EF
ASA IV	A patient with a severe systemic disease that is a constant threat to life	MI, CVA, TIA, or stent placement within 3 months, cardiac ischemia, severely reduced EF, shock, sepsis, DIC, ESRD not on dialysis
ASA V	A moribund patient who is not expected to survive without an operation	Ruptured aneurysm, massive trauma, ICH with mass effect, and ischemic bowel with multiorgan dysfunction
ASA VI	A brain-dead patient whose organs are being removed to transplant into another patient	

(CVA: cerebral vascular accident; DIC: disseminated intravascular coagulation; DM: diabetes mellitus; EF: ejection fraction; ESRD: end-stage renal disease; HTN: hypertension; ICH: intracerebral hemorrhage; MI: myocardial infarction; TIA: transient ischemic attack)

BOX 1: Increased risk in elderly patients with chronic kidney disease.[33,35,36]

- A creatinine clearance of <65 mL/min in the setting of osteoporosis increases the risk of traumatic falls and subsequent hip fractures in elderly patients
- Decreased neuromuscular function due to decreased vitamin D concentrations
- Increased bone fragility due to dysfunctional bone and mineral metabolism and parathyroid hormone imbalances

KIDNEY DISEASE

Chronic kidney disease (CKD) is seen in 7.4–18.5% of hip fracture patients and poses a substantially increased risk for morbidity and mortality.[5] End-stage renal disease (ESRD) patients are between 4 and 17 times more susceptible to hip fractures.[33] Patients with diabetic nephropathy are estimated to have a nearly threefold more significant risk of hip fracture.[34] Numerous explanations for this increased risk in elderly patients with CKD have been proposed **(Box 1)**.[33,35,36]

In elderly hip fracture patients, CKD increases twofold the risk of postoperative cardiovascular events, pneumonia, respiratory failure, and gastrointestinal bleeding.[5] The association between CKD and postoperative complications is even stronger in the face of concomitant underlying coronary vascular disease.[37] Chronic kidney disease has also been associated with more extended stays [longer length of stay (LOS)] and higher hospital costs after hip fracture surgery.[33]

Dialysis is associated with an increased risk of hip fractures and morbidity and mortality following postoperative repair.[38] The risk of hip fracture increases with the length of time on dialysis, with a cumulative increase in risk by 2% for every month that the patient requires dialysis.[34] Potential causes of this increased risk might be β2-microglobulin amyloidosis and chronic uremic osteodystrophy.[39] The risk of myocardial infarction (MI) within 30 days following hip fracture repair is two times greater in patients requiring dialysis.[40] Dialysis patients taking adrenal cortical steroids, benzodiazepines, narcotics, or selective serotonin reuptake inhibitors (SSRIs) are shown to be at an increased risk for hip and other bone fractures.[39] Needing immediate postoperative dialysis is associated with higher mortality in any fracture repair, even in patients who are on maintenance dialysis.[41] Overall, in-hospital mortality of hip fracture patients on dialysis ranges from 7 to 17%.[33,42]

The timing of dialysis before surgery may impact postoperative outcomes. General guidelines dictate when to dialyze a patient, though not specific to the geriatric populations, should be used as recommended **(Box 2)**.[43,44]

Dialysis patients tend to bleed more because of uremic platelet dysfunction caused by excess uremia and elevated parathyroid hormone. Strategies to reduce bleeding in such patients include desmopressin or

BOX 2: General guidelines for dialysis.[43,44]

When to dialyze?: General guidelines
- Dialysis should be done the day before surgery.
- Surgery should not be scheduled on Monday if a patient is on a Tuesday, Thursday, or Saturday dialysis schedule.
- If a surgery is urgent and must be performed on the day of dialysis, holding heparin in the dialysate should be considered, or surgery should be delayed 4 hours postdialysis to allow heparin clearance.
- Ideally, the patient should be euvolemic before surgery.

BOX 3: Anesthetic considerations in dialysis patients.[43]

- Avoid succinylcholine in patients with elevated serum potassium
- Appropriate ventilatory settings to correct or compensate for acid–base disturbances
- Use of fluids appropriate to the surgical procedure and perioperative volume status

cryoprecipitate to improve platelet dysfunction. Waiting for 4 hours after dialysis is recommended before operating because heparin is frequently used during dialysis.[43] Before surgery, a comprehensive assessment of glomerular filtration rate (GFR), potassium and hemoglobin levels, and acid-base and volume status should be performed to help avoid drugs or strategies that may negatively impact the outcomes **(Box 3)**.

CHRONIC OBSTRUCTIVE PULMONARY DISEASE

Like CKD, elderly patients with a history of COPD are at a higher risk of postoperative morbidity and mortality.[40] Typically, regional anesthesia is preferred in COPD patients undergoing hip fracture repair to eliminate the risk of barotrauma and airway injury during endotracheal intubation. However, if general anesthesia is required, lung recruitment maneuvers and low tidal volume ventilation decrease intraoperative lung injury, decreasing postoperative pulmonary complications.[40] Furthermore, intramedullary nailing of the fracture, as opposed to hip arthroplasty, is preferred due to reduced time under anesthesia and increased ability for remobilization.[40]

COGNITIVE IMPAIRMENT

Cognitive impairment (commonly caused by dementia, Alzheimer's disease, and Parkinson's disease) is significantly associated with postoperative mortality. Patients with cognitive impairment before admission face a 91% greater risk of death.[14] In the preoperative scenario, this increased mortality may be due to the correlation between cognitive decline, advancing age, and declining overall health. Postoperative cognitive impairment (delirium or dementia) makes it challenging to comply with rehabilitation regimens, thereby increasing morbidity and mortality risk.[14] Antidepressant use, positively correlated with comorbid conditions and growing age, is also associated with increased fracture risk.[45] Selective serotonin reuptake inhibitors and tricyclic antidepressants (TCAs) have increased the risk of geriatric hip fractures.[46] This risk is most significant within 6 weeks of starting antidepressant treatment. It is thought to be due to the inadvertent effect on serotonin transporters in osteocytes, osteoblasts, and osteoclasts.[45] Additionally, in the initial stages of antidepressant therapy, balance is negatively affected, and elderly users are twice as likely to experience a clinically significant fall after starting this class of medication.[47] Postural instability and reduced muscle strength are potential causal factors for the association between antidepressants and increased fall risk.[45,48,49]

■ INFECTION

The association between viral infections and hip fracture incidence in elderly patients has been investigated. The influenza virus and other flu-like illnesses have increased the risk of hip fractures, particularly in nursing home residents.[50,51] More recently, coronavirus disease 2019 (COVID-19) infection was seen in 21% of the hip fracture patients[52] and is associated with an increased LOS, 30-day mortality, and a seven-fold increase in the risk of overall mortality following hip fractures.[1] The leading causes of death include respiratory failure, COVID-19-associated pneumonia, and multiorgan failure.[52] Moreover, there is also an increased risk of venous thrombotic events secondary to COVID-19's inflammatory effect on endothelial cell dysfunction, fibrinolysis impairment, and excessive thrombin generation.[1]

■ CAUSES OF MORTALITY

The 1-year mortality following untreated hip fracture is 70%. Even when fracture repair is performed, 1-year mortality is roughly 20%.[53] For over 8 years following the index injury, the mortality continues to be higher than the baseline in all the elderly patients.[54] Any modifiable cause of mortality should be addressed proactively, recognizing that this patient subset already brings many nonmodifiable preoperative frailties.

Overall, short-term causes of death following hip fracture repair (in order of prevalence) are respiratory complications (bronchopneumonia and respiratory failure), cardiac complications [cardiac failure, MI, ischemic heart disease, pulmonary embolism (PE), and stroke], multiorgan failure, and septic shock.[17,31]

Sepsis and septic shock occur in roughly 2% of the hip fracture surgeries; still they can increase the risk of 30-day mortality by three times and 11 times compared to patients without sepsis or septic shock, respectively. Urinary tract infections, pneumonia, and surgical site infections typically precede most cases of postoperative sepsis and septic shock. Risk factors for postoperative sepsis include long-term steroid use, congestive heart failure (CHF), and preoperative ventilator dependence. The link between ventilator use and septic shock is likely due to the risk of developing ventilator-associated pneumonia and subsequent progression to septic shock. Both anemia and hypoalbuminemia are also associated with an increased risk of sepsis and septic shock following hip fracture repair. Preoperative administration of iron supplements and erythropoietin, even with its known time lag to efficacy, may improve recovery times and reduce hospital LOS. Although intuitive and used frequently, it is yet to be statistically validated.[55] Both surgical repair within 24 hours following the initial injury and early mobilization have decreased the risk of bronchopneumonia and pulmonary embolism.[56] The impact of time to hip fracture repair on postoperative mortality has been well studied, with delays over 48 hours resulting in a 30-day postoperative mortality rising to 50% and 1-year mortality increasing by 32%.[7,11,24,30,57,58] Surgery within 6 hours has decreased overall hospital LOS and incidence of postoperative delirium (POD), still it does not reduce mortality or nonfatal complications such as MI, stroke, VTE, sepsis, and pneumonia.[24]

Long-term causes of mortality include (in order of prevalence) cardiac complications, respiratory complications, dementia, and Alzheimer's disease.[4] Men are more likely to die from respiratory and circulatory illness following hip fracture fixation. This is speculated to be due to the increased prevalence of smoking and the earlier development of chronic heart disease in the male population, resulting in a greater incidence of respiratory and cardiac disorders.[4]

Cardiac Complications

Preoperative heart failure significantly correlates with LOS following surgery, increased risk of postoperative heart failure as a surgical complication, and increased 1-year mortality.[59] History of peripheral vascular disease (PVD), stroke, COPD, and cardiac disease are all significant predictors of postoperative cardiac events in all hip fracture patients.[40] Patients with CKD double their risk of cardiovascular events, including pulmonary embolism, angina pectoris, MI, heart failure, arrhythmia, CVA, and death, following hip fracture surgery than those without CKD.[5] Stress-induced hyperglycemia in nondiabetic patients is another predictor of postoperative MI.[60] Elevated perioperative troponin levels effectively predict 30-day and long-term mortality from hip fractures.[60] Between 30 and 70% of the hip fracture patients present with a high troponin level at admission secondary to catecholamine surge and thrombotic processes in the setting of pain.[60] It is difficult to assess a patient's preoperative cardiac status due to a lack of pretrauma cardiac data.[61] Obtaining preoperative troponins, B-type natriuretic peptide (BNP) levels, and perioperative echocardiograms provide a valuable tool for risk assessment and helps guide intraoperative anesthetic management.

Vascular Complications

Venous thromboembolism (VTE), specifically deep venous thrombosis (DVT), is among the principal causes of perioperative morbidity and mortality following total hip arthroplasty (THA).[62,63] The prevalence of DVTs in hip replacements performed without anticoagulation prophylaxis can reach up to 75%, while that of pulmonary embolism ranges between 0.5 and 3.5%.[64] When early surgical intervention and mobilization are challenging to achieve, thromboprophylaxis use can effectively reduce the risk of VTE by up to 60%.[65] Numerous agents currently exist for thromboembolism prophylaxis **(Flowchart 1)**.

Fondaparinux, a selective factor Xa inhibitor in the coagulation cascade, is commonly used in hip fracture cases and considered one of the more effective prophylactic agents, shown to reduce the risk of VTE by as much as 56.4%.[10] Heparin is another effective anticoagulant agent that rapidly works to block multiple factors in the coagulation cascade by augmenting the action of antithrombin III.[66] Available in two different preparations via intravenous injection; heparin exhibits other clearance mechanisms, making each preparation better suited for specific patient populations **(Table 4)**.[67]

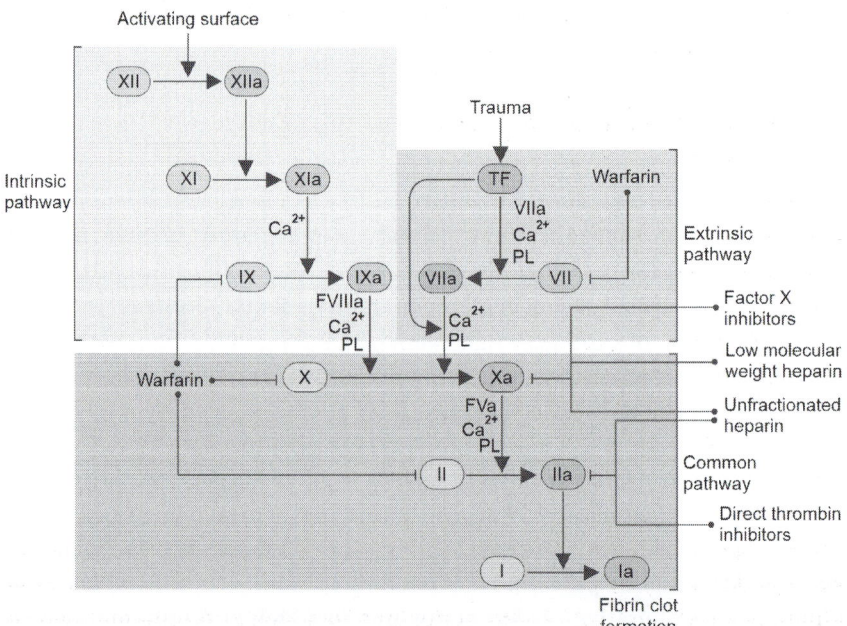

Flowchart 1: Multiple therapeutic targets of the coagulation cascade.

(PL: platelet membrane phospholipid; TF: tissue factor)

TABLE 4: Clearance of heparins.[67]

Mechanism	*Saturable*: Clearance through the reticuloendothelial system and endothelial cells	*Nonsaturable*: Clearance through renal excretion
Clearance	Rapidly increases at low doses, then plateaus	Increases linearly with dosage
Example	Low-dose unfractionated heparin	High-dose unfractionated heparin Low-molecular-weight heparin

Low-molecular-weight heparin (LMWH) such as dalteparin and enoxaparin may be preferable for some situations due to their better side effect profiles but should be avoided in patients with decreased renal function.[10,68] Instead, low dose unfractionated heparin (LDUH) is a safer option in patients with creatinine clearance <30 mL/min.[12] Overall, perioperative heparin administration is significantly effective in reducing the incidence of DVT in hip fracture repair.[69]

Mechanical calf/foot pumping devices and compression stockings are also proven to reduce DVT incidence during these surgeries.[10,69] In addition, regional anesthesia has been shown to help lower the risk of VTE, likely due to increased peripheral vasodilation and the inhibition of platelet aggregation and stabilization of endothelial cells.[70]

Before any injury, up to 40% of the hip fracture patients are on anticoagulant or antiplatelet regimens. This proportion increases when considering the prevalence of long-term treatment of thrombotic conditions such as atrial fibrillation, acute coronary syndrome (ACS), intrinsic hypercoagulable states, previous VTE, and prolonged immobility in the elderly patients.[24,71] Thus, clinicians must balance decreasing the risk of intraoperative hemorrhage with an elderly patient's underlying hypercoagulable state.[63]

Among the most common long-term anticoagulants used to prevent VTE are vitamin K antagonists (VKAs) such as warfarin, which contain the production of numerous factors in the coagulation cascade. Sufficient reversal of the effects of VKAs for hip fracture surgery, as measured by an international normalized ratio (INR) value of around 1.5, may take anywhere from 3 to 5 days.[71-73] In urgent hip fracture surgery, where delayed repair is associated with adverse outcomes, omitting anticoagulating agents may not be enough to reverse antithrombotic effects. Considerations are enumerated in **Table 5**.[71-73]

Antiplatelet therapy, including aspirin (ASA), clopidogrel, and ticagrelor are another anticoagulation treatments commonly used to prevent VTE. Platelet transfusion may be an effective reversal therapy for most antiplatelet regimens.[72] Some studies have indicated that delays in surgery to reverse

TABLE 5: Considerations for anticoagulant use in the hip fractures.[71-73]

IV infusion of vitamin K and halting VKAs	Administration of PCC
Effect within 12–36 hours of administration, depending on the preoperative dose of vitamin K*	It has been shown to reverse INR values to an average of 1.3 from therapeutic levels within 30 minutes of administration
INR <1.8 under general anesthesia INR <1.5 under spinal anesthesia	
Disadvantages: • Anaphylaxis (dose-dependent) • Acute thrombosis • Warfarin resistance	*Disadvantages*: • Allergic reaction • Heparin-induced thrombocytopenia • Disseminated intravascular coagulopathy • Thromboembolic events • High cost

*Additional research is necessary to elucidate the ideal utilization for VKA reversal in hip fracture repair.

(INR: international normalized ratio; IV: intravenous; PCC: prothrombin complex concentrate; VKAs: vitamin K antagonists)

antiplatelet therapy from aspirin and clopidogrel are unnecessary, as no difference in bleeding complications, blood loss, or transfusion requirements was found when compared to patients not on aspirin or clopidogrel.[72] The risk of vertebral canal hematoma (VCH) with spinal anesthesia in hip fracture repair for patients on anticoagulant regimens is well known. However, recent guidelines have advised that this risk may be lower than general anesthesia or delaying repair.[71]

Current recommendations for patients on anticoagulants undergoing hip fracture with spinal anesthesia are being depicted in **Flowchart 2**.

Bleeding is a common complication in hip fracture repair, with blood transfusion required in up to 30% of the cases.[74] There is some concern, however, that most of the blood loss associated with traumatic hip fractures occurred postinjury and before the repair itself, with average hemoglobin decrease of 1.5 units and 2.0 units of blood for intracapsular and extracapsular hip fractures, respectively.[75] Elderly patients undergoing hip fracture repair may present to the hospital already in a hypovolemic state due to chronic dehydration, blood loss after the initial trauma, or decreased ability to intake fluids due to fracture-related immobility, all of which emphasize the need for an assessment of preoperative volume status.[75] Methods of measuring intraoperative blood loss are inaccurate. They cannot provide immediate feedback on patient volume status,[76] requiring anesthesiologists to use their best judgment when deciding when to give blood or fluids based on the alternate criteria, such as heart rate, blood pressure, and pain control.

Flowchart 2: Decision-making for using spinal anesthesia in hip fracture repair for patients on direct oral anticoagulation therapy.[71]

```
Spinal anesthesia in hip fracture repair of patients on direct oral
                    anticoagulant therapy
         │                                    │
         ▼                                    ▼
 Thrombin inhibitors                   Factor Xa inhibitors
         │                          ┌───────────┴───────────┐
         ▼                          ▼                       ▼
 Schedule afternoon         Creatinine clearance:   Creatinine clearance:
 surgery the day after          ≥30 mL/min              <30 mL/min
   the last dose                    │                       │
         │                          ▼                       ▼
         ▼                      Proceed              Measure antifactor
 Measure thrombin               with                 Xa levels and
 levels the morning             surgery 24           discuss with
   of surgery                   hours after          hematologist before
         │                      last                 proceeding with
   ┌─────┴─────┐                dose                 surgery
   ▼           ▼                                     or
 Normal    Prolonged                                 delay surgery
   │           │
   ▼           ▼
Proceed with  Consider
 surgery      reversal with
              Idarucizumab
```

Tranexamic acid (TXA) is a pharmacologic agent that inhibits the normal breakdown of fibrin clots by preventing plasminogen activation.[77] The administration of TXA in urgent hip fracture surgery should be used cautiously in an elderly patient population that is frequently hypercoagulable. However, some studies have shown that TXA administration for hip fracture repair is not associated with an increased risk of thromboembolic events, does not increase 90-day mortality, and decreases the need for blood transfusions by up to 42%.[74,78] Reducing blood transfusions decrease the risk of transfusion reactions, infections, and anaphylaxis. Patients who had received TXA have also been shown to have higher hemoglobin concentrations postoperatively, further reducing the risk of complications such as sepsis and acute kidney injury (AKI).[74]

Pulmonary Complications

Postoperative pneumonia is one of the most common complications following hip fracture, resulting in severe morbidity and mortality due to altered immunity and susceptibility to infection in older patients **(Fig. 2)**.[79-83]

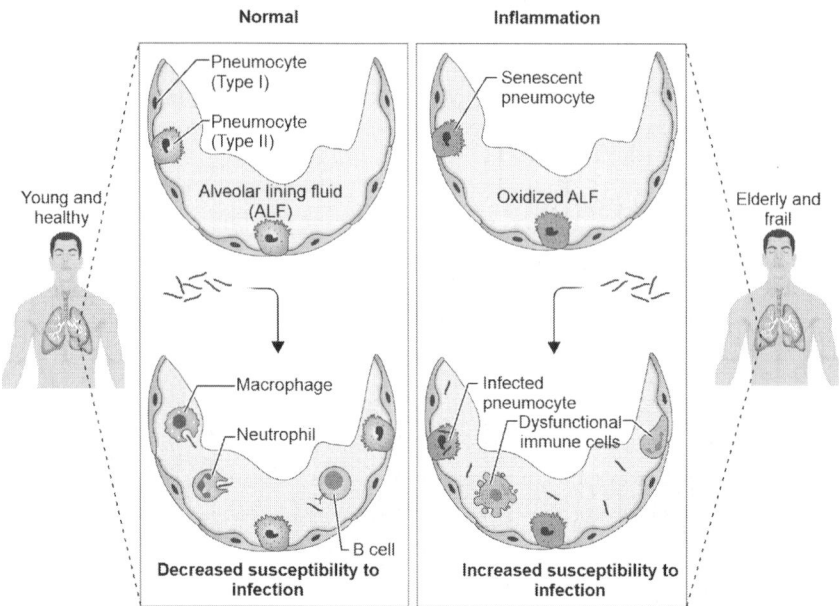

Fig. 2: Difference in immune responsiveness between a healthy adult immune response and an elderly individual.
Source: Available at BioRender.com

BOX 4: Age-related factors predisposing for pulmonary complications.

- Impaired effective cough decreases airway clearance
- Increased alveolar dead space
- Decreased responsiveness to drugs
- Poor dental and oral hygiene
- Diminished ventilatory response to hypoxia and hypercapnia
- Weakened immunity
- Poor nutritional status

Advanced age is associated with an increased risk of pulmonary conditions and infections such as pneumonia and atelectasis, due to numerous age-related factors **(Box 4)**.

Elderly patients presenting for the hip fracture repair with preoperative atelectasis or pulmonary consolidation were shown to have a greater propensity for postoperative pulmonary complications.[30] The incidence of such complications can be seen in up to a third of the patients, prompting the need for preventative practices **(Box 5)**.[30,84]

Prolonged bed rest is well-known to result in deterioration of muscle strength, insulin resistance, increased risk of thrombosis, and impaired respiration, all of which increase the risk of insufficient oxygenation and atelectasis.[87]

BOX 5: Methods of decreasing postoperative pneumonia incidence.[30,82,84-86]

- Implementing thorough oral care in daily nursing protocol and appropriate use of antibiotics can decrease the risk of aspirating bacterial microorganisms from the oral cavity and subsequent pulmonary infection
- Observing appropriate patient positioning for swallowing and preventing gastroesophageal reflux decreases the likelihood of aspiration
- Early remobilization through intense physiotherapy to promote mobility
- Postoperative chest physiotherapy using positive expiratory pressure devices and proper deep breathing techniques may help to improve oxygenation and facilitate mucous clearance

In addition to an increased risk of hip fracture, osteoporosis also contributes to decreased chest wall expansion due to calcification of the osteochondral joints.[80] The resultant reduced lung compliance leads to external cardiac compression and collapse of the inferior vena cava (IVC) as it passes through the diaphragm.[88,89] The reduced venous return to the right heart causes decreases in the left ventricular preload, stroke volume, and cardiac output.[88,89] In insufficient physiologic compensation, the reduced venous return can increase the risk of hypotension in elderly patients, compounded by age-related increases in closing volume. Increased closing volumes result in hyperinflated lungs, while decreased lung compliance creates increased intrathoracic pressure, which directly compresses the heart, reduces cardiac compliance and performance, and contributes to an increased risk of perioperative hypotension in the elderly patients. This increases the risk of hypoperfusion of end organs, increasing postoperative mortality and morbidity.[89-91]

Renal Complications

The sudden drop in renal function, also known as AKI, following surgery occurs in up to 28% of hip fracture repairs and is associated with prolonged hospital LOS and increased rates of postoperative morbidity and mortality.[92] The 30-day and 1-year mortality of patients with AKI after hip fracture is higher than that of patients without AKI (7 and 3 times higher, respectively).[92] The development of postoperative AKI is multifactorial **(Table 6)**.[92-96]

Intraoperative hypotension is a significant concern for the development of AKI as each additional hour where mean arterial pressure (MAP) is <70, 60, and 50 mm Hg increases the risk of AKI by 2, 5, and 22% respectively.[97] Postoperative hypoalbuminemia is a marker of decreased colloid osmotic pressure, which results in inadequate circulating volume and decreased glomerular filtration and renal function.[98]

Studies have investigated using the RRI to predict postoperative AKI and the early detection of renal microvascular damage following altered hemodynamics. The RRI is a noninvasive method of evaluating kidney

TABLE 6: Risk factors for acute kidney injury in hip fracture patients.[92-96]

Preoperative	Intraoperative	Postoperative
Advanced age	Hypotension time	Hypoalbuminemia
Male	Hypotension degree	Anemia
ASA >3	Massive bleed	Blood transfusion**
History • Peripheral vascular disease • COPD • Chronic kidney disease • Diabetes mellitus • Congestive heart disease • Tobacco use		
Low body mass index*		
Low GFR		
High creatinine		
Use of nephrotoxic drugs		

*Low BMIs may play a role in renal complications, although it is unclear what the role BMI plays in developing AKI.
**Blood transfusions are usually a consequence of severe illness. The association between blood transfusion and AKI is likely due to acute illness in patients rather than AKI compounded by the blood transfusion itself.
(ASA: American Society of Anesthesiologists; AKI: acute kidney injury; BMI: body mass index; COPD: chronic obstructive pulmonary disease; GFR: glomerular filtration rate)

perfusion, using Doppler waveforms at the level of arcuate or interlobar arteries.[99] RRI is calculated as:

$$RRI = \frac{(\text{Peak systolic velocity} - \text{end diastolic velocity})}{\text{Peak systolic velocity}}$$

Equation 1: Renal resistive index

Renal resistive index is inversely related to MAP, diastolic blood pressure, and heart rate and is directly associated with pulse pressure.[99] Regarding hip fracture repair, both preoperative and postoperative RRI are independent predictive factors of postoperative AKI. Postoperative RRI has shown value in detecting AKI up to a day earlier than serum creatinine levels or urine output.[94,100] An RRI higher than a cut-off threshold of 0.71 has been shown to predict AKI following hip fracture surgery, while values <0.70 demonstrate improved renal outcomes **(Table 7)**.[100,101] Current studies have emphasized the need for randomized control trials to better establish the value of RRI in managing AKI prevention.

Early fluid resuscitation, avoidance of nephrotoxic drugs, replenishment of albumin and hemoglobin, and strict maintenance of MAP above predetermined relative thresholds may all work to reduce the incidence of postoperative AKI.

TABLE 7: The renal resistive index can help predict AKI following hip fracture surgery.[100,101]

	p-value
Preoperative RRI values	0.014
No perioperative AKI	0.68 (0.67–0.71)
Presence of perioperative AKI	0.72 (0.70–0.73)
Postoperative RRI values	<0.0001
No perioperative AKI	0.6 (0.58–0.68)
Presence of perioperative AKI	0.74 (0.71–0.76)

(AKI: acute kidney injury; RRI: renal resistive index)

TABLE 8: Risk factors for postoperative delirium in hip fracture patients.[18,22,30,103,104]

Preoperative risk factors	Intraoperative risk factors
ASA class	Increased time under anesthesia
Male	Lability in blood pressure
COPD history	Blood transfusion
High frailty scores	Late surgery*
Dementia history	
Anemia	

*Observed particularly in patients with displaced femoral neck fractures, requiring hip bipolar hemiarthroplasty.

(ASA: American Society of Anesthesiologists; COPD: chronic obstructive pulmonary disease)

■ POSTOPERATIVE DELIRIUM

Postoperative delirium is the most common complication, reported in up to a third of these patients.[102] Postoperative delirium is also correlated with increased frailty, 1-year mortality, LOS, discharge destination, sepsis, and rate of 1-month readmission.[3,14,18,22,102] The risk of 6-month mortality increases by 10% with every additional day with POD.[18,102] Risk factors for postoperative delirium are shown in **Table 8**.[18,22,30,103,104]

Notably, the risk factors of POD are additive, stressing early recognition and prompt implementation of therapeutic measures.[105] Patients with POD have hospital costs increased by 2.5-fold, causing an additional economic burden of $16,000-64,000 per patient-year.[106] Although the underlying mechanism behind POD has not yet been discerned, neurotransmitter imbalance, systemic inflammation, and electrolyte/metabolic derangements are speculated as causes of POD.[18]

Multimodal pain control is effective in preventing and treating POD as it decreases the use of opioids and cholinesterase inhibitors.[18] Other vital maneuvers include optimizing hemodynamic stability and acid–base status, providing adequate oxygenation, and minimizing electrolyte abnormalities.[105] The choice of regional compared to general anesthesia does not change the incidence of POD.[107] Overall, close collaboration with intensivists, hospitalists, geriatricians, and orthopedists is essential in minimizing the risk of POD and improving functional recovery.[108]

GENERAL VERSUS REGIONAL ANESTHESIA

Whether general anesthesia is superior to regional anesthesia in the context of geriatric hip fracture repair is yet to be answered. Historically, the presence of multiple comorbidities in elderly patients makes it difficult to quantify the benefits of any mode of anesthesia over the other. However, hypotension is a significant concern in both methods due to impaired blood pressure regulation in elderly patients under anesthesia. Geriatric patients have decreased arterial compliance and cardiac cholinergic responsiveness, resulting in diminished responses to the acute changes in blood pressure caused by general or spinal anesthesia.[68,109,110] Some studies find that regional anesthesia (including spinal anesthesia and nerve blocks) is correlated with better outcomes and decreased risk of morbidity than general anesthesia. However, this correlation has been subject to debate given conflicting reports by studies, flaws in the study methodology, poorly defined measures of "outcome," and varying times between inciting event (use of anesthesia) and measured outcome (30-day postoperative mortality).[7,16,24,27,30,103,104,109,111-113] General guidelines suggest that it is not the choice of anesthesia crucial to decreasing mortality but the provider's comfort with that mode of anesthesia.[26]

HYPOTENSION

Hypotension has been cited as a decisive factor in postoperative morbidity and mortality, including myocardial injury after noncardiac surgery (MINS), stroke, AKI, MI, and POD in geriatric hip fracture repair.[7,27,61,103,104,112,114,115] Intraoperative hypotension is seen in over 50% of the elderly hip fracture surgeries. This is why 20% of the patients failed to meet the remobilization performance indicator on the Nottingham Hip Fracture Score (NHFS). This is likely because intraoperative hypotension may lead to brain hypoperfusion and an increased risk of developing POD.[3,18,24,112] Several preoperative risk factors for developing intraoperative hypotension include advanced age, preinduction hypotension, chronic hypertension and antihypertensive drugs, ASA status, and hypovolemia.[112] Historically, the lack of universally accepted perioperative blood pressure thresholds to define hypotension has made determining an optimal treatment plan complex, with cut-offs utilizing multiple measurements[7,112,114] **(Table 9).**

TABLE 9: Suggested thresholds for defining hypotension.[7,112,114]

MAP	SBP
Between 55 and 75 mm Hg	<100 mm Hg
	20–30% decrease

Note: Although no standardized definition of hypotension exists, increased cumulative time under any established hypotensive threshold is associated with an increased risk of postoperative morbidity and mortality, with organ injury occurring when MAP decreases < 55 mm Hg for ≥10 minutes.[7,103]

(MAP: mean arterial pressure; SBP: systolic blood pressure)

The risk of AKI or MI increases as MAP drops below 65 mm Hg, while mortality risk is postulated to increase at a MAP of 80 mm Hg. These risks cumulatively increase as time and degree of hypotension increase.[61] Mortality was significantly increased at 30 days, 60 days, and 1-year marks after surgical repair when a patient received a vasopressor infusion for over 3 hours, possibly due to decreased myocardial perfusion resulting in increased oxygen demand and eventual MINS.[103] Vasopressors that promote vasoconstriction may play a role in myocardial hypoperfusion and the development of MINS.[103]

Risk stratification based on the preoperative evaluation and early identification of hypotension is crucial in the timely and aggressive management of intraoperative hypotension. Absolute thresholds for hypotension may not be effective in geriatric populations as they assume all individuals within that category can autoregulate equally. There is a great degree of variation in autoregulatory ability amongst the aging population due to varying frailty, polypharmacy, and comorbidities.[104] However, using relative thresholds using preoperative blood pressure readings as a reference may also be flawed due to the potential for artificial inflation of such values secondary to the patient anxiety, stress, and pain.[104] Nonetheless, anesthesiologists should be urged to decrease hypotensive duration by treating patients promptly on a relative threshold formed by preoperative conditions and trendlines, as opposed to absolute threshold criteria.[114]

CONCLUSION

Hip fractures in the geriatric population have long been seen as harbingers of increased short-term mortality. Increased frailty and decreased mobility, in conjunction with co-existing kidney and cardiac disease, pulmonary pathology, and mental impairment increase the risk of falls and subsequent hip fracture requiring surgery. Perioperative respiratory compromise, hypotension, thrombotic events, blood loss, delirium, and infection pose significant barriers to good patient outcomes. Timely orthopedic intervention, a thorough assessment of cardiac and renal function prior to and following surgery, as well as early postoperative remobilization and physical therapy can all aid in decreasing the risk of morbidity and mortality following hip fractures in elderly patients.

REFERENCES

1. Lim MA, Pranata R. Coronavirus disease 2019 (COVID-19) markedly increased mortality in patients with hip fracture—A systematic review and meta-analysis. J Clin Orthop Trauma. 2021;12(1):187-93.
2. Gomez M, Marc C, Talha A, Ruiz N, Noublanche S, Gillibert A, et al. Fast track care for pertrochanteric hip fractures: How does it impact length of stay and complications? Orthop Traumatol Surg Res. 2019;105(5):979-84.
3. Shelton C, White S. Anaesthesia for hip fracture repair. BJA Educ. 2020;20(5):142-9.
4. Panula J, Pihlajamäki H, Mattila VM, Jaatinen P, Vahlberg T, Aarnio P, et al. Mortality and cause of death in hip fracture patients aged 65 or older: A population-based study. BMC Musculoskelet Disord. 2011;12:105.
5. Jiang Y, Luo Y, Li J, Jiang Y, Zhao J, Gu S, et al. Chronic kidney disease and risk of postoperative cardiovascular events in elderly patients receiving hip fracture surgery. Injury. 2022;53(2):596-602.
6. Dhanwal DK, Dennison EM, Harvey NC, Cooper C. Epidemiology of hip fracture: Worldwide geographic variation. Indian J Orthop. 2011;45(1):15-22.
7. Beecham G, Cusack R, Vencken S, Crilly G, Buggy DJ. Hypotension during hip fracture surgery and postoperative morbidity. Ir J Med Sci. 2020;189(3):1087-96.
8. Burge R, Dawson-Hughes B, Solomon DH, Wong JB, King A, Tosteson A. Incidence and economic burden of osteoporosis-related fractures in the United States, 2005-2025. J Bone Miner Res. 2007;22(3):465-75.
9. Kates SL. CORR Insights®: Surgery for Hip Fracture Yields Societal Benefits That Exceed the Direct Medical Costs. Clin Orthop Relat Res. 2014;472(11):3547-8.
10. Bateman L, Vuppala S, Porada P, Carter W, Baijnath C, Burman K, et al. Medical management in the acute hip fracture patient: A comprehensive review for the internist. Ochsner J. 2012 Summer;12(2):101-10.
11. Daugaard CL, Jorgensen HL, Riis T, Lauritzen JB, Duus BR, Van Der Mark S. Is mortality after hip fracture associated with surgical delay or admission during weekends and public holidays? A retrospective study of 38,020 patients. Acta Orthop. 2012;83(6):609-13.
12. Cornwall R, Gilbert MS, Koval KJ, Strauss E, Siu AL. Functional outcomes and mortality vary among different types of hip fractures: A function of patient characteristics. Clin Orthop Relat Res. 2004;(425):64-71.
13. Dayama A, Olorunfemi O, Greenbaum S, Stone ME, McNelis J. Impact of frailty on outcomes in geriatric femoral neck fracture management: An analysis of national surgical quality improvement program dataset. Int J Surg. 2016;28:185-90.
14. Smith T, Pelpola K, Ball M, Ong A, Myint PK. Pre-operative indicators for mortality following hip fracture surgery: A systematic review and meta-analysis. Age Ageing. 2014;43(4):464-71.
15. Dyer SM, Crotty M, Fairhall N, Magaziner J, Beaupre LA, Cameron ID, et al. A critical review of the long-term disability outcomes following hip fracture. BMC Geriatr. 2016;16(1):158.
16. Holt G, Smith R, Duncan K, Finlayson DF, Gregori A. Early mortality after surgical fixation of hip fractures in the elderly: An analysis of data from the Scottish hip fracture audit. J Bone Joint Surg Br. 2008;90(10):1357-63.

17. Groff H, Kheir MM, George J, Azboy I, Higuera CA, Parvizi J. Causes of in-hospital mortality after hip fractures in the elderly. Hip International. 2020;30(2):204-9.
18. Albanese AM, Ramazani N, Greene N, Bruse L. Review of Postoperative Delirium in Geriatric Patients After Hip Fracture Treatment. Geriatr Orthop Surg Rehabil. 2022;13:21514593211058947.
19. Dolenc E, Rotar-Pavlič D. Frailty assessment scales for the elderly and their application in primary care: A systematic literature review. Zdr Varst. 2019;58(2):91-100.
20. Mendiratta P, Schoo C, Latif R. Clinical Frailty Scale. Treasure Island (FL): StatPearls Publishing; 2023.
21. Huh JY, Matsuoka Y, Kinoshita H, Ikenoue T, Yamamoto Y, Ariyoshi K. Premorbid Clinical Frailty Score and 30-day mortality among older adults in the emergency department. J Am Coll Emerg Physicians Open. 2022;3(1):e122677.
22. Kistler EA, Nicholas JA, Kates SL, Friedman SM. Frailty and Short-Term Outcomes in Patients With Hip Fracture. Geriatr Orthop Surg Rehabil. 2015;6(3):209-14.
23. Krishnan M, Beck S, Havelock W, Eeles E, Hubbard RE, Johansen A. Predicting outcome after hip fracture: Using a frailty index to integrate comprehensive geriatric assessment results. Age Ageing. 2014;43(1):122-6.
24. Griffiths R, Babu S, Dixon P, Freeman N, Hurford D, Kelleher E, et al. Guideline for the management of hip fractures 2020: Guideline by the Association of Anaesthetists. Anaesthesia. 2021;76(2):225-37.
25. Aprato A, Bechis M, Buzzone M, Bistolfi A, Daghino W, Massè A. No rest for elderly femur fracture patients: early surgery and early ambulation decrease mortality. J Orthop Traumatol. 2020;21(1):12.
26. Divo MJ, Martinez CH, Mannino DM. Ageing and the epidemiology of multimorbidity. Eur Respir J. 2014;44(4):1055-68.
27. White SM, Moppett IK, Griffiths R. Outcome by mode of anaesthesia for hip fracture surgery. An observational audit of 65 535 patients in a national dataset. Anaesthesia. 2014;69(3):224-30.
28. Donegan DJ, Gay AN, Baldwin K, Morales EE, Esterhai JL, Mehta S. Use of medical comorbidities to predict complications after hip fracture surgery in the elderly. J Bone Joint Surg Am. 2010;92(4):807-13.
29. Cher EWL, Allen JC, Howe T Sen, Koh JSB. Comorbidity as the dominant predictor of mortality after hip fracture surgeries. Osteoporosis Int. 2019;30(12):2477-83.
30. Kim SD, Park SJ, Lee DH, Jee DL. Risk factors of morbidity and mortality following hip fracture surgery. Korean J Anesthesiol. 2013;64(6):505-10.
31. Chatterton BD, Moores TS, Ahmad S, Cattell A, Roberts PJ. Cause of death and factors associated with early in-hospital mortality after hip fracture. Bone Joint J. 2015;97-B(2):246-51.
32. Doyle DJ, Hendrix JM, Garmon EH. American Society of Anesthesiologists Classification. In: StatPearls [Internet]. Treasure Island (FL): StatPearls Publishing; 2023.
33. Kim SM, Long J, Montez-Rath M, Leonard M, Chertow GM. Hip Fracture in Patients With Non-Dialysis-Requiring Chronic Kidney Disease. J Bone Miner Res. 2016;31(10):1803-9.
34. Ball AM, Gillen DL, Sherrard D, Weiss NS, Emerson SS, Seliger SL, et al. Risk of hip fracture among dialysis and renal transplant recipients. JAMA. 2002;288(23):3014-8.

35. Dukas L, Schacht E, Stähelin HB. In elderly men and women treated for osteoporosis a low creatinine clearance of <65 ml/min is a risk factor for falls and fractures. Osteoporos Int. 2005;16(12):1683-90.
36. Covino M, Vitiello R, De Matteis G, Bonadia N, Piccioni A, Carbone L, et al. Hip Fracture Risk in Elderly With Non-End-Stage Chronic Kidney Disease: A Fall Related Analysis. Am J Med Sci. 2022;363(1):48-54.
37. Hsiue PP, Seo LJ, Sanaiha Y, Chen CJ, Khoshbin A, Stavrakis AI. Effect of Kidney Disease on Hemiarthroplasty Outcomes after Femoral Neck Fractures. J Orthop Trauma. 2019;33(11):583-9.
38. Karaeminogullari O, Demirors H, Sahin O, Ozalay M, Ozdemir N, Tandogan RN. Analysis of outcomes for surgically treated hip fractures in patients undergoing chronic hemodialysis. J Bone Joint Surg. 2007;89(2):324-31.
39. Jadoul M, Albert JM, Akiba T, Akizawa T, Arab L, Bragg-Gresham JL, et al. Incidence and risk factors for hip or other bone fractures among hemodialysis patients in the Dialysis Outcomes and Practice Patterns Study. Kidney Int. 2006;70(7):1358-66.
40. Sathiyakumar V, Avilucea FR, Whiting PS, Jahangir AA, Mir HR, Obremskey WT, et al. Risk factors for adverse cardiac events in hip fracture patients: an analysis of NSQIP data. Int Orthop. 2016;40(3):439-45.
41. Nakano Y, Mandai S, Genma T, Akagi Y, Fujiki T, Ando F, et al. Nationwide mortality associated with perioperative acute dialysis requirement in major surgeries. Int J Surg. 2022;104:106816.
42. Belmont PJ, Garcia EJ, Romano D, Bader JO, Nelson KJ, Schoenfeld AJ. Risk factors for complications and in-hospital mortality following hip fractures: A study using the National Trauma Data Bank. Arch Orthop Trauma Surg. 2014;134(5):597-604.
43. Nasr R, Chilimuri S. Preoperative Evaluation in Patients With End-Stage Renal Disease and Chronic Kidney Disease. Health Serv Insights. 2017;10:1178632917713020.
44. Harrak H, René E, Alsalemi N, Elftouh N, Lafrance JP. Osteoporotic fracture rates in chronic hemodialysis and effect of heparin exposure: A retrospective cohort study. BMC Nephrol. 2020;21(1):261.
45. Vangala C, Niu J, Montez-Rath ME, Yan J, Navaneethan SD, Winkelmayer WC. Selective Serotonin Reuptake Inhibitor Use and Hip Fracture Risk Among Patients on Hemodialysis. Am J Kidney Dis. 2020;75(3):351-60.
46. Liu B, Anderson G, Mittmann N, To T, Axcell T, Shear N. Use of selective serotonin-reuptake inhibitors or tricyclic antidepressants and risk of hip fractures in elderly people. Lancet. 1998;351(9112):1303-7.
47. Macri JC, Iaboni A, Kirkham JG, Maxwell C, Gill SS, Vasudev A, et al. Association between Antidepressants and Fall-Related Injuries among Long-Term Care Residents. Am J Geriatr Psychiatry. 2017;25(12):1326-36.
48. Kristjansdottir HL, Lewerin C, Lerner UH, Waern E, Johansson H, Sundh D, et al. High Serum Serotonin Predicts Increased Risk for Hip Fracture and Nonvertebral Osteoporotic Fractures: The MrOS Sweden Study. J Bone Miner Res. 2018;33(9):1560-7.
49. Hegeman J, Van Den Bemt B, Weerdesteyn V, Nienhuis B, Van Limbeek J, Duysens J. Unraveling the association between SSRI Use and falls: An experimental study of risk factors for accidental falls in long-term paroxetine users. Clin Neuropharmacol. 2011;34(6):210-5.

50. McConeghy KW, Lee Y, Zullo AR, Banerjee G, Daiello L, Dosa D, et al. Influenza illness and hip fracture hospitalizations in nursing home residents: Are they related? J Gerontol A Biol Sci Med Sci. 2018;73(12):1638-42.
51. Fraenkel M, Yitshak-Sade M, Beacher L, Carmeli M, Mandelboim M, Siris E, et al. Is the association between hip fractures and seasonality modified by influenza vaccination? An ecological study. Osteoporos Int. 2017;28(9):2611-7.
52. Ding L, Wei J, Wang B. The Impact of COVID-19 on the Prevalence, Mortality, and Associated Risk Factors for Mortality in Patients with Hip Fractures: A Meta-Analysis. J Am Med Dir Assoc. 2023;24(6):846-54.
53. Mundi S, Pindiprolu B, Simunovic N, Bhandari M. Similar mortality rates in hip fracture patients over the past 31 years. Acta Orthop. 2014;85(1):54-9.
54. Katsoulis M, Benetou V, Karapetyan T, Feskanich D, Grodstein F, Pettersson-Kymmer U, et al. Excess mortality after hip fracture in elderly persons from Europe and the USA: the CHANCES project. J Intern Med. 2017;281(3): 300-10.
55. Gonzalez CA, O'Mara A, Cruz JP, Roth D, Van Rysselberghe NL, Gardner MJ. Postoperative sepsis and septic shock after hip fracture surgery. Injury. 2023;54(8):110833.
56. Perez JV, Warwick DJ, Case CP, Bannister GC. Death after proximal femoral fracture—an autopsy study. Injury. 1995;26(4):237-40.
57. Carretta E, Bochicchio V, Rucci P, Fabbri G, Laus M, Fantini MP. Hip fracture: Effectiveness of early surgery to prevent 30-day mortality. Int Orthop. 2011;35(3):419-24.
58. Riggs BL, Melton LJ 3rd. The worldwide problem of osteoporosis: Insights afforded by epidemiology. Bone. 1995;17(5 Suppl):505S-511S.
59. Cullen MW, Gullerud RE, Larson DR, Melton LJ, Huddleston JM. Impact of heart failure on hip fracture outcomes: A population-based study. J Hosp Med. 2011;6(9):507-12.
60. Hietala P, Strandberg M, Strandberg N, Gullichsen E, Airaksinen KEJ. Perioperative myocardial infarctions are common and often unrecognized in patients undergoing hip fracture surgery. J Trauma Acute Care Surg. 2013;74(4):1087-91.
61. Wesselink EM, Kappen TH, Torn HM, Slooter AJC, van Klei WA. Intraoperative hypotension and the risk of postoperative adverse outcomes: a systematic review. Br J Anaesth. 2018;121(4):706-21.
62. Carpintero P, Caeiro JR, Carpintero R, Morales A, Silva S, Mesa M. Complications of hip fractures: A review. World J Orthop. 2014;5(4):402-11.
63. Santana DC, Hadad MJ, Emara A, Klika AK, Barsoum W, Molloy RM, et al. Perioperative management of chronic antithrombotic agents in elective hip and knee arthroplasty. Medicina (Kaunas). 2021;57(2):188.
64. Yen D, Weiss W. Results of adjusted-dose heparin for thromboembolism prophylaxis in knee replacement compared to those found for its use in hip fracture surgery and elective hip replacement. Iowa Orthop J. 2007;27:47-51.
65. Geerts WH, Bergqvist D, Pineo GF, Heit JA, Samama CM, Lassen MR, et al. Prevention of venous thromboembolism: American College of Chest Physicians evidence-based clinical practice guidelines (8th edition). Chest. 2008;133 (6 Suppl):381S-453S.
66. Hirsh J, Warkentin TE, Shaughnessy SG, Anand SS, Halperin JL, Raschke R, et al. Heparin and low-molecular-weight heparin: Mechanisms of action, pharmacokinetics, dosing, monitoring, efficacy, and safety. Chest. 2001;119 (1 Suppl):64S-94S.

67. Boneu B, Caranobe C, Sie P. Pharmacokinetics of heparin and low molecular weight heparin. Baillieres Clin Haematol. 1990;3(3):531-44.
68. Lim HH, Ho KM, Choi WY, Teoh GS, Chiu KY. The use of intravenous atropine after a saline infusion in the prevention of spinal anesthesia-induced hypotension in elderly patients. Anesth Analg. 2000;91(5):1203-6.
69. Handoll HHG, Farrar MJ, McBirnie J, Tytherleigh-Strong GM, Milne AA, Gillespie WJ. Heparin, low molecular weight heparin and physical methods for preventing deep vein thrombosis and pulmonary embolism following surgery for hip fractures. Cochrane Database Sys Rev. 2002;(4):CD000305.
70. Ho HH, Lau TW, Leung F, Tse HF, Siu CW. Peri-operative management of anti-platelet agents and anti-thrombotic agents in geriatric patients undergoing semi-urgent hip fracture surgery. Osteoporos Int. 2010;21(Suppl 4):S573-7.
71. Ashken T, West S. Regional anaesthesia in patients at risk of bleeding. BJA Educ. 2021;21(3):84-94.
72. Yassa R, Khalfaoui MY, Hujazi I, Sevenoaks H, Dunkow P. Management of anticoagulation in hip fractures: A pragmatic approach. EFORT Open Rev. 2017;2(9):394-402.
73. White RH, McKittrick T, Hutchinson R, Twitchell J. Temporary discontinuation of warfarin therapy: Changes in the international normalized ratio. Ann Intern Med. 1995;122(1):40-2.
74. Leverett GD, Marriott A. Intravenous tranexamic acid and thromboembolic events in hip fracture surgery: A systematic review and meta-analysis. Orthop Traumatol Sur Res. 2023;109(2):103337.
75. Smith GH, Tsang J, Molyneux SG, White TO. The hidden blood loss after hip fracture. Injury. 2011;42(2):133-5.
76. Nowicki PD, Ndika A, Kemppainen J, Cassidy J, Forness M, Satish S, et al. Measurement of Intraoperative Blood Loss in Pediatric Orthopaedic Patients: Evaluation of a New Method. J Am Acad Orthop Surg Glob Res Rev. 2018;2(5):e014.
77. Dunn CJ, Goa KL. Tranexamic acid: a review of its use in surgery and other indications. Drugs. 1999;57(6):1005-32.
78. Farrow LS, Smith TO, Ashcroft GP, Myint PK. A systematic review of tranexamic acid in hip fracture surgery. Br J Clin Pharmacol. 2016;82(6):1458-70.
79. Ji JY, Chung JH, Kim NS, Seo YH, Jung HS, Chun HR, et al. Causes and treatment of hypoxia during total hip arthroplasty in elderly patients: A case report. Int J Environ Res Public Health. 2021;18(24):12931.
80. Sharma G, Goodwin J. Effect of aging on respiratory system physiology and immunology. Clin Interv Aging. 2006;1(3):253-60.
81. Janssens JP, Krause KH. Pneumonia in the very old. Lancet Infect Dis. 2004;4(2):112-24.
82. Barceló M, Torres OH, Mascaró J, Casademont J. Hip fracture and mortality: study of specific causes of death and risk factors. Arch Osteoporos. 2021;16(1):15.
83. Wehren LE, Hawkes WG, Orwig DL, Hebel JR, Zimmerman SI, Magaziner J. Gender Differences in Mortality after Hip Fracture: The Role of Infection. J Bone Miner Res. 2003;18(12):2231-7.
84. Lawrence VA, Hilsenbeck SG, Noveck H, Poses RM, Carson JL. Medical complications and outcomes after hip fracture repair. Arch Intern Med. 2002;162(18):2053-7.

85. Quinn B, Giuliano KK, Baker D. Non-ventilator health care-associated pneumonia (NV-HAP): Best practices for prevention of NV-HAP. Am J Infect Control. 2020;48(5S):A23-27.
86. Ståhl A, Westerdahl E. Postoperative Physical Therapy to Prevent Hospital-acquired Pneumonia in Patients Over 80 Years Undergoing Hip Fracture Surgery-A Quasi-experimental Study. Clin Interv Aging. 2020;15:1821-9.
87. Brower RG. Consequences of bed rest. Crit Care Med. 2009;37(10 Suppl):S422-8.
88. Gelfman DM. The Valsalva Maneuver, Set in Stone. Am J Med. 2021;134(6):823-4.
89. Alian AA, Shelley KH. Respiratory physiology and the impact of different modes of ventilation on the photoplethysmographic waveform. Sensors (Basel). 2012;12(2):2236-54.
90. Oskvig RM. Special problems in the elderly. Chest. 1999;115(5 Suppl):158S-64S.
91. Kyhl K, Ahtarovski KA, Iversen K, Thomsen C, Vejlstrup N, Engstrøm T, et al. The decrease of cardiac chamber volumes and output during positive-pressure ventilation. Am J Physiol Heart Circ Physiol. 2013;305(7):H1004-9.
92. Wang H, Cao X, Li B, Wu H, Ning T, Cao Y. Incidence and predictors of postoperative acute kidney injury in older adults with hip fractures. Arch Gerontol Geriatr. 2023;112:105023.
93. Jang WY, Jung JK, Lee DK, Han SB. Intraoperative hypotension is a risk factor for postoperative acute kidney injury after femoral neck fracture surgery: A retrospective study. BMC Musculoskelet Disord. 2019;20(1):131.
94. Kipnis E. Predicting acute kidney injury after hip-fracture surgery: Join the (renal) resistance! Anaesth Crit Care Pain Med. 2016;35(6):369-70.
95. Christensen JB, Aasbrenn M, Castillo LS, Ekmann A, Jensen TG, Pressel E, et al. Predictors of Acute Kidney Injury After Hip Fracture in Older Adults. Geriatr Orthop Surg Rehabil. 2020;11:2151459320920088.
96. Zhan S, Xie W, Yang M, Zhang D, Jiang B. Incidence and risk factors of acute kidney injury after femoral neck fracture in elderly patients: a retrospective case-control study. BMC Musculoskelet Disord. 2022;23(1):7.
97. Lehman LW, Saeed M, Moody G, Mark R. Hypotension as a risk factor for acute kidney injury in ICU patients. Comput Cardiol (2010). 2010;37:1095-8.
98. Agar A, Gulabi D, Sahin A, Gunes O, Hancerli CO, Kılıc B, et al. Acute kidney injury after hip fracture surgery in patients over 80 years of age. Arch Orthop Trauma Surg. 2022;142(9):2245-52.
99. Cauwenberghs N, Kuznetsova T. Determinants and Prognostic Significance of the Renal Resistive Index. Pulse (Basel). 2015;3(3-4):172-8.
100. Marty P, Ferre F, Labaste F, Jacques L, Luzi A, Conil JM, et al. The Doppler renal resistive index for early detection of acute kidney injury after hip fracture. Anaesth Crit Care Pain Med. 2016;35(6):377-82.
101. Ferré F, Marty P, Folcher C, Kurrek M, Minville V. Effect of fluid challenge on renal resistive index after major orthopaedic surgery: A prospective observational study using Doppler ultrasonography. Anaesth Crit Care Pain Med. 2019;38(2):147-52.
102. Lee DH, Chang CH, Chang CW, Chen YC, Tai TW. Postoperative Delirium in Patients Receiving Hip Bipolar Hemiarthroplasty for Displaced Femoral Neck Fractures: The Risk Factors and Further Clinical Outcomes. J Arthroplasty. 2023;38(4):737-42.

103. Kristiansson J, Olsen F, Hagberg E, Dutkiewicz R, Nellgård B. Prolonged vasopressor support during hip-fracture surgery is a risk factor for enhanced mortality. Acta Anaesthesiol Scand. 2019;63(1):46-54.
104. White SM, Moppett IK, Griffiths R, Johansen A, Wakeman R, Boulton C, et al. Secondary analysis of outcomes after 11,085 hip fracture operations from the prospective UK Anaesthesia Sprint Audit of Practice (ASAP-2). Anaesthesia. 2016;71(5):506-14.
105. Robinson TN, Eiseman B. Postoperative delirium in the elderly: Diagnosis and management. Clin Interv Aging. 2008;3(2):351-5.
106. Oosterhoff JHF, Karhade AV, Oberai T, Franco-Garcia E, Doornberg JN, Schwab JH. Prediction of Postoperative Delirium in Geriatric Hip Fracture Patients: A Clinical Prediction Model Using Machine Learning Algorithms. Geriatr Orthop Surg Rehabil. 2021;12:21514593211062277.
107. Bhushan S, Huang X, Duan Y, Xiao Z. The impact of regional versus general anesthesia on postoperative neurocognitive outcomes in elderly patients undergoing hip fracture surgery: A systematic review and meta-analysis. Int J Surg. 2022;105:106854.
108. Shields L, Henderson V, Caslake R. Comprehensive Geriatric Assessment for Prevention of Delirium After Hip Fracture: A Systematic Review of Randomized Controlled Trials. J Am Geriatr Soc. 2017;65(7):1559-65.
109. Wood RJ, White SM. Anaesthesia for 1131 patients undergoing proximal femoral fracture repair: A retrospective, observational study of effects on blood pressure, fluid administration and perioperative anaemia. Anaesthesia. 2011;66(11):1017-22.
110. Monahan KD. Effect of aging on baroreflex function in humans. Am J Physiol Regul Integr Comp Physiol. 2007;293(1):R3-12.
111. Neuman MD, Feng R, Carson JL, Gaskins LJ, Dillane D, Sessler DI, et al. Spinal Anesthesia or General Anesthesia for Hip Surgery in Older Adults. N Engl J Med. 2021;385(22):2025-35.
112. Guarracino F, Bertini P. Perioperative hypotension: causes and remedies. Anaesth Crit Care Pain Med. 2022;2(1):17.
113. Shih YJ, Hsieh CH, Kang TW, Peng SY, Fan KT, Wang LM. General versus spinal anesthesia: Which is a risk factor for octogenarian hip fracture repair patients? Int J Gerontol. 2010;4(1):37-42.
114. Wickham AJ, Highton DT, Clark S, Fallaha D, Wong DJN, Martin DS. Treatment threshold for intra-operative hypotension in clinical practice-a prospective cohort study in older patients in the UK. Anaesthesia. 2022;77(2):153-63.
115. Davies SJ, Yates DR, Wilson RJT, Murphy Z, Gibson A, Allgar V, et al. A randomised trial of non-invasive cardiac output monitoring to guide haemodynamic optimisation in high risk patients undergoing urgent surgical repair of proximal femoral fractures (ClearNOF trial NCT02382185). Perioper Med (Lond). 2019;8(1):8.

CHAPTER 6

Anesthesia for Spine Surgeries

*Balavenkatasubramanian Jagannathan,
Vivekanandan Natarajan, Sathish
Rajaselvam Parameswaran*

ABSTRACT

Spine surgeries have become refined over the years by introducing advancements such as minimally invasive surgeries, computed tomography navigation instrumentation, neural integrity monitors, etc. Advances in management have led to more and more difficult spine deformities getting operated which would have been considered dangerous and inoperable in the yesteryears. Anesthesia for spine surgeries as such is fraught with risks and dangers due to the altered physiology the patient is exposed to when prone. A better understanding of the physiology of the prone position and modifying the anesthetic technique to cater to the needs of modern spine surgical methods have led to better outcomes and a significant reduction in perioperative complications. This chapter tries to give a brief account of the best practices associated with anesthetizing a patient planned for spine surgery.

Keywords: Prone position; TCI; MEP; SSEP; Spine surgery anesthesia; POVL; Cell saver; Anesthesia for scoliosis; Blood conservation strategies

■ KEY POINTS

- Preanesthetic assessment of a patient presenting for any spine surgery should include *general and spine-specific assessments.* There is a gradual progression of restrictive lung disease with an increase in the Cobb angle, and at angles >100°, there is an alveolar hypoventilation and ventilation-perfusion mismatch.
- Bleeding is a particular concern in these surgeries. Many blood conservation strategies are employed in the pre- and intraoperative periods.
- Compared to the supine position, there is a better matching of ventilation-perfusion in the prone position, leading to an increase in the arterial partial pressure of oxygen. The architecture of pulmonary vascular and bronchiolar systems becomes more conducive for matching ventilation-perfusion in the prone position.

- Careful attention to specific details, while making a patient prone, helps prevent complications. These include but are not limited to how the endotracheal tube (ETT) fastening, padding of extremities to prevent injuries to soft tissues and peripheral nerves, the relative position of the heart to the head, free and hanging abdomen, and prevention of abnormal traction or rotation on the major vessels and nerves of the neck.
- Halogenated inhalational agents and nitrous oxide inhibit the amplitude and latency of motor-evoked potential (MEP) and somatosensory evoked potentials (SSEP) in a dose-dependent manner. Propofol can inhibit both MEP and SSEP at higher doses. However, neural transmission is preserved at clinically relevant doses.
- Conventional direct laryngoscopy involves extension at the atlantoaxial joint and flexion at the rest of the cervical spine. Such a movement might cause or aggravate neurological deficits in a predisposed cervical spine.
- Target-controlled infusion (TCI) pumps use computed algorithms to achieve desired concentrations of propofol at target sites such as plasma and brain.
- Spine surgeries account for significant postoperative vision loss (POVL). It is devastating to the patient, as the injury is generally irreversible. Two commonly described modes of injury for POVL are: (1) Central retinal artery occlusion (CRAO), and (2) ischemic optic neuropathy (ION).

INTRODUCTION

Anesthesia for spine surgeries can vary from a minimalist technique like monitored anesthesia care with intravenous sedation, for a biopsy, to a full general anesthetic with an endotracheal tube and the use of advanced hemodynamic monitors and sophisticated drugs, for an extended segment scoliosis correction. A bloodless surgical field and precise instrumentation leading to a fully awake-oriented patient soon after waking up from the anesthetic, adequately moving his limbs to the surgeon's commands, are endpoints that satisfy the surgeon and the anesthesiologist. However, the conduct of an anesthetic is complex, requiring deliberate techniques and interventions at multiple stages throughout the surgery to ensure that the surgery progresses without any complications. This involves clear communication with the surgeon at specific time points of the surgery.

PREANESTHETIC CONSIDERATIONS AND ASSESSMENT

Preanesthetic assessment of a patient presenting for any spine surgery should include general and spine-specific assessments.
- *General assessment* will include asking for a history of any chronic illnesses, evaluation of functional capacity, airway examination, systemic examination, and ordering for basic investigations such as hemogram,

chest radiograph, electrocardiograph, and metabolic profile and for specific investigations depending on specific systems involved from the progression of comorbidity.

In elective surgeries, optimization of any physiological derangement, such as control of blood sugars, recalibration of antihypertensive medications, titration of medications for a compensated heart, or nutritional and pharmacological intervention to improve anemia, can be undertaken, whereas in emergencies, most are bypassed. Risk is stratified, and after informed consent, surgery proceeded, with optimization measures initiated in the limited time available before surgery commences.

- *Spine-specific assessment*: Anesthetic considerations specific to the spine surgery depends on the pathology involved, functional impairment due to the spine pathology per se, and invasiveness of the surgical procedure.[1] Here is a brief discussion of the preanesthetic assessment and anesthetic considerations in commonly performed spine surgeries.
- *Scoliosis correction*: Cobb angle on the anteroposterior X-ray of the spine measures the severity of the scoliosis curvature and correlates with the underlying respiratory system involvement.[2] There is a minimal interference in gas exchange at angles of 35°. Arterial blood gas analysis (ABG) might reveal a slight decrease in arterial oxygen tension [arterial partial pressure of oxygen (PaO_2)], and partial pressure of carbon dioxide ($PaCO_2$) is expected at this stage. There is a gradual progression of restrictive lung disease with an increase in the Cobb angle, and at angles >100°, there is an alveolar hypoventilation, and ventilation–perfusion mismatch, which are reflected on the ABG by a decrease in PaO_2 and an increase in $PaCO_2$.[2-4]

  Pulmonary function test (PFT) becomes a necessity with severe curves and curves with thoracic apex. PFT is advised in case of dyspnea or if the Cobb angle is >80°. Restrictive lung disease decreases forced vital capacity (FVC) and forced expiratory volume at 1 second (FEV_1). FVC of <35% predicted predicts risk for postoperative pulmonary compromise and the need for mechanical ventilation.[5]

  Respiratory symptoms, poor effort tolerance, or signs of right heart failure should entail an echocardiogram to quantify pulmonary hypertension and assess ventricular functions. Mitral valve prolapse is a frequent finding, and echocardiography helps rule out valvular lesions and septal defects in patients with congenital scoliosis.

  Unlike the clinical progression seen in patients with idiopathic scoliosis described earlier, patients with neuromuscular scoliosis have a much more acute deterioration in the respiratory system. Hence, they would require corrective surgery much earlier than their idiopathic scoliosis counterparts. This is best exemplified by the indication of surgery at a

Cobb angle of 20° in patients with Duchenne muscular dystrophy, as further progression is considered inevitable after this stage.

Scoliosis involving the cervical or the upper thoracic spine may interfere with the movements of the neck, which can lead to difficulty in managing the airway. Some patients have a halo traction device fixed to their skull, which may interfere with securing the airway. Duchenne muscular dystrophy is associated with tongue hypertrophy.

Bleeding is a particular concern in these surgeries. Hemoglobin must be optimized with iron supplements and erythropoietin. Preoperative autologous donation (PAD) is a blood conservation strategy initiated in the preoperative period. PAD is discussed later in the chapter.

- *Surgeries for traumatic spine fractures*: Associated neurological injuries, level of spine injury, and presence of other organ system injuries dictate further clinical management. In polytrauma, other systems injuries are ascertained by clinical examination, supplemented by whole-body computed tomography (CT) or magnetic resonance imaging (MRI) investigations. These injuries must be managed according to existing local protocols.

  Anesthetic goals in managing spine fractures include preventing neurological deterioration during intubation or positioning and establishing measures to limit secondary neurologic injury that invariably follows a traumatic primary injury. Adequate intravascular volume, optimal mean arterial pressure, and adequate tissue oxygenation help limit this secondary injury process and can improve the long-term prognosis of these patients.

  The act of intubation can deteriorate spinal cord trauma associated with cervical fractures.[6] Techniques to prevent such injuries are discussed further. Fractures above C4 can involve the diaphragm, requiring early mechanical ventilation.[1] Lower cervical or upper thoracic fractures may not involve the diaphragm but can impair respiration by interfering with the nerve supply to intercostal and accessory respiration muscles. Fractures around T5 interfere with sympathetic outflow, which can result in neurogenic shock.[1]

- *Thoracotomy and videoassisted thoracoscopic surgeries for the anterior approach to the thoracic spine*: One-lung ventilation (OLV) is required to gain surgical access to the anterior thoracic spine. Comorbidities such as smoking and obstructive sleep apnea negatively affect the feasibility of OLV. Pulmonary function test can reveal restrictive lung disease and echocardiography helps assess pulmonary hypertension and the right and left heart. Airway examination and chest CT help choose appropriate equipment for lung isolation.[7]

- *Decompression surgeries for radiculopathy/myelopathy*: Anesthetic assessment is based on the level of spine involvement, as discussed for fracture spine, and the presence of comorbidities.

PHYSIOLOGICAL CHANGES OF POSITIONING IN SPINE SURGERIES

Most spine surgeries happen in the prone position. A brief description of the associated physiological changes is given underneath. Changes associated with lateral, supine, and sitting positions are not discussed here.

- *Cardiovascular changes*: The heart is at a hydrostatic level above the head and the limbs. This leads to a reduction in preload. Inferior vena cava (IVC) compression, increased intrathoracic pressures, and use of positive end-expiratory pressure (PEEP) during intermittent positive pressure ventilation (IPPV) lead to further fall in preload.[8] This leads to a decrease in cardiac output. Baroreceptors mediate the increase in systemic vascular resistance to the maintain blood pressure. Change in the heart rate is minimal. Anesthetic techniques can influence the fall in cardiac index. Total intravenous anesthesia (TIVA) has been found to cause a more significant fall in the cardiac index compared to inhalational anesthesia.[8]
- *Respiratory changes*: Functional residual capacity is increased in the prone position. The free abdomen reduces the cephalad pressure on the diaphragm and reopens atelectatic segments.[8] The prone position does not lead to any change in the chest wall or lung compliance.

Compared to the supine position, there is a better matching of ventilation-perfusion in the prone position. This leads to an increase in the arterial partial pressure of oxygen. The architecture of pulmonary vascular and bronchiolar systems becomes more conducive for matching ventilation-perfusion in the prone position.[8,9]

POSITIONING—ANESTHETIC CONSIDERATIONS

Careful attention to specific details while making patient prone helps prevent complications **(Fig. 1)**.

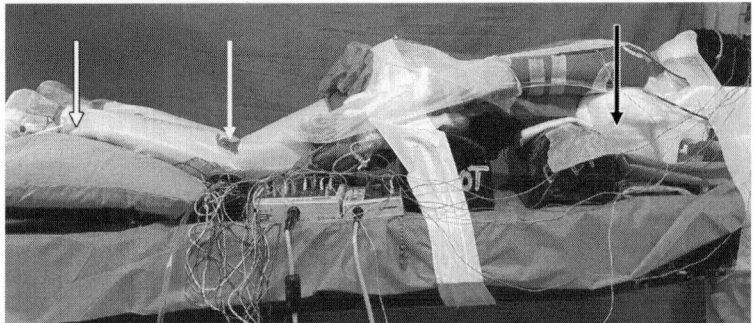

Fig. 1: A patient anesthetized, positioned prone and ready for T3-L3 posterior instrumented deformity correction of scoliosis. The black arrow shows support below the shoulder to prevent excessive traction on the brachial plexus. White arrow shows padding and support beneath the knees and ankles to prevent pressure injuries. The figure also shows the position being secured to the table to prevent inadvertent movement. Equipment of neural integrity monitor (NIM) can be seen lying by the side of the patient.

The endotracheal tube is adequately fastened and secured to prevent accidental dislodgment.[9] Corrugated extensions can be used to attach the breathing circuit to the ETT. This minimizes the chances of the ETT getting kinked as it comes out of a headrest.

The patient might be positioned on a frame or a pair of bolsters **(Figs. 2A and B)**. The chest is placed on the cranial half of the frame or the upper bolster so that the shoulders remain free and the clavicles are about 2–3 cm from the edge of the frame. The breasts should be pushed medially to prevent any pressure on the nipples. The lower half of the frame or the lower bolster supports the pelvis at the level of the anterior superior iliac spine.[10] This allows the abdomen to hang free, which minimizes the pressure on the inferior vena cava, decreasing bleeding at the operating site.

The head can be placed on a surgical pillow, a head ring, or a specifically designed headrest **(Figs. 3A to F)** or fixed in a rigid three-pin fixation. The cervical spine is maintained neutral with the rest, except in a few cases where flexion might be required.[8]

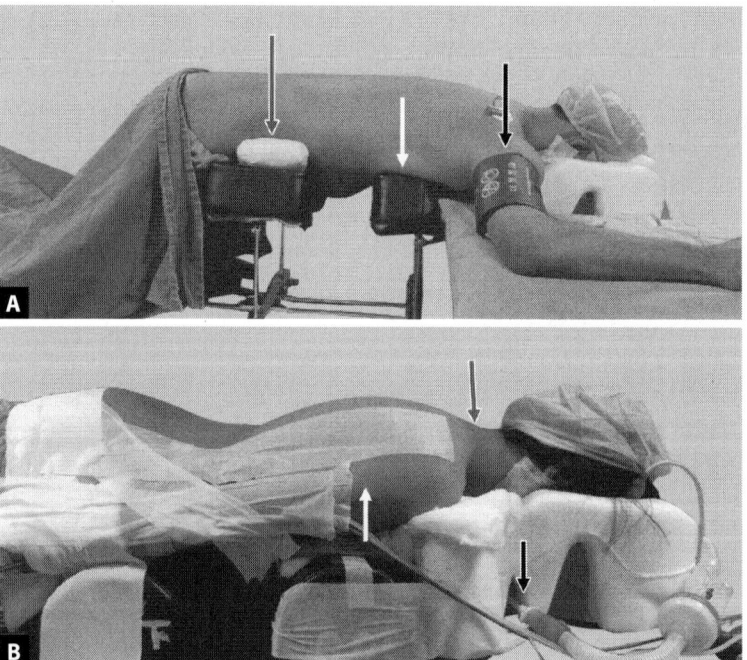

Figs. 2A and B: (A) Patient positioned on the R-H frame in the prone "Superman" position. The black arrow indicates the arm's position, not abducted >90° relative to the chest. White and gray arrows show the pillars of the R-H frame allowing the abdomen to hang freely. The sandbag below the ASIS further helps this purpose; (B) Patient positioned prone on bolsters, the arms placed by the side of the torso (white arrow). The gray arrow indicates that the cervical spine is maintained neutral to the rest of the spine. (R-H: Relton-Hall; ASIS: anterior superior iliac spine)

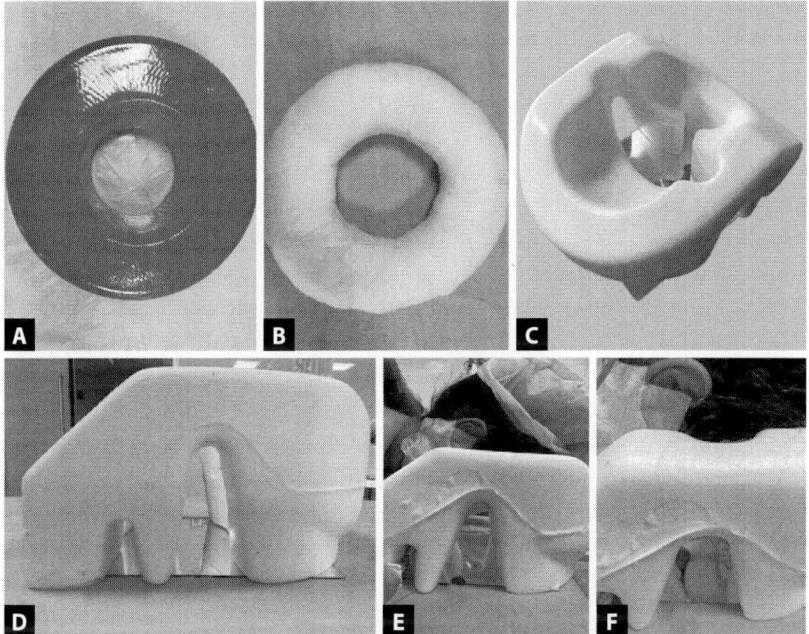

Figs. 3A to F: Headrests used during prone position surgeries. (A) Gel head ring; (B) Head ring made of a gauze pad wrapped around the cotton, the size of this ring can be customized to fit the patient's facial anatomy; (C) The effectiveness of the foam headrest. The foam supports the bony parts of the face, such as the forehead, malar regions, and chin, while leaving gaps for the eyes, nose, and lips; (E and F) The endotracheal tube (ETT) comes out through a designated space without kinking, and there is a mirror to allow periodic inspection of soft structures (D and F).

Eyes are covered, and the face is adequately placed on a headrest so there is no pressure on the eyes, lips, or nose. The face should be observed at frequent intervals during the surgery to prevent any pressure on the soft structures that might occur due to inadvertent movements.

The arms are positioned by the side of the patient's body (*see* **Figs. 2A and B**). This has been observed to cause the slightest pressure on the brachial plexus. Also, this position of the arms allows adequate space for the surgeon and his assistant while operating on the cervical or thoracic spine.[8]

The arms can be brought upward beside the patient's ears for surgeries involving the lower thoracic, lumbar, or sacral regions. Abduction beyond 90° is avoided to limit pressure on the brachial plexus.[8]

Pressure points such as the elbows, shoulders, knees, hips, and ankles should be adequately padded and safeguarded against pressure injuries.[9] The ulnar nerve and lateral cutaneous nerve of the thigh are known to frequently get affected in the prone position.[8]

Vascular access and probes to monitors are appropriately secured to prevent any accidental dislodgment leading to any difficulty during the conduct of anesthesia or surgery.

ANESTHETIC DRUGS

Most spine surgeries are undertaken with a general anesthetic technique, including an induction agent, analgesic drugs, which can be opioids or nonopioids, and a neuromuscular blocking agent **(Figs. 4A to D)**.

Drugs that specifically cater to the needs of spine surgeries can be understood based on the purpose they serve, i.e., (1) drugs that help in hypotensive anesthesia and (2) drugs that help in the smooth conduct of neural integrity monitoring (NIM) during certain surgeries.

Hypotensive anesthesia is associated with lesser blood loss **(Figs. 5A to D)**. Primary anesthetic agents, such as halogenated inhalational agents such as sevoflurane and isoflurane, or intravenous hypnotics such as propofol or thiopentone, can be titrated to produce hypotension. Other drugs used include vasodilators such as nitroglycerin and sodium nitroprusside, β-blockers such as metoprolol and esmolol, ganglionic blockers such as trimethaphan, dopamine agonists like fenoldopam, alpha agonists such as clonidine and dexmedetomidine, and α-blockers such as prazosin.[1]

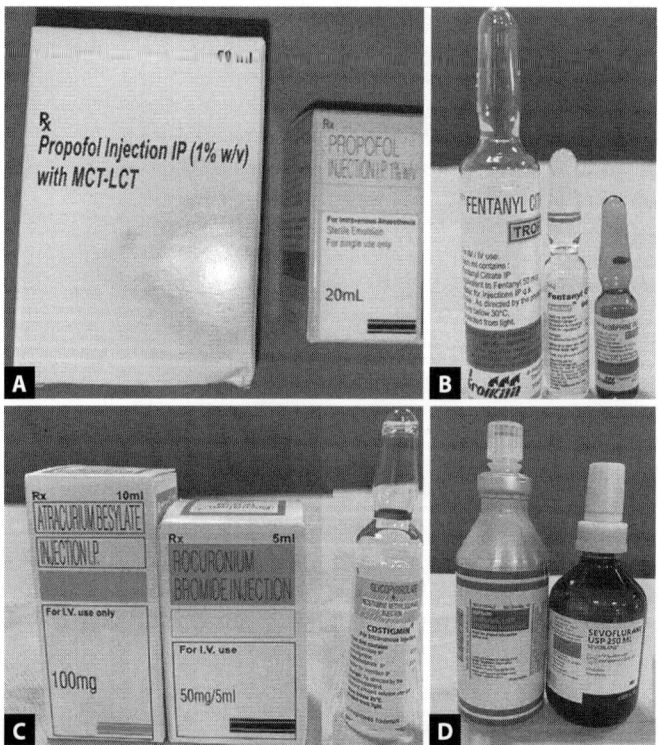

Figs. 4A to D: Drugs commonly used to conduct general anesthesia. Enhanced recovery after surgery (ERAS) protocols have made emphasis on the use of short-acting agents.

Anesthesia for Spine Surgeries

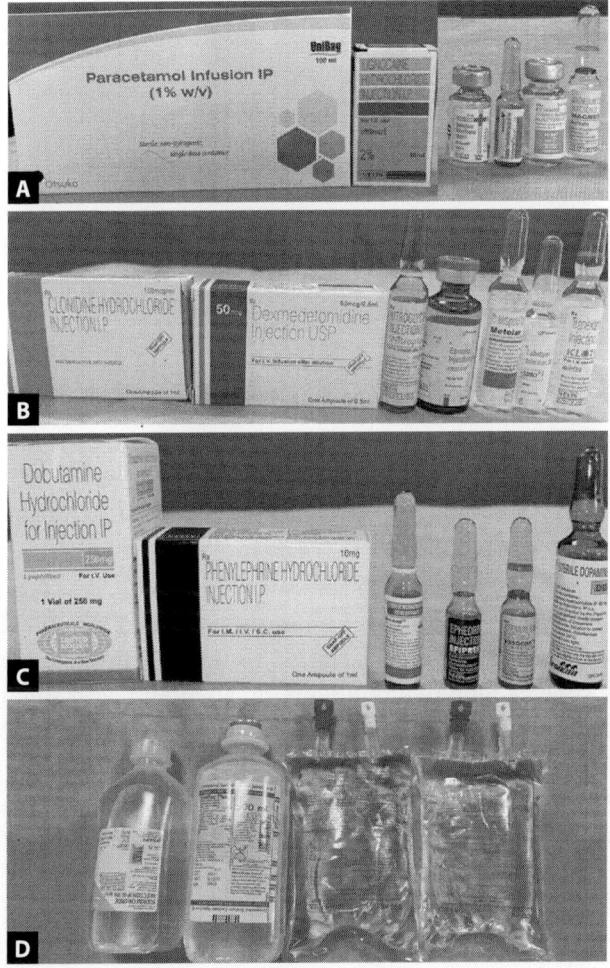

Figs. 5A to D: (A) Nonopioid techniques try to avoid short-term and long-term adverse effects associated with opioids; (B) Drugs commonly used in hypotensive anesthesia. Hypotensive anesthesia can cause a disastrous decrease in perfusion pressure; (C) These drugs help to maintain a minimum mean arterial pressure; (D) Large volumes of crystalloids are associated with complications such as postoperative visual loss (POVL). A higher colloid-to-crystalloid ratio is advocated for the use in prone-position surgeries associated with significant blood loss.

Halogenated inhalational agents and nitrous oxide have been found to inhibit the amplitude and latency of motor-evoked potential and somatosensory evoked potential (discussed further) in a dose-dependent manner. They are used with satisfactory neural integrity monitoring when minimum alveolar concentration (MAC) is kept at or <0.5.[11] Amnesia in this setting is augmented with intravenous infusions of hypnotic agents such as propofol or midazolam.[12]

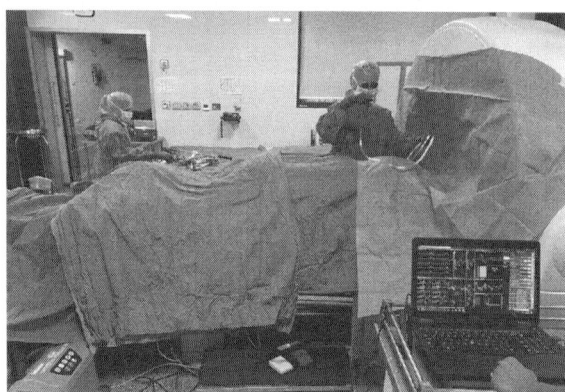

Fig. 6: Patient is anesthetized, positioned, cleaned, draped, and ready for incision. A baseline recording of SSEP/MEP is taken soon after positioning (right lower corner of the figure). A forced air warmer can be seen on the left lower corner of the figure. (MEP: motor-evoked potential; SSEP: somatosensory evoked potential)

Propofol can inhibit both MEP and SSEP at higher doses **(Fig. 6)**, but the neural transmission is preserved at clinically relevant doses.[1] Most centers perform corrective surgeries with a target-controlled infusion of propofol.[13]

Opioids such as fentanyl, remifentanil, alfentanil, and sufentanil have minimal effect on MEP and SSEP. Fentanyl can be used as intermittent boluses or as a continuous infusion. Careful titration of the total dose consumed is required to prevent delayed awakening after surgery.

Motor-evoked potential is abolished by neuromuscular blocking agents.

ANESTHETIC EQUIPMENT

The minimum requirements would be an anesthesia workstation, an airway trolley carrying basic airway instruments, and a drug trolley carrying emergency and routine drugs. The anesthesia workstation incorporates a ventilator, gases/vapors delivering systems, a multipara monitor, and an auxiliary oxygen reserve. Certain spine surgeries will require the use of some other specific equipment to cater to specific needs.

- *Airway equipment*: Conventional direct laryngoscopy involves extension at the atlantoaxial joint and flexion at the rest of the cervical spine. Such a movement might cause or aggravate neurological deficits in a predisposed cervical spine.[6,14] Specific techniques and advanced airway equipment have been used to limit movement at the cervical spine as much as possible **(Fig. 7)**.
    - *Manual in-line stabilization* during laryngoscopy requires two personnel. One person stabilizes the cervical spine by applying firm pressure on the mastoid processes from the head end, while the second person performs a laryngoscopy. This method may decrease the

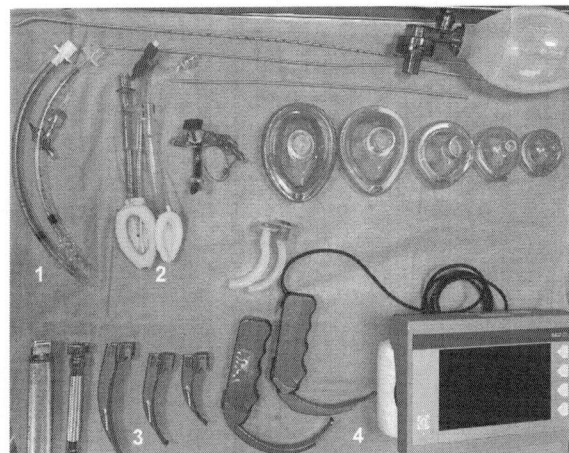

Fig. 7: Airway equipment used frequently in spine surgeries. (1) Endotracheal tube; (2) Laryngeal mask airway; (3) Direct laryngoscopes with blades of different sizes; (4) Videolaryngoscopes of different sizes.

Note: Facemasks, bougies, stylet, Guedel's airways, and an artificial manual breathing unit (AMBU) bag can also be seen in the picture.

laryngeal view by one grade, making intubation difficult. Eschmann stylet or gum elastic bougie is used under such circumstances to gain access to the airway way.[15]

- *Videolaryngoscopes (VL) and fiberoptic bronchoscopes (FOB)* help in limiting movement at the cervical spine. FOBs can be used to intubate the trachea with the neck in the neutral position. FOBs can be used in a spontaneously breathing awake patient after thorough airway anesthesia through regional techniques when the airway has been deemed difficult and at a risk of collapse after induction.[1,8]
- *Laryngeal mask airway (LMA)* can be used as rescue airway devices when other measures fail in intubating the trachea. They can also be used as a conduit through which an endotracheal tube or a FOB can be passed. It is of particular use is during accidental extubation in the prone position. LMAs can be used to ventilate the patient in such dreaded scenarios.[8] Many factors are to be considered to continue the surgery with the LMA, and the same is discussed with the surgeon.
- *TCI:* TIVA administered using standard infusion pumps required the anesthesiologist to calculate and alter the infusion rates based on the time since induction, the intensity of the noxious stimuli from surgery, and the expected time of closure and extubation.[16] This leads to problems of under-dosing or over-dosing of propofol, which creates problems such as inadequate plane of anesthesia, unstable hemodynamics, or delayed awakening from surgery.

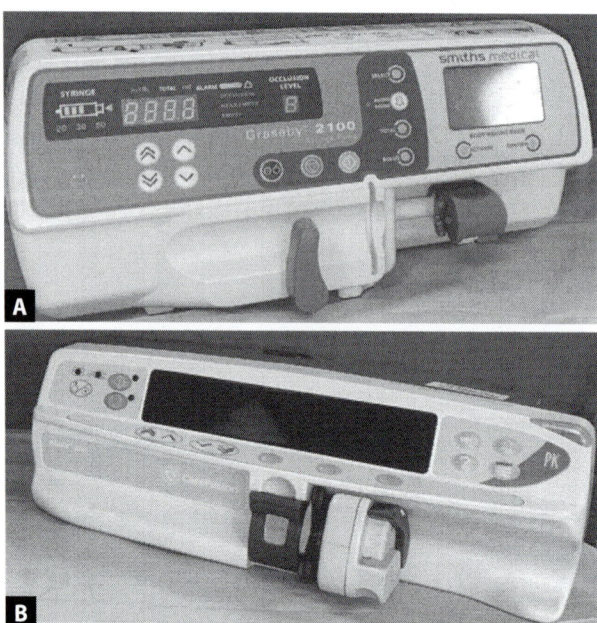

Figs. 8A and B: Major spine surgeries necessitate multiple infusions accomplished with (A) automated pumps and (B) pump equipped to provide a target-controlled infusion.

Target-controlled infusion pumps **(Figs. 8A and B)** use computed algorithms to achieve desired concentrations of propofol at target sites such as plasma and brain. The machine calculates the estimated target concentration of propofol based on age, body weight, time since the start of infusion, and previous infusion rates. Propofol is then infused at estimated rates to achieve the target concentrations desired by the anesthesiologist.[16]

- *Depth of anesthesia monitoring (DoA):* Intraoperative awareness is a concern with any form of general anesthetic. In spine surgeries involving NIM, DoA has a role, as too deep a plane has been shown to interfere with MEP and SSEP monitoring. An inadequate plane of anesthesia can cause involuntary movements to noxious surgical stimuli or cause increased bleeding at the surgical site.[11,17]
    - *Bispectral index (BIS)* is commonly used. Electroencephalogram inputs, derived from frontal leads, are processed through an algorithm to a dimensionless numerical value on a continuous scale of 0–100. The number 100 represents regular cortical electrical activity in a completely awake patient, and 0 represents cortical electrical silence, i.e., deep anesthetic plane. BIS maintained between 40 and 50, is associated with an adequate anesthetic plane with minimal interaction with NIM.[17]
    - *Entropy, narcotrend, and near-infrared spectroscopy (NIRS)* are other forms of DoA monitoring equipment available in the market. Many of these are yet to be validated clinically.

ANESTHETIC TECHNIQUES

Spine surgeries are commonly performed under balanced general anesthesia, preferably an opioid-based technique. Recently, there has been interest in nonopioid techniques, which try to replace opioid analgesia with a combination of two or more drugs such as lignocaine, ketamine, magnesium, and dexmedetomidine, with or without a regional anesthetic block. Erector spinae block has been found to provide satisfactory intraoperative and postoperative analgesia in spine surgeries.[18]

There are reports of lumbar spine surgeries such as single-level or two-level laminectomies/discectomies, being performed under a subarachnoid block. Less blood loss, less nausea and vomiting, improved pain scores, and prevention of pressure/nerve injuries are some of the benefits associated with subarachnoid block.[19]

Specific techniques are employed for necessities of spine surgeries, such as blood conservation strategies for corrective surgeries involving multiple segments, TIVA to facilitate neural integrity monitoring, or use of lung isolation ventilation during anterior approaches to the thoracic spine. Target-controlled infusion has been discussed already. A brief note on blood conservation strategies and OLV is given underneath.

- *Blood conservation strategies*: These include a preoperative autologous donation, acute normovolemic hemodilution (ANH), intraoperative cell salvage, use of controlled hypotension, and use of antifibrinolytic agents.[1,20-22]
  - *Preoperative autologous donation*: Blood is collected from the patient and stored for 3–5 weeks before surgery. This blood is transfused intraoperatively, should there be a requirement. Hematocrit is improved in this period by administering iron supplements and erythropoietin. Preoperative autologous donation prevents risks associated with allogenic blood transfusion. PAD-related complications include weight <50 kg, anemia, coronary artery disease, and severe aortic stenosis.[1]
  - *Acute normovolemic hemodilution*: Blood is withdrawn from the patient early in the operative period and replaced with crystalloids or colloids to maintain intravascular volume. Blood loss early in the surgery results in a lower hematocrit. The autologous blood can be transfused to the patient when blood loss exceeds the set threshold.[1]
  - *Intraoperative cell salvage*: Blood is collected from the operative field through suction, anticoagulated, filtered, and stored in a reservoir. This blood is centrifuged into packed red cells and plasma components. The red cells are washed with a crystalloid solution and transfused to the patient when needed. The use of cell salvage has low evidence of benefit in spine surgeries, probably due to low recovery rates associated with smaller suction devices, contamination with bone and fat, and liberal use of sponges.

- *Controlled hypotension*: Studies have demonstrated lower blood loss with controlled hypotension. Persistent hypotension is associated with end-organ hypoperfusion and should be carefully titrated or avoided in high-risk patients, such as hypertension, diabetes, coronary insufficiency, carotid stenosis, cerebral ischemia, and chronic kidney disease.[1]
- *Antifibrinolytic agents*: Aprotinin, tranexamic acid, and epsilon aminocaproic acid are some of the antifibrinolytic agents used and studied extensively to minimize bleeding in spine surgeries. Aprotinin is not used nowadays due to its association with renal failure. Tranexamic acid and epsilon aminocaproic acid have established safety profiles. They act by inhibiting the conversion of plasminogen to plasmin and directly suppressing plasmin's ability to degrade fibrinogen. Tranexamic acid has been used at a loading dose of 10 mg/kg, followed by an infusion at 1–10 mg/kg/h.[1]

ANTERIOR APPROACH FOR THORACIC SPINE SURGERIES

Anterior approaches to the thoracic spine, particularly video-assisted thoracoscopic surgeries, will require lung isolation by OLV techniques. One-lung ventilation is required in these cases to allow adequate spine visualization and increase the surgeon's operative space.

Planning for OLV will include specific assessment in the preoperative period, including pulmonary function testing and a study of the patient's airway anatomy to understand the feasibility of carrying out such a technique and to evolve a plan to execute lung isolation, which involves preparing equipment such as a double-lumen tube and a bronchial blocker. An explanation of the lung isolation technique is beyond this chapter's scope.

Extubation and postoperative period: Most patients can be extubated at the end of the surgery. The decision to continue elective ventilation in the postoperative period is made based on the extensiveness of the surgery, amount of blood loss and fluid shifts, absence of any complications,[1] adequacy of expansion of the deflated lung when OLV was used, and fulfillment of other conventional criteria for extubation.

Prone position for extended durations can cause facial and airway edema, which may delay extubation. Leak test and airway ultrasound can be used to detect potential airway-compromising edema. Cervical canal decompression can lead to reperfusion-associated cord edema, requiring elective ventilation and treatment with steroids, head elevation, and diuretics.

Postoperative pain can be severe in patients undergoing spine surgeries. Various techniques have been used with varied results. These include intrathecal opioids, an epidural catheter placed by the surgeon at the end of the surgery, erector spinae plane block, and various multimodal analgesia regimens,[23] which may or may not include opioids. Opioids can be administered as boluses or continuous infusions. Patient-controlled epidural analgesia and patient-controlled intravenous opioid analgesia are the other options.[1]

■ COMPLICATIONS AND THEIR PREVENTION

Anesthesia in the prone position is inherently associated with some complications. Most are self-limiting and gets resolved with the passage of time, but a few are potentially devastating. Careful attention to positioning, meticulous planning, and conduct of anesthesia helps prevent most of these complications.

- *Airway problems:* These include kinking of ETT, endobronchial migration of ETT, obstruction by inspissated sputum, blood clots, or accidental extubation of ETT.

  Obstruction in the ETT can be relieved by suctioning. Endobronchial migration of the ETT leads to an increase in the airway pressures and desaturation. A recurrent increase in airway pressure or accidental tracheal extubation would necessitate the patient to be supine to reestablish the airway. This requires discussion with the surgeon about the stage at which the surgery is on and the feasibility of continuing the surgery with a rescue airway. As previously discussed, LMAs can rescue ventilation in patients with accidentally extubated trachea in the prone position.

- *Neurological injuries:* Neurological deficits such as depressed consciousness, quadriparesis, paraparesis, and aphasia have been reported. Causes include arterial or venous occlusion to the central nervous system, dislocation of an unstable spine causing direct trauma to the spinal cord, pneumocephalus, and paradoxical embolism. Peripheral nerve injury is thought to occur due to undue stretching or direct pressure.[8]

  Careful neck positioning ensures adequate flow in the carotid, vertebral arteries, and jugular veins. Maintaining adequate mean arterial pressure during surgery helps prevent cerebral infarcts and hypoperfusion-related injuries. The neutral position of the neck ensures adequate flow in the mentioned vessels. The use of invasive arterial blood pressure monitoring and aids such as BIS and SSEP/MEP monitors help identify global hypoperfusion due to reduced mean arterial pressure (MAP).[8]

  Some surgeries require a certain degree of cervical flexion, such as when accessing the atlantoaxial joint or the foramen magnum. Rigid three-pin fixation, such as a Mayfield head holder, can be used in such cases. It is necessary to ensure a minimum of two finger-breadth between the patient's chin and sternum.[8]

  Motor-evoked potential/SSEP measurement immediately after intubation or positioning helps detect direct spinal cord trauma early, which can help adjust the position or fast-track a surgical exploration.

Surgeries in the cervical spine or the foramen magnum can allow air entrainment, leading to pneumocephalus or pneumorrachis, mainly when the head is higher than the heart. Nursing in a head-down position has less likelihood of such complications.[8]

- *Embolism:* Embolisms of blood clots, fat, and bone particles have been reported. Pulmonary embolism leads to respiratory distress and hemodynamic compromise. Migration of the embolus from the right heart to the left heart through a patent foramen ovale or a septal defect results in the generation of a systemic embolus, which can lodge in the coronary or cerebral circulation or any other end organ circulation.[8]

  Preoperative assessment by history and Doppler study of the lower limb vessels in at-risk patients can elicit the presence of deep vein thromboses. Risk assessment, prognostication, treatment with anticoagulation therapy, and deployment of an IVC filter are measures to be initiated in the presence of deep vein thrombosis. Echocardiography to look for a patent foramen ovale or a septal defect is not recommended routinely.

- *Venous air embolism (VAE):* Subnormal central venous pressure, hypovolemia, higher hydrostatic position, and valveless nature of the epidural veins lead to an increased negative pressure gradient between the veins at the operative site and the right atrium. This gradient can lead to venous air embolism.[8]

  Venous air embolism is characterized by a decrease in end-tidal carbon dioxide ($EtCO_2$), reflecting a decrease in cardiac output. Hemodynamic catastrophe can ensue. Alertness and suspicion help in the early identification of such episodes. The surgeon sutures opened vessels and floods the surgical field with saline to prevent further air entrainment.

  Intraoperative transesophageal echocardiography is recommended in patients at a high risk for VAE. A multiorifice central venous catheter with its tip placed just below the junction of the right atrium and the superior vena cava can help aspirate the entrained air.

  Ensuring adequate intravascular hydration and the use of vasopressors help maintain tissue perfusion. Large VAE can cause rapid hemodynamic collapse and cardiac arrest. Below is a brief discussion about managing cardiac arrest in the prone position.

- *Peripheral nervous system injury:* Brachial plexus, ulnar nerve, and lateral femoral cutaneous nerve injuries have been infrequently reported to be associated with prone positioning. Flexion of the neck and rotation to the opposite side leads to traction on the brachial plexus. The lateral femoral cutaneous nerve of the thigh is much more commonly involved in patients undergoing prone positioning on a Relton–Hall frame.

  Neutral head and neck position, avoiding abduction of arms to >90°, avoiding extension of the arm, and adequate padding of pressure points throughout the body, are vital to prevent injuries to the peripheral nerves.

- *Ophthalmic complications:* Spine surgeries account for many postoperative visual loss reported so far. It is devastating to the patient, as the injury is generally irreversible.

    Two commonly described modes of injury for POVL are: (1) Central retinal artery occlusion, and (2) ischemic optic neuropathy.[8]

    Direct external pressure on the orbits by a headrest or other supports leads to increased intra-orbital pressure, resulting in retinal ischemia and visual loss. Ophthalmic examination findings in such cases are consistent with CRAO.

    Postoperative vision loss also occurred without direct external pressure on the orbits, such as when the head had been supported on pins.[9] The proposed mechanism for such cases is ION.

    Ischemic optic neuropathy is characterized by inadequate optic nerve oxygenation with subsequent impulse transmission failure. Perfusion to the optic nerve depends on the MAP and intraocular pressure. A decrease in mean arterial pressure or an increase in intraocular pressure leads to a decrease in optic nerve perfusion.

    Mean arterial pressure decrease can happen in deliberate hypotensive anesthesia, significant blood loss, or preexisting cardiac dysfunction. Extended durations in the prone position lead to an increase in the intraocular pressure. Replacement of blood loss by large amounts of crystalloids leads to increased intraocular pressure. Over-zealous use of crystalloids also leads to relative anemia, which can interfere with optic nerve oxygenation.[8]

    Not surprisingly, studies have associated POVL with long surgical duration, extensive blood loss, and administration of large volumes of crystalloids. Other risk factors include atherosclerosis, diabetes, and preexisting hypertension.

    Preventing any external compression on the eyes is of paramount importance. A neutral neck position allows free drainage of venous blood from the head. A slight head-up tilt of the entire table to keep the head above the heart helps in this regard. Maintaining a minimum mean arterial pressure, increasing transfusion trigger for blood loss, and judicious use of crystalloids and colloids are some measures proposed to correct potential causes of decreased oxygen delivery in POVL.[8]

- *Advanced cardiac life support (ACLS) in the prone position*: Returning to the supine position helps in the effective administration of ACLS for obvious reasons such as direct access to the airway, precordium, and familiarity in conducting ACLS in a supine position. Having the patient's trolley inside the operating room throughout the surgery has been recommended for high-risk patients. This helps in early supination in an unstable clinical situation.[8]

When turning the patient supine is not immediately possible, chest compression can be provided by placing the palms in the upper back, between the scapulae. Counter-pressure from under the chest is advocated to make the compressions effective. In cases of surgical incision extending through the upper back, one-hand or two-hands technique in the vicinity of the upper back has been recommended.[8]

Anterior–posterior placement of paddles on the thoracic cage is used to administer defibrillation in the prone position. Paddle placement can be a problem in a patient with an open upper back. Right-left paddle placement on the lateral chest walls is advised in these situations. Even before the commencement of surgery, fixing adhesive defibrillation pads is advised in high-risk patients.[8]

■ CONCLUSION

Adequate hemoglobin is a prerequisite for significant spine surgeries. Patients with low hemoglobin are prescribed iron supplements and erythropoietin during the preanesthetic checkup. Preoperative autologous donation starts 3–5 weeks before the surgery.

Increasing Cobb angle or a Cobb angle with a high thoracic apex is associated with restrictive lung disease, reflected by decreased PaO_2 and increased PCO_2 in the ABG. Pulmonary function testing helps assess the severity of restrictive lung disease, which can predict the need for postoperative mechanical ventilation.

The intubation involves flexion at the cervical spine and extension of the atlantoaxial joint. Direct or videolaryngoscopy with manual in-line stabilization or fiberoptic bronchoscopy can prevent significant movements in the cervical spine. Using a laryngeal mask airway as a rescue airway device is invaluable.

Prone positioning of a patient is associated with predictable changes in the cardiovascular and respiratory systems. Anesthetic technique and due precaution to certain practices during positioning can limit these changes. Some essential practice points include a neutral neck, free eyes, hanging abdomen, arms by the side, and padding of pressure points. Also, correct positioning prevents significant complications inherently associated with the prone position.

The integrity of neural pathways is assessed during surgery using SSEP/MEP monitoring. All anesthetic agents interfere with SSEP/MEP signals. Propofol has minimal effect on SSEP/MEP at clinically relevant doses. TIVA through TCI has become a standard practice for spine surgeries involving NIM.

Blood loss is significant in major spine surgeries. Blood conservation strategies are frequently used. Deliberate hypotension is associated with lesser blood loss but is also associated with complications such as POVL. Acute normovolemic hemodilution, PAD, cell salvage, and antifibrinolytics are other strategies to control blood loss.

Prone position predisposes the patient to complications such as POVL, venous air embolism, deep vein thrombosis and pulmonary embolism, cerebrovascular accidents, macroglossia and swelling of other oropharyngeal structures, and peripheral nervous system injury. Prolonged surgical time is a common denominator in many of these complications. Optimal positioning, adequate intravascular volume, optimal mean arterial pressure, and minimizing crystalloid use for blood loss have all been found to help prevent these complications.

Note: This chapter has already been published in the book "ASSI theater manual" 2022. This is reproduced here with due permission from previous editors and publishers.

REFERENCES

1. Raw DA, Beattie JK, Hunter JM. Anaesthesia for spinal surgery in adults. Br J Anaesth. 2003;91(6):886-904.
2. Kulkarni AH, Ambareesha M. Scoliosis and anesthetic considerations. Indian J Anaesth. 2007;51(6):486-95.
3. Huh S, Eun LY, Kim NK, Jung JW, Choi JY, Kim HS. Cardiopulmonary function and scoliosis severity in idiopathic scoliosis children. Korean J Pediatr. 2015;58(6):218-23.
4. Weinstein SL, Dolan LA, Spratt KF, Peterson KK, Spoonamore MJ, Ponseti IV. Health and function of patients with untreated idiopathic scoliosis: a 50-year natural history study. JAMA. 2003;289(5):559-67.
5. Lao L, Weng X, Qiu G, Shen J. The role of preoperative pulmonary function tests in the surgical treatment of extremely severe scoliosis. J Orthop Surg Res. 2013;8(1):32.
6. Durga P, Sahu BP. Neurological deterioration during intubation in cervical spine disorders. Indian J Anaesth. 2014;58(6):684-92.
7. Ashok V, Francis J. A practical approach to adult one-lung ventilation. BJA Educ. 2018;18(3):69-74.
8. Edgcombe H, Carter K, Yarrow S. Anaesthesia in the prone position. Br J Anaesth. 2008;100(2):165-83.
9. Feix B, Sturgess J. Anaesthesia in the prone position. Contin Educ Anaesthesia, Crit Care Pain. 2014;14(6):291-7.
10. Soundararajan N, Cunliffe M. Anaesthesia for spinal surgery in children. Br J Anaesth. 2007;99(1):86-94.
11. Sloan TB, Toleikis JR, Toleikis SC, Koht A. Intraoperative neurophysiological monitoring during spine surgery with total intravenous anesthesia or balanced anesthesia with 3% desflurane. J Clin Monit Comput. 2015;29(1):77-85.
12. Pajewski TN, Arlet V, Phillips LH. Current approach on spinal cord monitoring: the point of view of the neurologist, the anesthesiologist and the spine surgeon. Eur Spine J. 2007;16(Suppl 2):S115-29.

13. Lu CH, Wu ZF, Lin B-F, Lee MS, Lin C, Huang YS, et al. Faster extubation time with more stable hemodynamics during extubation and shorter total surgical suite time after propofol-based total intravenous anesthesia compared with desflurane anesthesia in lengthy lumbar spine surgery. J Neurosurg Spine. 2016;24(2):268-74.
14. Austin N, Krishnamoorthy V, Dagal A. Airway management in cervical spine injury. Int J Crit Illn Inj Sci. 2014;4(1):50-6.
15. Thiboutot F, Nicole PC, Trépanier CA, Turgeon AF, Lessard MR. Effect of manual in-line stabilization of the cervical spine in adults on the rate of difficult orotracheal intubation by direct laryngoscopy: a randomized controlled trial. Can J Anaesth. 2009;56(6):412-8.
16. Nimmo AF, Absalom AR, Bagshaw O, Biswas A, Cook TM, Costello A, et al. Guidelines for the safe practice of total intravenous anaesthesia (TIVA): Joint Guidelines from the Association of Anaesthetists and the Society for Intravenous Anaesthesia. Anaesthesia. 2019;74(2):211-24.
17. Sudhakaran R, Makkar JK, Jain D, Wig J, Chabra R. Comparison of bispectral index and end-tidal anaesthetic concentration monitoring on recovery profile of desflurane in patients undergoing lumbar spine surgery. Indian J Anaesth. 2018;62(7):516-23.
18. Singh S, Choudhary NK, Lalin D, Verma VK. Bilateral ultrasound-guided erector spinae plane block for postoperative analgesia in lumbar spine surgery: a randomized control trial. J Neurosurg Anesthesiol. 2020;32(4):330-4.
19. McLain RF, Kalfas I, Bell GR, Tetzlaff JE, Yoon HJ, Rana M. Comparison of spinal and general anesthesia in lumbar laminectomy surgery: a case-controlled analysis of 400 patients. J Neurosurg Spine. 2005;2(1):17-22.
20. Verma R. Blood conservation in scoliosis surgery. J Postgrad Med Educ Res. 2017;51(2):68-73.
21. Tate DE Jr, Friedman RJ. Blood conservation in spinal surgery. Review of current techniques. Spine (Phila Pa 1976). 1992;17(12):1450-6.
22. Joseph SA, Berekashvili K, Mariller MM, Rivlin M, Sharma K, Casden A, et al. Blood conservation techniques in spinal deformity surgery: a retrospective review of patients refusing blood transfusion. Spine (Phila Pa 1976). 2008;33(21):2310-5.
23. Alboog A, Bae S, Chui J. Anesthetic management of complex spine surgery in adult patients: a review based on outcome evidence. Curr Opin Anaesthesiol. 2019;32(5):600-8.

CHAPTER 7

Total Intravenous Anesthesia: Basic Principles and Practical Aspects

Gaurav Kakkar

ABSTRACT

Total intravenous anesthesia (TIVA) is an essential anesthetic skill required to look after patients who specifically require TIVA due to its core benefits or the contraindications of a volatile-based anesthetic. TIVA requires a specific knowledge and skill set for which curriculum-based training should be introduced at all anesthesia training institutes. The terms TIVA and target-controlled infusion (TCI) are not mutually interchangeable. TCI stands for the target-controlled drug infusion using a specific syringe pump, while TIVA is the entire process of intravenous anesthetic delivery using TCI pumps. The basic pharmacological and multicompartmental pharmacokinetics of drugs and pharmacological models should be well understood before any attempts at TCI or TIVA. The key TCI models for propofol are Marsh and Schneider, while the main remifentanil model is the Minto model. Specific safety recommendations, as advised by the Society for Intravenous Anaesthesia (SIVA) and the Association of Anaesthetists, must be followed to deliver TIVA and safely minimize any incidences of awareness. The mandatory use of TIVA/TCI pumps and specific intravenous sets with the Luer-lock and antisiphon mechanisms are predominant amongst them. TIVA is a core anesthetic technique that provides multiple patient benefits and minimum environmental damage and has a huge potential for the future.

Keywords: Total intravenous anesthesia; Target-controlled infusion; Remifentanil; Marsh model; Minto model; Kataria model; Bristol regimen; 10-8-6 regimen; Three-compartment model; Volatile free; Closed-loop system; Awareness prevention; Patient safety

KEY POINTS

- Total intravenous anesthesia (TIVA) as a technique is a preferred anesthetic technique for various scenarios.
- Dedicated TIVA/TCI pumps are available, which should be used for all the TIVA cases.
- Comprehensive curriculum-based training is imperative for a safe TIVA service.

- Dedicated and specific TIVA sets should be used as suggested by international guidelines to ensure patient safety.
- Basic pharmacological principles of the drugs and pharmacological models should be well grasped and followed.
- Standards of the TIVA service should be the same even for locations requiring TIVA outside the operating theaters.

INTRODUCTION

Total intravenous anesthesia is an anesthetic technique that delivers general anesthesia entirely by the intravenous (IV) route by combining a hypnotic agent and an analgesic sedative without any volatile anesthetic agents. The intravenous hypnotic agent used is propofol, and the most common intravenous analgesic sedative used is remifentanil, with other options being alfentanil or sufentanil. These pharmacological agents are used due to the available pharmacokinetic models of these drugs, which are incorporated into microprocessor-guided infusion pumps. The terms TIVA and target-controlled infusion (TCI) are sometimes interchangeably used, which should not be the case. TCI is a mechanism to give a specific drug at a desired plasma or effect-site concentration through a microprocessor-controlled infusion pump with the drug's pharmacokinetic model installed in the pump. On the other hand, TIVA is the broader mechanism of intravenous delivery of the general anesthetic using the two specific drugs through their TCI-driven pumps. TIVA has gained popularity over the years due to its proven benefits in day case surgery and in surgeries requiring intraoperative evoked potential monitoring. A basic understanding of the pharmacokinetic principles of intravenous drugs and their pharmacokinetic models, along with certain practical safety principles, are essential for a safe and effective TIVA practice.[1]

HISTORY

The first historical attempt at intravenous drug administration was in the 17th century when Christopher Wren injected opium into a dog using a goose quill. Subsequently, in the mid-19th century, the hollow needle (1845) and the syringe (1853) were developed by Francis Rynd and Charles Gabriel Pravaz, respectively, as the essential equipment required to deliver intravenous drugs. Using this new mode of drug delivery, Pierre Cyprian Ore pioneered the use of Chloral Hydrate as an intravenous agent in 1872. In 1909, intravenous hedonal was used for general anesthesia, but the long duration of action had limited its use. Subsequently, various new compounds such as paraldehyde, magnesium sulfate, and ethanol were tried in the mid-20th century with limited success, and their use was truncated due to high morbidity and mortality. It was in the 1970s that the first propofol (diisopropylphenol) was synthesized and trialed by Glenn et al. in the preliminary clinical studies, which had to be stopped due to adverse drug reactions. In 1986, the first lipid emulsion of propofol was formulated and used safely for the first time as an intravenous agent, and this was further leveraged by the introduction of the Diprifusor pump in the 1990s that enabled the initial and safe use of target-controlled propofol infusion. The introduction of remifentanil as a potent ultrashort-acting opioid and its programmable pharmacokinetic modeling by Dr Charles Minto, an Australian anesthetist, in the late 1990s, facilitated the evolution of TIVA using the synergistic properties of both propofol and remifentanil. Since then, various pharmacokinetic models have been made for propofol and remifentanil for both adult and pediatric age groups. Also, principles of safe, practical delivery of TIVA have evolved over the years from the learnings of reported incidents, and this has culminated in the formulation of basic guidelines for the safe delivery of TIVA practices from the major anesthesia societies of the world.

TIVA OR TCI: WHAT IS THE DIFFERENCE? OR ARE THEY IDENTICAL?

Both terms are used interchangeably, but there is a difference.

Total intravenous anesthesia is an anesthetic with no volatile anesthetic gases such as sevoflurane and desflurane, while it can be given using a TCI pump, this is unnecessary and can be delivered by hand or a simple mL per hour pump or even as a bolus. However, dedicated TCI pumps are highly recommended for the safe delivery of TIVA in the 21st century to minimize clinical errors resulting in accidental awareness.[2]

Target controlled infusion, on the other hand, is giving an intravenous anesthetic using a specialized microprocessor-controlled syringe driver. With a TCI pump, the anesthetist enters the patient's details, selects the target concentration (plasma or effect site), and the pump calculates the appropriate infusion rate.

BENEFITS OF TOTAL INTRAVENOUS ANESTHESIA

The use of TIVA has gained popularity worldwide amongst anesthetists due to certain advantages and also due to its necessary use in certain medical conditions. The key benefits or advantages of TIVA over a volatile-based anesthetic are as follows:[3]

- Smooth onset
- Intraoperative cardiovascular stability
- Predictable, rapid, and clearer recovery
- Reduced incidence of postoperative nausea vomiting (PONV)
- Minimizing greenhouse gas effect of volatile anesthetics.

The use of TIVA becomes essential when the volatile-based anesthesia is either contraindicated or is inappropriate, such as in the following instances:
- Known or suspected malignant hyperthermia (MH)
- Intraoperative use of motor and sensory evoked potentials (neuromonitoring)
- Anesthesia for airways surgery/procedure
- Anesthesia requirements outside the operating room
- Anesthesia requirements during the transfer of patients.

All anesthetists should be trained and competent in the safe use of TIVA as specific conditions such as MH and the requirement to use neuromonitoring can arise for any individual. The use of TIVA, thus, cannot be a rarely practiced technique for any anesthetist.

■ DISADVANTAGES OF TOTAL INTRAVENOUS ANESTHESIA

The most significant risk of TIVA, as confirmed by the National Audit Project-5 (NAP-5) audit of the Royal College of Anaesthetists (RCoA), is that of accidental awareness in patients primarily due to improper practical use of TIVA and its equipment.[2,3] It highlights the flawed use of the technique and the improper kit or the improper use of the kit required to deliver it rather than the technique itself. Consensus guidelines for the safe delivery of TIVA were thus constituted by the Association of Anaesthetists (AAGBI) and the Society for Intravenous Anaesthetists (SIVA) group. In the absence of a "closed-loop" TIVA system, which has yet to evolve beyond the research stage, conformity to the aforementioned guidelines becomes ever more critical to ensure the patients safety.

A significant indirect disadvantage of TIVA is the inadvertent or even negligent use of 2% propofol. All pharmacokinetic modeling done in various propofol models is based on 1% propofol; hence, using 2% propofol is not justified as a simpler alternative. Moreover, there are serious concerns due to the actual quantity of propofol used and its lipid load in 2% based propofol practices, leading to excessive use related to propofol infusion syndrome and even mortality. Most of the guidelines and practices on TIVA advocate using 1% propofol as a rule and encourage uniformity in practice across departments.

There have been some concerns regarding hyperalgesia after excessive use of remifentanil. However, no significant evidence exists to link any causality to remifentanil.

Dedicated TIVA pumps and their related equipment such as dedicated TIVA lines, nonreturn valves, and depth of anesthesia monitoring, are the minimum equipment required to deliver TIVA safely. All this has an expense attached to it and thus becomes a disadvantage for smaller units trying to run a TIVA service.

The nonavailability of suitable opioids such as remifentanil, sufentanil, or alfentanil makes it unattractive to run a TIVA service, as the primary advantage of doing a TIVA is lost in the absence of the above drugs. India is a prime example, where the need for regulatory approval for any of the aforementioned medications makes TIVA an unscientific and unsafe technique to be practiced or even advocated.

PHARMACOKINETICS

After intravenous administration, a drug is redistributed throughout the body to the tissues, muscles, organs, and fat, and eliminated from the body by the kidneys, liver, etc., thus a bolus of propofol after acting at its site of action, i.e., the brain has an effect for a few minutes as it is quickly redistributed through the whole body, as displayed in **Figure 1**. The duration of action of a drug depends on its pharmacokinetic properties and also on the physiological characteristics of the patients.[4]

- The three-compartment pharmacological model **(Fig. 2)** is the fundamental model that describes the distribution and elimination of a drug from the body after an intravenous injection.
- Let us take the example of propofol:
  - Propofol is initially injected/infused into the central compartment, primarily plasma. Then, some of it is distributed to the two other compartments (C2 and C3) and the brain, which is considered a separate compartment in this model.
- (These compartments are theoretical and do not represent actual body compartments)
  - *C1*: Central blood compartment for instant action of the drug
  - *C2*: Highly perfused tissues where the movement of the drug is fast, e.g., muscles
  - *C3*: Less well-perfused tissue that has slower drug movement, e.g., fat
- *The effect site:* Brain

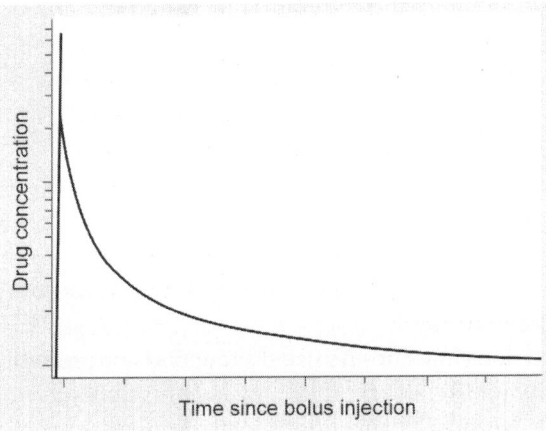

Fig. 1: Concentration: Time graph after a single bolus of propofol.

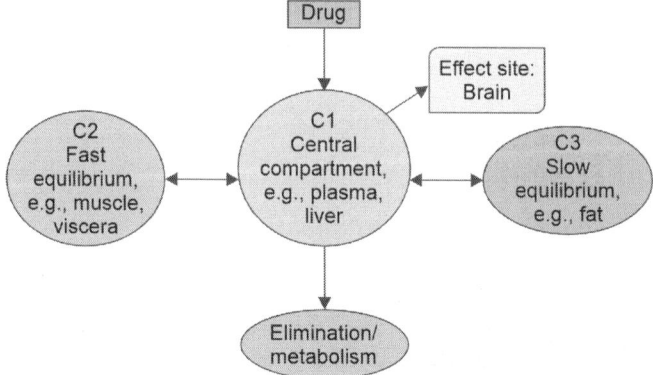

Fig. 2: The three-compartment model—*C1:* Central compartment, *C2:* Rapid equilibrium, and *C3:* Slow equilibrium.

At the initiation of the infusion, the rate of the propofol is high to compensate for the uptake of the drug in the peripheral compartments. Once the equilibrium is reached, the infusion rate is reduced to maintain a steady state.

The removal of the drug from the body is only from the central compartment via either elimination or metabolization. If the level of the drug drops in the central compartment, like when an infusion is stopped, then the redistribution of the drug happens from peripheral compartments to the central compartment for further elimination from the central compartment.[4] For this reason, there is a decremental reduction in the propofol infusion rate in TCI models. When it is not done in manually controlled TIVA techniques, there is a delay in the emergence of the patient from the intravenous anesthesia.

Pharmacokinetics and the Infusion Rate of TIVA/TCI Pumps

After the target concentration is set using the patient's demographics, the pump calculates the total infusion rate by combining the three separate infusion rates, using the bolus, elimination, and transfer (BET) principle. An initial bolus is given to fill the central compartment immediately. Then there is an infusion at a constant rate to replace the drug lost through elimination from the central compartment (*see* **Fig. 2**). This infusion compensates for the loss through distribution to the peripheral compartments (C2 and C3). This reduces over time as the levels equilibrate between the compartments.[4]

Total intravenous anesthesia's usual induction concentration is between 3 and 6 µg/mL, but like all anesthetic agents, this depends on the patient's characteristics. No single concentration is appropriate for all the patients, and titration to patient response and surgical stimulus is recommended.[4]

The starting concentration of propofol may be as high as 8 µg/mL in a young, anxious patient. It would have to be lower in an elderly, frail, or unwell patient, where induction levels of two to three are targeted and revised if required. Proficient users of TIVA would carefully observe the effect-site concentration at which the patient loses response to verbal or noxious stimulus and subsequently use this to tailor TIVA levels.

Propofol maintenance levels are kept at 3–4 µg/mL while remifentanil levels are kept at 6–7 ng/mL, provided both infusions run synergistically.

Plasma and Effect Site Concentrations

In plasma concentration models, the pump calculates and maintains an estimated drug concentration in the plasma (C1). Since the site of action of the intravenous anesthetics is in the brain, it takes a longer time for the brain concentration to equilibrate with that in the plasma, especially since propofol moves slowly between the compartments.

On the other hand, effect site concentrations give a larger initial bolus than the plasma concentration models so that the effect site, i.e., brain levels of the drug, rise faster, leading to a rapid induction.

It is worth noting that both these concentrations are estimated concentrations, and in practice, the actual concentrations cannot be measured. Hence, closed-loop TIVA/TCI systems are not available in clinical practice.

■ COMMONLY USED MODELS

Bristol Model (10-8-6 Model)

It was the first pharmacokinetic model used to deliver TIVA/TCIA before the advent of the TCI pumps. It still forms the fundamental basis of most of the current TCI models. It is also known as the *10-8-6 model*. It is based on the three-compartment model of healthy patients. The patients in the above model were premedicated with temazepam and fentanyl 3 µg/kg was given at induction along with nitrous oxide. Propofol was given at induction using a 1 mg/kg induction bolus followed by a 10-8-6 maintenance as follows:[5]
- 10 mg/kg/h for first 10 minutes
- 8 mg/kg/h for the next 10 minutes
- 6 mg/kg/h after that, as maintenance.

Marsh Model

The Marsh model is one of the most popular models used, and it uses the body weight to calculate the infusion rate and autoadjusts the infusion rate every 10 seconds. Though an age is entered, it is only used to ensure that the patient is over 16 years of age, or else the pump will not operate. It uses a smaller induction dose than the Schneider model, but overall, a larger volume is given throughout the case. The smaller induction dose can lead to a lag in induction time.[5]

Schneider Model

The Schneider model came after the Marsh model, and its infusion rates are based on the patient's weight, height, age, and sex. It initially gives a larger bolus (overshoot) that leads to a faster induction, and then less propofol is given during the rest of the case.

Minto Model

The Minto model is used for remifentanil and uses a specific lean body mass for individuals over 12 years. Both plasma and effect site concentrations can be used. Target remifentanil concentrations of 6–7 ng/mL are usually used for synergistic action with propofol during TIVA.

■ COMMONLY USED TERMINOLOGIES

Some of the commonly used terms are described here and are also highlighted in **Figure 3**.
- *Cpt:* Target plasma concentration
- *Cet:* Target effect site concentration
- *Cp:* Actual/observed plasma concentration
- *Ce:* Actual/observed effect site concentration
- *Flow rate:* Infusion rate of the drug
- *Total dose given:* Total dose of the drug delivered till that time
- *Decrement time:* Time to 1 µg/mL or estimated "wake-up" time
- *Graphic plasma levels:* Descriptive graphs of plasma levels.

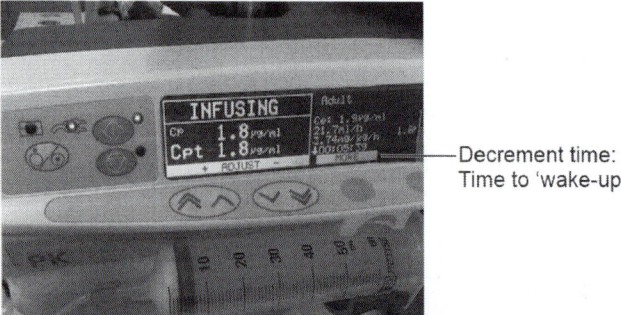

Fig. 3: A TIVA/TCI (Alaris) pump using propofol. (TCI: target-controlled infusion; TIVA: total intravenous anesthesia)

Note: Display legend: *Cpt:* Target plasma concentration, *Cp:* Plasma concentration, *Cet:* Target effect site concentration, mg/kg/h infusion rate (10-8-6)

TIVA IN SPECIAL CIRCUMSTANCES: ELDERLY/PEDIATRICS/OBESE

Elderly

Usually, in many areas of anesthesia, there is debate over the ideal model for elderly or frail patients. Though the Marsh model uses age, it is not used in the calculations. An 85-year-old weighing 65 kg will receive the same infusion rate as a 25-year-old of the same weight, which could be better. Some may consider the Schneider model to be better in this regard, although it delivers a larger induction bolus, it delivers a reduced total volume throughout the case, which may benefit frail patients. Irrespective of the mode used, a lower target concentration should be used (initially 1–2 µg/mL) with incremental increases every few minutes or as per the cardiovascular stability.

Pediatrics

Target-controlled infusion in children is a specialized area of practice. The two model-specific models for pediatrics are the Paedfusor and the Kataria models, which can be used for ages up to 16 years and weighing up to 61 kg. Adult models can be used if the patients are above these limits.

For propofol infusions during extended periods (i.e., >15–20 hours) in children, there is a very small risk of propofol infusion syndrome, which can cause fatal complications such as cardiac failure, rhabdomyolysis, metabolic acidosis, and kidney failure.

Obese

Like the elderly, neither the Schneider nor the Marsh models are accurate for obese patients. The maximum body weight accepted by the Marsh model is 150 kg, which bases infusion rates on actual body weight. This may result in a relative overdose in obese patients. The Schneider model only accepts a body mass index (BMI) < 35 for females or <42 for males and calculates a lean body mass for its infusions.

Thus for TIVA in obese patients, it is recommended to titrate to clinical parameters and overall monitoring.

PRACTICAL ASPECTS: FIFTEEN RULES FOR TIVA

1. The TIVA should only be delivered using dedicated TIVA pumps for both the drugs under all circumstances and locations. There should be no exception to this rule, even for experienced operators, as the risk of human errors is huge, especially in cases of longer duration.[6]
2. The models for the TIVA were developed on individuals with average weight, age, and normal physiology. Adjustments must be made for extremes of height, weight, age, or altered physiology as per the given

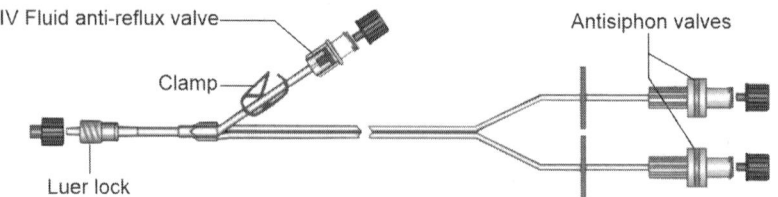

Fig. 4: A typical total intravenous anesthesia (TIVA) set connector.

situations in the respective scenarios. This is akin to the concept of a certain percentage of people falling outside the range of a safe minimum alveolar concentration (MAC) for a volatile-based anesthetic.

3. The syringe pumps should be programmed only after loading the respective drug syringes onto the pumps. This is to prevent exchange errors in the loading of wrong syringes.[7]
4. To minimize the risk of awareness, proper equipment and precautions should be used to ensure the delivery of TIVA to the patient. Most of the cases of awareness can be prevented by using proper delivery techniques of TIVA.[7] A typical TIVA set connector with a Luer-lock and antisiphon valve is shown in **Figure 4**.
5. The TIVA delivery sets with syringes and infusion lines must have Luer-lock connectors to reduce the risk of accidental disconnection.
6. There should also be an antisiphon valve on the drug delivery lines to prevent uncontrolled infusion from an erroneous line.[8]
7. An antireflux valve should be present, especially on the intravenous line, to prevent the backward flow of the drug if multiple infusions are running on the same intravenous cannula. This is also true in most multidrug giving connectors like the octopus connectors.[8]
8. Intravenous access should be in sight to act as a visual check for the connection of the lines.
9. Bispectral index (BIS) monitoring or any other depth of anesthesia monitoring is recommended but is not mandatory. It should be noted that using a depth of anesthesia monitor does not prevent awareness on its own and should be used to complement overall multimodal monitoring.[9]
10. Most TIVA anesthetists would recommend against the use of a neuromuscular blocking infusion during a routine TIVA. The reason for this is twofold; firstly, the use of remifentanil almost negates the requirement of a paralytic agent due to its superior potency. Secondly, it acts as a safety net to prevent awareness, as a patient with a lighter depth of anesthesia will generally respond with some movement to a painful stimulus before it is long enough for the risk of awareness to set in. The use of neuromuscular paralysis would take away this advantage.[10]

11. TIVA should also be used for the patient's induction in all cases. Given the estimated target concentrations, this acts like an individual control for that patient.
12. Most TIVA anesthetists would recommend a high remifentanil and low propofol technique to exploit the maximal benefits of TIVA. The usual maintenance level for remifentanil should be around 6–7 ng/mL, and that for propofol should be around 3–4 µg/mL for any TCI model. Usually, propofol levels below 3 µg/mL are not recommended.
13. The target concentration can be gradually reduced toward the end of the case, although the effect site concentration should not be dropped below 2.0 µg/mL. Due to the use of remifentanil, a longer-acting opioid such as morphine should be administered around 20 minutes before the end of the procedure to prevent gaps in analgesia requirements.[10]
14. The decrement time on most pumps will give an estimated time for the concentration to drop to 1.0 µg/mL. This is a rough estimate of wake-up time. Routine TIVA users would often note at the effect-site concentration the patient loses response to a verbal or noxious stimulus and use this as an indicator of the wake-up time. This can be very variable, though, and thus caution is advised.
15. Flushing all infusion lines before leaving the operating room is mandatory to prevent unsupervised boluses of unused residual drugs, especially remifentanil.

TOTAL INTRAVENOUS ANESTHESIA OUTSIDE THE OPERATING ROOM

The benefits of TIVA enable it to be an attractive option for procedures performed outside of the operating theater (OT) environment, e.g., procedures in specialties such as interventional neurology, bronchoscopy, gastrointestinal endoscopy or colonoscopy, radiation suite biopsy, etc., are increasingly being performed under TIVA. However, the minimum standards required for TIVA are usually not considered while delivering this service. It is of utmost importance that the standards of TIVA safety observed and followed in OT should be applicable and followed diligently in the TIVA practices outside of the OT. Failure to follow the basic safety rules like nonuse of dedicated TIVA pumps or TIVA lines, etc., have led to documented cases of awareness or patients coming to harm. Thus, the basic competencies of the TIVA practice, along with the basic equipment required, are a minimum prerequisite for initiating or delivering TIVA outside of the OT environment.[6]

TOTAL INTRAVENOUS ANESTHESIA IN INDIA

The potential for TIVA as an anesthetic technique in India is huge. Much interest has been generated recently in the practice and use of TIVA in India.

However, certain key challenges are currently faced by the anesthetists practicing in India about TIVA.

First and foremost is the need for more structure or training toward the basic principle of TIVA. No (or minimal, if any) curriculum offers the basic fundamental training for the TIVA practice in anesthesia training programs or postgraduate courses. Competency-based training for TIVA must be included in anesthesia curriculums in the country. Ad hoc and conference-based training should differ from the standard for delivering TIVA or TCI.

Secondly and equally important is the lack of availability of a suitable opioid in India that is required for TIVA. The three suitable opioids, i.e., remifentanil, sufentanil, and alfentanil, are unavailable in India. Remifentanil has been awaiting regulatory approval in India for a while and is expected to be available shortly. However, it is extremely important that suitable and appropriate training is available and made mandatory before the patients are exposed to this fantastic agent, which can have complications if improperly used, e.g., the concentrations and dilutions, the infusion practices, the strict "no manual bolus" strategies, etc. Training is needed for any institution before using remifentanil, either in anesthesia or as a drug for sedation in intensive care.[6]

The availability of advanced TCI/TIVA pumps in the Indian market has led to a peculiar situation where the key drug to be used in these pumps is missing. With the nonavailability of the key opioids, the only use of the pumps would be to administer TCI propofol. No intended benefit of TIVA is justified by using any other opioid or by giving TIVA manually using intravenous propofol in various prevalent ways. All these prevailing practices are unscientific, unproven, and unsafe. The international guidelines for the safe delivery of TIVA were made to reduce the burden of harm in patients with all the key ingredients available. In light of the nonavailability of key drugs and training, practicing anesthesiologists should reconsider using TIVA in India. They should also refrain from giving local, unproven, unscientific intravenous delivery techniques the nomenclature of TIVA. The effectiveness and safety of all such practices should be analyzed as any previously published techniques before validating and calling them TIVA techniques.

There is immense scope for TIVA as a technique in India, provided adequate structured training, availability of key opioids, and a robust reporting mechanism of possible complications arising from improper or inadvertent practices.

■ CONCLUSION

Total intravenous anesthesia or TCI are not interchangeable terminologies. TIVA is the technique of delivering anesthesia entirely by the intravenous route using dedicated TIVA or TCI pumps. TCI uses microprocessor-controlled, pharmacokinetically-enabled infusion pumps to deliver propofol or other specific drugs using their estimated plasma levels as desired targets. The benefits of TIVA make it an attractive technique for specific procedures, especially those involving evoked potential-based neuromonitoring, day case procedures, and conditions where volatile-based anesthetics are contraindicated. The key prerequisites of appropriate training and availability of essential medications/equipment must be met to ensure a safe and effective TIVA service initiation and delivery.[11]

REFERENCES

1. Al-Rifai Z, Mulvey D. Principles of total intravenous anaesthesia: basic pharmacokinetics and model descriptions. BJA Educ. 2016;16(3):92-7.
2. Association of Anaesthetists of Great Britain and Ireland (AAGBI) and the Society for Intravenous Anaesthesia (SIVA). Total Intravenous Anaesthesia 2017: guidelines for safe practice. [online] Available from https://www.aagbi.org/sites [Last accessed September, 2023].
3. Miller RD, Eriksson LI, Fleisher LA, Wiener-Kronish JP, Cohen NH, Young WL. Miller's Anesthesia, 8th edition. Philadelphia, Pa: Elsevier, Saunders; 2015.
4. Miller T, Gan T. Total Intravenous Anesthesia and Anesthetic Outcomes. J Cardiothorac Vasc Anesth. 2015;29(Suppl 1):S11-5.
5. Life In The Fastlane. (2023). Total Intravenous Anaesthesia and Target-Controlled Infusion. [online] Available from: https://partone.litfl.com/tiva-and-tci.html [Last accessed September, 2023].
6. Sivasubramaniam S. (2007). Target controlled infusions in anaesthetic practice. Available from: https://resources.wfsahq.org/atotw/target-controlled-infusions-in-anaesthetic-practice-anaesthesia-tutorial-of-the-week-75/ [Last accessed September, 2023].
7. Aston D, Rivers A, Dharmadasa A. Equipment in Anaesthesia and Critical Care. United Kingdom: Scion Publishing Limited; 2014. p. 404.
8. Davey A, Diba A, Ward C. Ward's Anaesthetic equipment, 6th edition. Edinburgh: Saunders Elsevier; 2012.
9. Davey A, Ince CS. Fundamentals of operating department practice. London: Cambridge University Press; 1999.
10. Harrington J, Strong E, Carragher L. (2019). Total Intravenous Anaesthesia for Adults. St. John's Hospital, Lothian NHS. [online] Available from: https://www.periopcpd.com/wp-content/uploads/TCI-12.pdf [Last accessed September, 2023].
11. Nimmo AF, Absalom AR, Bagshaw O, Biswas A, Cook TM, Costello A, et al. Guidelines for the safe practice of total intravenous anaesthesia (TIVA): Joint Guidelines from the Association of Anaesthetists and the Society for Intravenous Anaesthesia. Anaesthesia. 2019;74(2):211-24.

CHAPTER 8

The Contemporary Perioperative Management of Pheochromocytoma

A Kumar, Venkatesan Thiruvenkatarajan

ABSTRACT

Pheochromocytomas are rare neuroendocrine tumors arising from chromaffin tissue that synthesize catecholamines. They are responsible for 0.2% of all cases of sustained hypertension. Once considered formidable, perioperative mortality rates have reduced substantially with an improved understanding of the preoperative pharmacological preparation, enhanced imaging techniques for accurate localization, and advances in intraoperative management. Surgical resection is the treatment of choice and poses significant challenges to the anesthesiologist. Laparoscopic and, the more recent, robotically assisted minimally invasive approaches facilitate improved analgesia and enhanced recovery after surgery. Literature on perioperative management principles is predominantly derived from observational studies; thus, high-quality evidence is lacking as the condition is relatively uncommon. Institution-wise protocols should be implemented considering the availability of pharmacological agents and local expertise established from multidisciplinary interaction across endocrine, surgical, anesthesia, and intensive care specialties. This chapter aims to review the current perioperative management principles of pheochromocytoma and to emphasize the role of a multidisciplinary approach in its clinical management.

Keywords: Pheochromocytoma; Preoperative optimization; Anesthesia; Perioperative; Hemodynamic management

KEY POINTS

- Pheochromocytoma poses challenges to anesthesiologists throughout the perioperative period.
- Our understanding of pathophysiology, pharmacological principles, and surgical characteristics has improved perioperative outcomes.
- Preoperative pharmacological preparation and optimization should be based on international recommendations tailored to local resources and expertise.

- A thorough understanding of the pharmacological principles of medications used in hemodynamic management and an appreciation of their adverse effects are vital for everyone involved in the perioperative journey of these patients.

■ INTRODUCTION

Pheochromocytoma are rare catecholamine secreting neuroendocrine tumors arising from chromaffin tissues. Surgical resection is the treatment of choice, and their perioperative management is often challenging to the anesthesia team. This chapter will discuss the pathophysiology and perioperative management of pheochromocytomas, focusing on the contemporary aspects of preprocedural optimization and improving the surgical outcomes.

■ ETIOLOGY AND EPIDEMIOLOGY

Pheochromocytomas are catecholamine-secreting tumors that originate either from the chromaffin cells of the adrenal medulla or neural crest progenitors located in the extra-adrenal ganglia of the sympathetic system.[1,2] Adrenal origin accounts for nearly 80% of cases, and most are benign.[2,3] Rarely, these tumors can occur in atypical sites such as the head and neck, aortic bifurcation, pericardium, inferior mesenteric artery (the organ of Zuckerkandl), and chromaffin tissues in the abdomen, pelvis, and thorax.[2,4] The historical *"rule of 10"* to describe pheochromocytoma as 10% extra-adrenal, malignant, and bilateral is no longer applicable as contemporary evidence does not support this.[5]

These tumors peak in the fourth to fifth decade and occur equally in men and women.[6] Most occur sporadically, but an autosomal–dominant gene mutation may occur in one-third of cases.[1] These familial presentations may be associated with Von Hippel-Lindau disease, multiple endocrine neoplasia 2A and 2B, neurofibromatosis, and succinate dehydrogenase enzyme mutations.[1]

Pheochromocytomas are detected in 0.2–0.6% of patients with sustained hypertension.[7] The incidence derived from studies performed after 2010 is approximately 0.6/100,000 annually.[8]

■ CLINICAL FEATURES

The clinical features of the tumor are attributed to excess circulatory catecholamines and their metabolites. The classical symptom triad of headache, palpitations, and generalized inappropriate sweating may be present in up to 40% of patients.[9,10] Although hypertension is present in about 90% of cases, it can be paroxysmal in up to 50% of presentations.[1] Other nonspecific manifestations include lethargy, nausea, constipation, weight loss, fever, pallor, tremors, and hyperglycemia.[1,11] Prolonged catecholamine exposure may result in dilated cardiomyopathy, arrhythmia, heart failure, myocardial infarction, stroke, or vascular ischemic events in the form of bowel ischemia.[2] Malignant hypertension may induce papilledema and associated visual disturbances. Half of these tumors are identified as incidental findings during work-up for an unrelated indication.[1]

■ BIOCHEMICAL INVESTIGATIONS AND IMAGING

The diagnosis of pheochromocytoma traditionally relied upon measuring plasma catecholamines and the 24-hour urinary catecholamines and vanillylmandelic acid.[1,11] However, the sporadic release of catecholamines and their short half-life reduce the sensitivity and specificity of these tests.[1,11] Current recommendations comprise measuring the breakdown products of catecholamines instead of their parent moieties.[1,11,12] Norepinephrine and epinephrine are metabolized to normetanephrine and metanephrine within the chromaffin tissues of the tumor, independent of the paroxysmal catecholamine release.[1,11,12] Elevated catecholamine metabolites suggest increased catecholamine tumoral production; hence, diagnostic tests based on these estimates yield a nearly 100% sensitivity.[11,12] Although the urinary fractionated metanephrine assay offers a reasonably good sensitivity, its specificity is low.[12]

Biochemical tests must be interpreted cautiously if patients are on medications that may interfere with catecholamine release. These include tricyclic antidepressants, selective norepinephrine reuptake inhibitors, monoamine oxidase inhibitors, and recreational drugs such as cocaine and amphetamines.[1,11] Dopamine antagonists, namely droperidol or haloperidol, may stimulate tumor catecholamine release.[11] These agents may need to be interrupted briefly to avoid false-positive results.[1]

The tumor's location and extent must be delineated after the diagnosis is established based on the clinical history and biochemical profile.[1,2,12] Furthermore, it is vital to investigate multiple primary tumors and metastatic lesions in those with genetic inheritance.[12] Both magnetic resonance imaging (MRI) and computed tomography (CT) are used in this respect, and these modalities are often supplemented with additional functional radiotracer imaging, such as scintigraphy.[1]

■ PREOPERATIVE EVALUATION AND PREPARATION

Perioperative mortality rates before the era of alpha-blockade were as high as 30–45%.[13] These have since declined to 0–3% after implementing alpha-adrenoceptor blockade regimens.[13-15] Poor outcomes were usually a result of hypertensive crisis, malignant arrhythmias, myocardial ischemia, and intraoperative multiple organ failure.[1] A meticulous preoperative planning and pharmacological preparation to control symptoms of excess catecholamines will play a decisive role in improving perioperative outcomes.[2] The goals of preoperative optimization are: (1) stabilization of blood pressure; (2) restoration of normovolemia; (3) heart rate and arrhythmia control; (4) assessment and optimization of myocardial function; (5) correction of blood glucose and electrolyte abnormalities.[1]

PHARMACOLOGICAL PREPARATION FOR BLOOD PRESSURE CONTROL

Pharmacological preoperative blockade against the effect of catecholamines is the cornerstone of achieving safe perioperative outcomes. Both blockade of catecholamine synthesis and the blockade of their downstream effects have been described in the literature.[11] The choice of medications is dictated by regional or international practices and their local availability.[11,16,17]

Numerous approaches to pharmacologic preparation have been proposed; however, to date, no randomized trials have compared the efficacy of these regimens.[11] As endocrinologists are involved in preoperative pharmacological optimization, outpatient and inpatient preparations are now feasible.[11] In most centers, alpha-adrenergic blockade, beta-adrenergic blockade, and sometimes calcium channel blockers are often used.

The alpha-adrenergic blockade is typically commenced 10-14 days preoperatively, facilitating blood pressure control and expansion of the intravascular volume.[16,17] Phenoxybenzamine is the preferred alpha-antagonist in most centers. It is an irreversible, long-acting, and nonspecific alpha-adrenergic blocking agent. The initial dose is 10 mg every 6-12 hours and is increased by 10-20 mg every 2-3 days up to a maximum dose of 240 mg/day. As it causes irreversible inactivation of alpha-1 and alpha-2 receptors, it may result in postoperative refractory hypotension. Hence, it must be ceased 24-48 hours before surgery.[1,12] Patients should be warned about potential side effects: headaches, drowsiness, orthostatic hypotension, dizziness, and tachycardia.

Specific short-acting and competitive alpha-1 antagonists include prazosin, terazosin, and doxazosin **(Table 1)**. These agents produce less reflex tachycardia as the alpha-2 receptors are spared and are associated with a lesser degree of postoperative hypotension.[1,12] They are used in patients who cannot tolerate phenoxybenzamine,[11] and the common side effects include malaise, dizziness, vertigo, headache, and nausea.[12] PRESCRIPT (Pheochromocytoma Randomized Study Comparing Adrenoreceptor Inhibiting Agents for Preoperative Treatment) is a recent trial that compared the efficacy of phenoxybenzamine versus doxazosin initiated 2-3 weeks before pheochromocytoma resection.[18] The results showed that doxazosin was comparable to phenoxybenzamine in maintaining intraoperative blood

TABLE 1: Drugs used in the preoperative preparation of pheochromocytoma.

Drug class	Doses	Comment	Adverse effects
Alpha-blockers			
Phenoxybenzamine	Commence 10 mg twice daily, usual dose 1 mg/kg/day	Start 10–14 days preoperatively	Postural hypotension and reflex tachycardia
Prazosin	2–5 mg twice or thrice daily	If the last dose is given the night before, the plasma levels drop significantly and impact intraoperative blood pressure control, due to its short half-life	
Doxazosin	2–8 mg daily		
Terazosin	2–5 mg daily		
Beta-blockers			
Propranolol	20–80 mg twice or thrice daily	Start only after establishing alpha-blockade	Caution in those with bronchial asthma, heart failure, and conduction defects
Metoprolol	25–50 mg twice or thrice daily		
Atenolol	12.5–25 mg twice or thrice daily		
Calcium channel blockers			
Amlodipine	10–20 mg/day	• Useful if other agents are inadequate or poorly tolerated • Beneficial in cardiomyopathy or coronary vasospasm	
Nifedipine	30–90 mg/day		
Nicardipine	60–90 mg/day		
Verapamil	180–540 mg/day		
Diltiazem	90–240 mg/day		
Catecholamine synthesis inhibitor			
Metyrosine	Initial dose 250 mg 6 hourly, titrate up to 4 g/day	Used in metastatic lesions, unresectable tumors, or intolerance to other medications	*Significant effects*: Anxiety, depression, sedation, nightmare, crystalluria, urolithiasis, galactorrhea, and extrapyramidal signs

pressure.[18] It was less effective in preventing intraoperative hemodynamic instability; however, this effect did not impact the clinical outcome.

The beta-adrenergic blockade should only be initiated with adequate alpha-blockade owing to the catastrophic hypertensive crisis that could ensue with unopposed alpha-receptor stimulation.[2] Beta-blockade also counteracts tachycardia precipitated by nonselective alpha-blockade or due to vasodilation.[12] Propranolol (nonselective beta-blocker), atenolol, metoprolol, and labetalol have been used successfully in varying doses and regimens (see **Table 1**). Cardioselective agents such as atenolol and metoprolol are preferred.

Calcium channel blockers are used as adjuncts and are less likely to cause orthostatic hypotension. They inhibit norepinephrine-induced intracellular calcium influx, thereby preventing coronary spasm and attenuating hypertensive responses.[2] They are indicated in those intolerant to phenoxybenzamine and in situations of inadequate combined alpha- and beta-adrenergic blockade.[11] They are also used in normotensive patients exhibiting paroxysmal hypertension bouts.[2,12] Amlodipine (5–20 mg/day), nicardipine (30–90 mg/day), verapamil (180–540 mg/day), and diltiazem (90–240 mg/day) are the commonly used agents.[12]

Alpha-methyl-para-tyrosine (metyrosine) is a competitive inhibitor of tyrosine hydroxylase enzyme, a rate-limiting step in catecholamine formation.[19] It can reduce catecholamine stores and their release on tumor stimulation.[2] It is helpful in those with extensive tumor metastasis or in those where conventional drugs were either ineffective or tolerated poorly.[2,11]

ASSESSMENT AND OPTIMIZATION OF MYOCARDIAL FUNCTION

Tachyarrhythmias can occur in this patient population as a secondary manifestation of alpha-2-receptor blockade or due to excess epinephrine or dopamine.[1] Selective beta-1 blockers are recommended to manage these cases, and they should be commenced only after establishing complete alpha-blockade.[1] This helps to prevent unopposed alpha-adrenoceptor-mediated vasoconstriction that could manifest after antagonism of beta-2 adrenergic receptor-mediated vasodilation.[1]

A thorough cardiovascular evaluation must be performed for preoperative risk stratification and optimization. A 12-lead electrocardiogram (ECG) may reveal the presence and extent of left ventricular strain, hypertrophy, bundle branch blocks, and ischemia.[1] Left ventricular systolic dysfunction can occur in 10% of the patients, along with a degree of diastolic dysfunction; hence preoperative echocardiography is essential. Moreover, chronic hypertension-induced hypertrophic cardiomyopathy is also frequent in these patients.[1] Echocardiography will also help delineate other types of cardiomyopathies, such as catecholamine-induced and Takotsubo cardiomyopathy, and rule out primary cardiac pheochromocytoma in select patients.[1] Primary cardiac tumors need further evaluation using an MRI and/or CT scan.

INTRAVASCULAR VOLUME OPTIMIZATION

Excess catecholamines cause vasoconstriction through alpha-1 receptor activation. This can be superimposed with alpha blockade-induced profound orthostatic hypotension. Increasing fluid intake and a high sodium diet are recommended to overcome this effect.[1]

Assessment of Adequacy of Optimization

The adequacy of the alpha-blockade has been defined by many authors, including Roizen, as: no inhospital blood pressure >160/90 mm Hg for 24 hours before surgery, no orthostatic hypotension with blood pressure <80/45 mm Hg, no ST- or T-wave changes for 1-week before surgery, no more than five premature ventricular contractions per minute.[20] Various other criteria have also been proposed, as shown in **Box 1**. Notably, these endpoints may need to be expressed more adequately from a clinical perspective due to the extreme heterogeneity of the disease.[12]

Serial hematocrit values gauge the effectiveness of volume expansion. A 5–10% drop in hematocrit is usually seen in well-prepared patients, but it is used only as an approximate guide to assessing volume expansion.[12]

SURGICAL APPROACH

Currently, laparoscopic resection with either a lateral transabdominal (**Fig. 1**) or posterior retroperitoneoscopic (**Fig. 2**) approach is the preferred technique across many centers for tumors that are <6 cm and under 100 g.[21,22] The benefits

BOX 1: Proposed targets of adequate alpha-receptor blockade.*

- Blood pressure <130/80 mm Hg
- Blood pressure control for a minimum of 3–5 days
- Heart rate <80 beats/min
- Orthostatic hypotension with blood pressure >80/45 mm Hg
- Hematocrit <45
- No ST- and T-wave changes in electrocardiogram (ECG)
- Ventricular arrhythmias <1 in 5 minutes

*Values are likely to vary based on the institutional protocols.

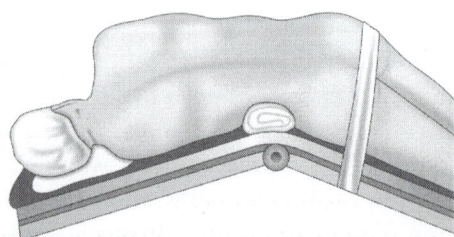

Fig. 1: A patient positioned for a laparoscopic transabdominal approach.

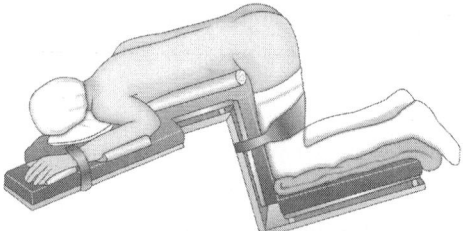

Fig. 2: A patient positioned for laparoscopic retroperitoneoscopic approach.

of laparoscopy are reduced catecholamine surges, better postoperative analgesia, early recovery, reduced incidence of thromboembolic and pulmonary complications, and shortened hospital stay.[23-26] Open procedures performed using a transperitoneal approach through a subcostal or midline incision are typically reserved for larger masses and extra-adrenal tumors with limited access.[15,22,27] Robotic-assisted minimally invasive approaches have also been used in some centers.[28] The most common approach at the author's institution is a posterior retroperitoneoscopic approach, where the patient is placed in a half-jack-knife position[22] (see **Fig. 2**). The surgical method of choice is usually based on the surgeons' expertise, preference, convenience, and complexity of the surgery.[12,22] These procedures should only be embarked in adequately equipped specialist centers and performed by experienced teams.

■ ANESTHESIA MANAGEMENT

As mentioned earlier, pheochromocytoma resection is widely considered to be among the most challenging in anesthetic practice. The goals of anesthetic management are: to avoid drug-induced catecholamine release, avert catecholamine surges related to anesthetic or surgical maneuvers and tumor manipulation, and be vigilant to treat hypotension after tumor devascularization.[1] High preoperative plasma norepinephrine levels, large tumors, hypotension after initiation of the alpha-blockade, and a preinduction mean arterial pressure (MAP) above 100 mm Hg are recognized risk factors for intraoperative hemodynamic instability.[29] Conscientious planning and preparation and multidisciplinary communication with endocrinology and surgical colleagues are paramount to achieving optimal perioperative outcomes.

General anesthesia with tracheal intubation is used in all patients regardless of the surgical approach. Many approaches using various combinations of anesthetic agents and adjuvants have been described in the literature. Nonetheless, there is little evidence to promote one intraoperative anesthetic approach over another.[11] Vigilant anticipation and management of hemodynamic instability and an appreciation of intravascular volume depletion are two fundamental principles of intraoperative management.

A laparoscopic approach has recently become more common, and low intra-abdominal pressure of 8-10 mm Hg has been shown to reduce catecholamine release and consequently fewer hemodynamic fluctuations.[30]

Avoid Drugs Implicated in Catecholamine Release

Many drugs used in the perioperative period may increase circulating catecholamine levels which should be avoided **(Table 2)**. Implicated mechanisms include stimulation of the presynaptic release of catecholamines, inhibition of neuronal reuptake, and stimulation of histamine release.

Preinduction

Short-acting alpha-1 antagonists can be continued on the morning of the procedure, whereas longer-acting agents such as phenoxybenzamine and doxazosin are usually ceased 12-24 hours preoperatively.[31] The administration of an anxiolytic to alleviate stress-induced catecholamine surge should be strongly considered as part of perianesthetic preparation.

TABLE 2: Agents deemed to be unsafe in patients with pheochromocytoma.

Agent class	Comments
Inhalational agents	
• Halothane	• Arrhythmogenic, myocardial sensitization to catecholamines
• Desflurane	• Sympathomimetic effects
Neuromuscular blockers	
• Succinylcholine	• Arrhythmias, fasciculations-induced catecholamine release
• Pancuronium	• Histamine release
• Atracurium	• Histamine release
Intravenous anesthetics	
Ketamine	Sympathomimetic effect
Opioid analgesics	
Morphine, pethidine	Histamine release
Dopamine-2 antagonists	
Metoclopramide, haloperidol, droperidol, olanzapine, chlorpromazine	Can induce hypertensive crisis
Tricyclic antidepressants	
Monoamine oxidase inhibitors, and serotonin reuptake inhibitors, e.g., amitriptyline, phenelzine, duloxetine	Can induce hypertensive crisis
Peptide hormones	
• Glucagon	• Catecholamine release
• Amphetamine, ephedrine, sibutramine, phentermine, cocaine	• Sympathomimetics

Options include long-acting oral benzodiazepines such as lorazepam or diazepam the night before and/or intravenous (IV) midazolam 1-2 mg titrated to effect during transfer to the operating room, placement of vascular access, and while performing neuraxial techniques.[15] Prolonged fasting times should be avoided as these patients manifest relative hypovolemia due to catecholamine-induced chronic vasoconstriction (Field 27).

The institution's dilution protocols should prepare vasoactive medications. The list includes but is not limited to, nitroglycerin (GTN), sodium nitroprusside (SNP), diltiazem, esmolol, magnesium sulfate, norepinephrine, and vasopressin.[15] Patients with catecholamine-induced cardiomyopathy may require epinephrine, dobutamine, and milrinone in the context of right ventricular impairment.[15] Rapid infusion systems may be required for cases with large tumors and tumors with major vascular involvement.[15]

Intraoperative Monitoring

Invasive arterial monitoring should be established before anesthetic induction with judicious infiltration of local anesthetics and adequate supplementation with anxiolytics; e.g., midazolam 1-3 mg IV and small doses of opioids, for instance, fentanyl 25-100 μg IV.[11] It is worth reiterating that even a trivial sympathetic stimulus may trigger a hypertensive crisis.[11] Central venous access is usually placed following induction of anesthesia and is indicated for the infusion of vasoactive medications and volume replacement.[11] Central venous pressure (CVP) monitoring should not be used to guide fluid resuscitation as it correlates poorly with left ventricular filling pressure.[27] There is no evidence to recommend an ideal technique to assess this surgery's circulatory volume and cardiac output.[1] Pulmonary artery catheters are no longer regarded as the standard of care for assessment of volume status.[11] They may be considered in patients with catecholamine-induced cardiomyopathy, preexisting severe cardiac disease, or pulmonary hypertension.[11,27] Technologies based on arterial pulse contour analysis and transpulmonary thermodilution systems such as LiDCOrapid™ (Medtronic, Minneapolis, MN, USA), FloTrac™ (Edwards Lifesciences, Irvine, CA, USA), and PiCCO™ (Pulsion Medical System, Feldkirchen, Germany) are less invasive and safer alternatives to monitor cardiac output.[1,32] However, algorithm-based cardiac output devices may be inaccurate due to fluctuating vascular tone and hemodynamic instability.[1] At the author's institution, the arterial pressure monitoring catheter is coupled to Philips Intellivue Monitor™ (Philips Medical Systems, Boeblingen, Germany) and the FloTrac™ (Edwards Lifesciences, Irvine, CA, USA) system. This enables continuous assessments of pulse pressure variation, stroke volume variation, and cardiac output parameters.

Systolic pressure variation is superior to CVP in assessing volume status and response to fluid challenges.[11] Reports suggest its usefulness in pheochromocytoma surgery, with the limitation being the need for sinus rhythm and a closed chest.[11]

Transesophageal echocardiography may be helpful to guide volume status, detect myocardial ischemia, and valvular abnormalities, and assist vasoactive therapy in the presence of cardiomyopathy.[11] Nonetheless, the setup may be expensive and requires expertise. It may be beneficial in cases of intracardiac pheochromocytoma, severe catecholamine-induced cardiomyopathy, or intraoperative cardiovascular collapse.[11]

Aside from standard guidelines endorsed monitoring, temperature, neuromuscular, and urine output assessments are essential. Additionally, serial blood gas estimates should be used to monitor acid–base status and blood sugar levels. During tumor manipulation, blood levels of inhaled and IV anesthetics may vary due to fluctuations in cardiac output.[33] Hence, the depth of anesthesia should be monitored using processed electroencephalography algorithms.

Anesthesia Induction and Tracheal Intubation

Two large-bore peripheral IV accesses should be established with adequate anxiolysis. Anesthetic induction and tracheal intubation may provoke a sympathetic response, and this should be moderated with adjuvant drugs such as esmolol, fentanyl, remifentanil, or lidocaine, to name a few.

Propofol, sodium thiopentone, and etomidate have all been used to induce anesthesia.[11] Propofol is preferred due to its vasodilating properties and ability to blunt the hemodynamic response during laryngoscopy and tracheal intubation.[2] At the same time, etomidate is known for its benefit in maintaining cardiovascular stability.[2] Ketamine is unsuitable due to its sympathomimetic properties.[11] A judicious dose of neuromuscular blocker should be used, and its adequacy should be quantified before tracheal intubation.

Inhalational and Intravenous Agents

Sevoflurane is likely to be the most frequently preferred inhalational agent in contemporary practice, while enflurane and isoflurane have been extensively used in the past.[15,34] Sevoflurane lacks arrhythmogenic properties and has a favorable hemodynamic profile compared with desflurane, isoflurane, and nitrous oxide. Halothane is contraindicated in this setting due to its propensity to sensitize the myocardium to the arrhythmogenic effects of circulating catecholamines.[35] Desflurane is not preferred as it can cause sympathetic stimulation.[36] While nitrous oxide has been safely used during routine resection and in those treated during pregnancy,[37-39] its application will be majorly curtailed in the future due to its recognized impact on carbon footprint.[40]

Total IV anesthetic regimes using propofol and a potent opioid such as remifentanil have been popular in many centers, including ours. Remifentanil can be rapidly titrated to both heart rate and MAP, effectively blunt sympathetic surge from laryngoscopy, and provide intraoperative analgesia.[1] However, it is ineffective in attenuating the hemodynamic response from tumor manipulation.[1] Target-controlled infusions (TCI) of propofol and remifentanil are the preferred approach at the author's institution. Dexmedetomidine, a centrally acting selective alpha-2 receptor agonist, has also been used as part of the general anesthetic armamentarium to supplement both inhalational and IV agents. Besides its sedative and analgesic properties, its central sympatholytic effect can lower plasma norepinephrine levels. Case reports and retrospective series describe its use in this surgical setting.[41-44]

Neuromuscular Blocking Agents

Neuromuscular blocking agents with a propensity for minimal or nil histamine release and autonomic effects are preferred. In this regard, rocuronium, vecuronium, and cisatracurium are ideal choices.[45] Atracurium and pancuronium can trigger sympathetic activity and potential arrhythmia and therefore, are better avoided.[46,47] Succinylcholine has inherent autonomic stimulating properties, and the fasciculations can mechanically provoke the tumor-induced catecholamine release. Hence, it should be used with caution if deemed necessary.

In patients requiring awake intubation, adequate topicalization, and anxiolysis should be ensured along with meticulous planning and execution with expertise to facilitate smooth passage and optimal positioning of the endotracheal tube.

Options for Analgesia

Opioids are routinely used for perioperative analgesia and to blunt responses during various phases of a sympathetic surge, such as tracheal intubation, peritoneal insufflation, and tumor manipulation. Fentanyl, remifentanil, and hydromorphone are routinely used, and large doses of morphine are better avoided given the risk of histamine release and the consequent vasodilation and hypotension.[11] On a similar note, pethidine should also be avoided.

Epidural catheters are recommended for open procedures and rarely employed for laparoscopic approaches. If used intraoperatively, the resultant sympathetic blockade and vasodilation may exacerbate hypotension after tumor devascularization. However, it does not attenuate the response to tumor manipulation and may contribute to postexcision hypotension.[48]

INTRAOPERATIVE HEMODYNAMIC RESPONSE

Management of Hypertension and Arrhythmias

Hypertension during resection may result from stimulating events/processes other than tumor manipulation, such as tracheal intubation, positioning, and surgical incision.[15] In these situations, the catecholamine release is from the nerve endings and is usually transient and responsive to quick interventions.[49] Conversely, manipulating the tumor bed can cause an intense pressure response attributed to increased plasma levels of circulating catecholamines.[50] Even in well-optimized patients, hemodynamic spells during resection are not uncommon and need immediate treatment.[11] The presentations partly depend on the predominant catecholamine secreted by the tumor.[15] Accordingly, the manifestation can be either severe bradycardia accompanied by hypertension in cases of norepinephrine preponderance or severe tachycardia and tachyarrhythmias in cases of epinephrine preponderance.[1] Tachycardia may also be a reflex response to vasodilator therapy.

Hypertensive responses are usually managed with a vasodilator, whereas tachyarrhythmias are treated with beta-blockers.[1] Beta-blockers can also modulate the excess inotropy seen with epinephrine-secreting tumors.[1] Amiodarone and lidocaine should be used as indicated.[51] The choice of drug administration is based on availability and familiarity, and there is little evidence to support using one agent over the other.[1,11] Adaptation of these drugs **(Table 3)** in the perioperative setting is based on their pharmacodynamic properties and proven efficacy in other acute care disciplines.[11] Standard intraoperative measures to mitigate hypertensive spikes include enhanced sympatholysis by deepening the plane of anesthesia, short-acting opioid administration such as fentanyl or remifentanil, and facilitation of surgical exposure by an adequate neuromuscular blockade. Although the blood pressure spikes are likely to be short-lived given the pharmacokinetic properties of catecholamines, treatment modalities should ideally match the anticipated duration of these spikes.[11] Accordingly, vasoactive drugs may be administered either as intermittent boluses or continuous infusions titrated to effect. While short-acting agents such as esmolol (10–50 mg IV), phentolamine (1–5 mg IV), and labetalol (5–20 mg IV) can be administered as intermittent boluses, potent vasodilators such as SNP and GTN needs to be delivered as continuous infusions.

Sodium nitroprusside and nitroglycerin are the commonly used vasodilators. Both drugs have a rapid onset of action and are easily titratable. These agents and an ultrashort-acting beta-blocker such as esmolol help manage hypertension and coexisting tachycardia. Magnesium sulfate has also been increasingly used to achieve hemodynamic control.

The benefit of a sole agent or isolated multidrug intraoperative approach is challenging to quantify as controlled trials do not exist in this regard.[11]

TABLE 3: Drugs used for intraoperative hemodynamic control.

Drug class	Doses	Comment
Vasodilators		
Sodium nitroprusside	*Infusion*: 0.3–1.5 μg/kg/min	Solution must be protected from light, metabolic product is cyanide, toxicity is unlikely at therapeutic doses
Nitroglycerin	10–200 μg/min or 0.1–3.0 μg/kg/min	Tachyphylaxis and reflex tachycardia
Esmolol	*Bolus*: 25–100 mg *Infusion*: 50–300 μg/kg/min	Caution with asthma, AV block, heart failure
Labetalol	5 mg bolus up to 100 mg *Infusion*: 20–160 mg/h (in glucose)	Start only after establishing alpha-blockade
Phentolamine	2–5 mg	
Magnesium sulfate	*Bolus*: 1–2 g IV or 40–60 mg/kg over 10 minutes *Infusion*: 1–2 g/h	• Useful if other agents are inadequate or poorly tolerated • Beneficial in cardiomyopathy or coronary vasospasm
Vasoconstrictors		
Norepinephrine	0.04–0.4 μg/kg/min	Used in metastatic lesions, unresectable tumors, or intolerance to other medications
Epinephrine	2–20 μg/min (0.04–0.4 μg/kg/min)	Can trigger myocardial ischemia
Phenylephrine	*Bolus*: 20–100 μg *Infusion*: 30–60 μg/min or 0.5–1.5 μg/kg/min	Use with caution in cardiac failure or cardiogenic shock
Vasopressin	0.03–0.04 units/min or 1–4 units/h	Non-adrenergic vasopressor, effective in refractory hypotension

(AV: atrioventricular; IV: intravenous)

Timely, clear, and effective communication with the surgical team will enable the anesthesiologist to foresee and preemptively manage the hypertensive crisis.

Management of Hypotension

Hypotension after tumor devascularization is commonly encountered, attributed to residual alpha-blockade and sudden catecholamine depletion in conjunction with catecholamine receptor downregulation.[1] This effect may be accentuated in the setting of a contracted plasma volume, uncorrected/

ongoing blood loss, and anesthetic-induced vasodilation.[15] A liberal prior fluid loading up to 2–3 L of crystalloid and colloid and discontinuation of vasodilators are routine practices during tumor ligation.[15]

Norepinephrine, vasopressin, and phenylephrine are the vasoactive agents used to counteract hypotension.[11,15] A transesophageal echocardiography (TEE) may be indicated for persistent hypotension to assess ventricular filling.[15] As the pressor effect of vasopressin is not dependent on peripheral adrenergic receptors, it is beneficial in cases of refractory hypotension.[15] Vasoactive infusions can usually be weaned over 2–12 hours and are rarely indicated beyond 24 hours. Exogenous steroid administration is recommended in bilateral adrenalectomies to manage hypotension. Blood glucose levels should be monitored frequently in anticipation of hyperglycemia coinciding with catecholamine surges and hypoglycemia post-devascularization.

POSTOPERATIVE MANAGEMENT

All patients need intensive postoperative monitoring either in intensive care or high-dependency unit.[1,12] The incidence of postoperative refractory hypotension secondary to catecholamine withdrawal and residual preoperative adrenergic blockade varies between 20 and 70%.[12,52] Vasopressor infusion or other vasoactive drugs may be required along with fluid loading for a short duration.[12] Persistent hypotension may indicate surgical bleeding, inadequate fluid resuscitation, or residual anesthetic-induced vasodilatation. Postprocedural hypertension usually reflects postoperative pain, underlying essential hypertension, urinary retention, or fluid overloaded.[1] Accidental ligation of the renal artery can provoke hyperreninism and subsequently delay hypertension.[1] Persistent hypertension may also indicate metastatic disease or incomplete tumor resection.[1] Abrupt catecholamine depletion can lead to rebound hyperinsulinemia which, together with depleted glycogen stores, can precipitate severe hypoglycemia. Vigilance in blood sugar and electrolyte monitoring, and acid–base parameters are, thus, mandatory in the immediate postoperative period.[12] Long-term follow-up is recommended for most patients as hypertension persists in 50% of patients at 10 years, even without tumor recurrence.[1]

SPECIFIC SCENARIOS

Pregnancy and Pheochromocytoma

Pheochromocytoma is a rare cause of hypertension during pregnancy, with an estimated incidence of 1 in 54,000 pregnancies.[31,53,54] The maternal and fetal mortality from undiagnosed and untreated cases is 48 and 54%, respectively,[55] but can be reduced to 4 and 11% with early detection and treatment.[56] Coexisting pregnancy-induced hypertension, gestational hypertension, and limitations in using specific imaging modalities and isotope testing make it difficult to diagnose this rare presentation.[15] Hypertensive spells can be stimulated by pressure from the gravid uterus, postural changes, and uterine contractions (Field 31). Commencement and progress of labor, vaginal delivery, and anesthesia can increase maternal and fetal complications, including mortality.[31] Fetal mortality is attributed to hypertension-induced placental abruption or rebound hypotension-induced hypoxia.[31] Pharmacological preparation usually comprises an alpha blocker and, if necessary, beta-blockers. Phenoxybenzamine is commonly used with the understanding that it can cross the placenta and precipitate transient hypotension in the fetus and neonate.[31] Hence, maternal blood pressure should be adequately maintained to preserve uteroplacental circulation. Methyldopa, a drug commonly used in gestational hypertension, is contraindicated as it can provoke a crisis.[31]

Surgery is the definitive treatment option, and the timing is based on the gestation. For gestations <24 weeks, adequate preparation followed by a laparoscopic resection is recommended. If the gestational age is >24 weeks, the recommendation is an elective cesarean section (C-section) followed by tumor resection[31] or a simultaneous resection and C-section.[57] The transperitoneal laparoscopic approach is recommended as prone positioning is contraindicated in pregnancy.[58]

Incidental Pheochromocytoma

Unexpected and undiagnosed cases can present with hypertension, tachyarrhythmia, or refractory hypotension during induction of anesthesia.[59] The unavailability of rapid or point-of-care investigations hampers intraoperative diagnosis. Vasodilator therapy is the mainstay of treatment, and since the mortality is high, the attempted procedure should be abandoned unless it is life-threatening.[1,59]

Areas of Uncertainty

The benefits of the alpha-blockade in reducing perioperative morbidity and mortality have been successfully documented by various sources over many decades.[51] However, as aforementioned, the evidence to support this practice could be much higher. Several investigators have questioned this practice, and consequently, a few comparative studies have been undertaken.[13,60-64] The results showed that pretreatment with alpha-blockers was not beneficial compared to patients who did not receive alpha-blockade. Further, the studies raised concerns about an increased risk of orthostatic hypotension and postoperative hypotension associated with alpha-blockers. Notably, all these studies were retrospective observational and had inherent shortcomings such as allocation bias, heterogeneity among patients, and numerous other confounding factors.[51] These studies were embarked at highly specialized centers with supervision from experienced teams.[13,51] It remains to be seen whether similar results will be reproducible or if those strategies are applicable in real-world conditions in centers with limited experience and resources. This can only be addressed by adequately designed randomized controlled trials. Until then, we reaffirm the recommendations the International Endocrine Society endorsed that all patients with a biochemically active pheochromocytoma should undergo preoperative pharmacological blockade, preferably with an alpha blocker.[21] These recommendations are still valid and reinforced by the vast clinical experience with these medications, their targeted mechanism of action, and the apparent methodological deficiencies in studies disputing their utility.[51]

CONCLUSION

Patients with pheochromocytoma pose a formidable challenge to multiple disciplines involved in their clinical management. Pharmacological preoperative optimization, understanding its impact on reducing perioperative morbidity and mortality, and perioperative hemodynamic management have resulted in improved outcomes after surgery. Specialists involved in managing these patients would benefit from a comprehensive understanding of the pathophysiology of the tumor and the pharmacology of the perioperative medications, including their adverse effects. This will enable them to manage the hemodynamic perturbations throughout the perioperative period appropriately. Clinicians should be vigilant about the hemodynamic instability in the postoperative period, and intensive monitoring should be continued until satisfactory hemodynamic control is achieved.

ACKNOWLEDGMENTS

We thank Dr Riya Jose (Lyell McEwin Hospital, South Australia) and Dr Jack Sharples (The Queen Elizabeth Hospital, South Australia) for their inputs during the editing process and Dr Amar Nandakumar (KMCH Hospital, Coimbatore, Tamil Nadu, India) for his valuable inputs.

REFERENCES

1. Connor D, Boumphrey S. Perioperative care of phaeochromocytoma. BJA Education. 2016;16:153-8.
2. Gupta A, Garg R, Gupta N. Update in perioperative anesthetic management of pheochromocytoma. World J Anesthesiol. 2015;4:83-90.
3. Lenders JW, Eisenhofer G, Mannelli M, Pacak K. Phaeochromocytoma. Lancet. 2005;366:665-75.
4. Manger WM, Gifford RW. Pheochromocytoma. J Clin Hypertens (Greenwich). 2002;4:62-72.

5. Elder EE, Elder G, Larsson C. Pheochromocytoma and functional paraganglioma syndrome: no longer the 10% tumor. J Surg Oncol. 2005;89:193-201.
6. Guerrero MA, Schreinemakers JM, Vriens MR, Suh I, Hwang J, Shen WT, et al. Clinical spectrum of pheochromocytoma. J Am Coll Surg. 2009;209:727-32.
7. Zuber SM, Kantorovich V, Pacak K. Hypertension in pheochromocytoma: characteristics and treatment. Endocrinol Metab Clin North Am. 2011;40:295-311,vii.
8. Al Subhi AR, Boyle V, Elston MS. Systematic review: incidence of pheochromocytoma and paraganglioma over 70 years. J Endocr Soc. 2022;6:bvac105.
9. Bravo EL. Pheochromocytoma: new concepts and future trends. Kidney Int. 1991;40:544-56.
10. Bravo EL, Tagle R. Pheochromocytoma: state-of-the-art and future prospects. Endocr Rev. 2003;24:539-53.
11. Woodrum DT, Kheterpal S. Anesthetic management of pheochromocytoma. World J Endocr Surg. 2010;2:111-7.
12. Ramachandran R, Rewari V. Current perioperative management of pheochromocytomas. Indian J Urol. 2017;33:19.
13. Keegan M. Preoperative α-blockade in catecholamine-secreting tumours: fight for it or take flight? Br J Anaesth. 2017;118(2):145-8.
14. Roizen MF, Schreider BD, Hassan SZ. Anesthesia for patients with pheochromocytoma. Anesthesiol Clin North America. 1987;5:269-75.
15. Ramakrishna H. Pheochromocytoma resection: Current concepts in anesthetic management. J Anaesthesiol Clin Pharmacol. 2015;31:317-23.
16. Pacak K. Preoperative Management of the pheochromocytoma patient. J Clin Endocrinol Metab. 2007;92:4069-79.
17. Pacak K, Eisenhofer G, Ahlman H, Bornstein SR, Gimenez-Roqueplo AP, Grossman AB, et al; International Symposium on Pheochromocytoma. Pheochromocytoma: recommendations for clinical practice from the First International Symposium, October 2005. Nat Clin Pract Endocrinol Metab. 2007;3:92-102.
18. Buitenwerf E, Osinga TE, Timmers HJLM, Lenders JWM, Feelders RA, Eekhoff EMW, et al. Efficacy of α-blockers on hemodynamic control during pheochromocytoma resection: a randomized controlled trial. J Clin Endocrinol Metab. 2019;105:2381-91.
19. Gruber LM, Jasim S, Ducharme-Smith A, Weingarten T, Young WF, Bancos I. The role for metyrosine in the treatment of patients with pheochromocytoma and paraganglioma. J Clin Endocrinol Metab. 2021;106:e2393-e401.
20. Roizen M, Horrigan R, Koike M, Eger EI, Mulroy MF, Frazer B, et al. A prospective randomized trial of four anesthetic techniques for resection of pheochromocytoma. Anesthesiology. 1982;57:A43.
21. Lenders JW, Duh QY, Eisenhofer G, Gimenez-Roqueplo AP, Grebe SK, Murad MH, et al; Endocrine Society. Pheochromocytoma and Paraganglioma: an Endocrine Society Clinical Practice Guideline. J Clin Endocrinol Metab. 2014;99:1915-42.
22. Patel D. Surgical approach to patients with pheochromocytoma. Gland Surg. 2020;9:32.
23. Conzo G, Musella M, Corcione F, De Palma M, Ferraro F, Palazzo A, et al. Laparoscopic adrenalectomy—a safe procedure for pheochromocytoma: a retrospective review of clinical series. Int J Surg. 2013;11:152-6.

24. Kulis T, Knezevic N, Pekez M, Kastelan D, Grkovic M, Kastelan Z. Laparoscopic adrenalectomy: lessons learned from 306 cases. J Laparoendosc Adv Surg Tech A. 2012;22:22-6.
25. Mellon MJ, Sundaram CP. Laparoscopic adrenalectomy for pheochromocytoma versus other surgical indications. JSLS. 2008;12:380.
26. Nguyen PH, Keller JE, Novitsky YW, Heniford BT, Kercher KW. Laparoscopic approach to adrenalectomy: review of perioperative outcomes in a single center. Am Surg. 2011;77:592-6.
27. Román-Conzález A, Padilla-Zambrano H, Vásquez Jiménez LF. Perioperative management of pheocromocytoma/paraganglioma: a comprehensive review. Rev Colomb Anestesiol. 2021;49.
28. Xia Z, Li J, Peng L, Yang X, Xu Y, Li X, et al. Comparison of perioperative outcomes of robotic-assisted vs laparoscopic adrenalectomy for pheochromocytoma: a meta-analysis. Front Oncol. 2021;11:724287.
29. Bruynzeel H, Feelders RA, Groenland TH, van den Meiracker AH, van Eijck CH, Lange JF, et al. Risk factors for hemodynamic instability during surgery for pheochromocytoma. J Clin Endocrinol Metab. 2010;95:678-85.
30. Sood J, Jayaraman L, Kumra VP, Chowbey PK. Laparoscopic approach to pheochromocytoma: is a lower intra-abdominal pressure helpful? Anesth Analg. 2006;102:637-41.
31. Subramaniam R. Pheochromocytoma: current concepts in diagnosis and management. Curr Anaesth Crit Care. 2011;1:104-10.
32. Grensemann J. Cardiac output monitoring by pulse contour analysis. the technical basics of less-invasive techniques. Front Med (Lausanne). 2018;5:64.
33. Watanabe T, Hiraoka H, Araki T, Nagano D, Aomori T, Nakamura T, et al. Significant decreases in blood propofol concentrations during adrenalectomy for phaeochromocytoma. Br J Clin Pharmacol. 2017;83:2205-13.
34. Janeczko GF, Ivankovich AD, Glisson SN, Heyman HJ, El-Etr AA, Albrecht RF. Enflurane anesthesia for surgical removal of pheochromocytoma. Anesth Analg. 1977;56:62-7.
35. Maze M, Smith CM. Identification of receptor mechanism mediating epinephrine-induced arrhythmias during halothane anesthesia in the dog. Anesthesiology. 1983;59:322-6.
36. Lippmann M, Ford M, Lee C, Ginsburg R, Foran W, Raum W, et al. Use of desflurane during resection of phaeochromocytoma. Br J Anaesth. 1994;72:707-9.
37. Hull CJ. Phaeochromocytoma: diagnosis, preoperative preparation and anaesthetic management. Br J Anaesth. 1986;58:1453-68.
38. Dimitriou V, Chantzi C, Zogogiannis I, Atsalakis J, Stranomiti J, Varveri M, et al. Remifentanil preventing hemodynamic changes during laparoscopic adrenalectomy for pheochromocytoma. Middle East J Anaesthesiol. 2006;18:947-54.
39. Hamilton A, Sirrs S, Schmidt N, Onrot J. Anaesthesia for phaeochromocytoma in pregnancy. Can J Anaesth. 1997;44:654-7.
40. Charlesworth M, Swinton F. Anaesthetic gases, climate change, and sustainable practice. Lancet Planet Health. 2017;1:e216-7.
41. Bryskin R, Weldon BC. Dexmedetomidine and magnesium sulfate in the perioperative management of a child undergoing laparoscopic resection of bilateral pheochromocytomas. J Clin Anesth. 2010;22:126-9.

42. Jung JW, Park JK, Jeon SY, Kim YH, Nam SH, Choi YG, et al. Dexmedetomidine and remifentanil in the perioperative management of an adolescent undergoing resection of pheochromocytoma: a case report. Korean J Anesthesiol. 2012;63:555-8.
43. Hegde HV, Maheshwari S, Pai BS, Ahmed S. Dexmedetomidine in anaesthesia for a high-risk case of pheochromocytoma with poor left ventricular function. Indian J Anaesth. 2016;60:146-8.
44. Sivrikoz N, Turhan Ö, Yavru HA, Altun D, Işcan Y, Sormaz IC, et al. Magnesium and dexmedetomidine combination reduces sodium nitroprusside requirement in laparoscopic pheochromocytoma. Ulus Travma Acil Cerrahi Derg. 2022;28:1563-9.
45. Naguib M, Samarkandi AH, Bakhamees HS, Magboul MA, el-Bakry AK. Histamine-release haemodynamic changes produced by rocuronium, vecuronium, mivacurium, atracurium and tubocurarine. Br J Anaesth. 1995;75:588-92.
46. Amaranath L, Zanettin GG, Bravo EL, Barnes A, Estafanous FG. Atracurium and pheochromocytoma: a report of three cases. Anesth Analg. 1988;67:1127-30.
47. Solares G, Ramos F, Blanco J, Blanco E. Alcuronium, pancuronium and phaeochromocytoma. Anaesthesia. 1987;42:77-8.
48. Jeon S, Cho AR, Ri HS, Lee HJ, Hong JM, Lee D, et al. The effect of combined epidural-general anesthesia on hemodynamic instability during pheochromocytoma and paraganglioma surgery: a multicenter retrospective cohort study. Int J Med Sci. 2020;17:1956.
49. Bravo EL, Tarazi RC, Gifford RW, Stewart BH. Circulating and urinary catecholamines in pheochromocytoma: diagnostic and pathophysiologic implications. N Engl J Med. 1979;301:682-6.
50. Vater M, Achola K, Smith G. Catecholamine responses during anaesthesia for phaeochromocytoma. Br J Anaesth. 1983;55:357-60.
51. Berends AMA, Kerstens MN, Lenders JWM, Timmers HJLM. Approach to the Patient: perioperative management of the patient with pheochromocytoma or sympathetic paraganglioma. J Clin Endocrinol Metab. 2020;105(9):dgaa441.
52. Agrawal R, Mishra SK, Bhatia E, Mishra A, Chand G, Agarwal G, et al. Prospective study to compare peri-operative hemodynamic alterations following preparation for pheochromocytoma surgery by phenoxybenzamine or prazosin. World J Surg. 2014;38:716-23.
53. Harrington JL, Farley DR, van Heerden JA, Ramin KD. Adrenal tumors and pregnancy. World J Surg. 1999;23:182-6.
54. Sarathi V, Lila AR, Bandgar TR, Menon PS, Shah NS. Pheochromocytoma and pregnancy: a rare but dangerous combination. Endocr Pract. 2010;16:300-9.
55. Schenker J, Chowers I. Pheochromocytoma and pregnancy: review of 89 cases. Obstet Gynecol Surv. 1971;26:739-47.
56. Ahlawat SK, Jain S, Kumari S, Varma S, Sharma BK. Pheochromocytoma associated with pregnancy: case report and review of the literature. Obstet Gynecol Surv. 1999;54:728.
57. Lenders JW. Pheochromocytoma and pregnancy: a deceptive connection. Eur J Endocrinol. 2012;166:143-50.
58. van der Weerd K, van Noord C, Loeve M, Knapen MFCM, Visser W, de Herder WW, et al. Endocrinology in pregnancy. Pheochromocytoma in pregnancy: case series and review of literature. Eur J Endocrinol. 2017;177:R49-58.

59. Sasidharan P, Johnston I. (2009). Phaeochromocytoma: Perioperative Management. Anaesthesia Tutorial of the Week 2009. [online] Available from: https://resources.wfsahq.org/atotw/phaeochromocytoma-perioperative-management/ [Last accessed September, 2023].
60. Boutros AR, Bravo EL, Zanettin G, Straffon RA. Perioperative management of 63 patients with pheochromocytoma. Cleve Clin J Med. 1990;57:613-7.
61. Ulchaker JC, Goldfarb DA, Bravo EL, Novick AC. Successful outcomes in pheochromocytoma surgery in the modern era. J Urol. 1999;161:764-7.
62. Groeben H, Nottebaum BJ, Alesina PF, Traut A, Neumann HP, Walz MK. Perioperative α-receptor blockade in phaeochromocytoma surgery: an observational case series. Br J Anaesth. 2017;118:182-9.
63. Groeben H, Walz MK, Nottebaum BJ, Alesina PF, Greenwald A, Schumann R, et al. International multicentre review of perioperative management and outcome for catecholamine-producing tumours. Br J Surg. 2020;107:e170-e8.
64. Buisset C, Guerin C, Cungi PJ, Gardette M, Paladino NC, Taïeb D, et al. Pheochromocytoma surgery without systematic preoperative pharmacological preparation: insights from a referral tertiary center experience. Surg Endosc. 2021;35:728-35.

CHAPTER 9

Sedation for Healthcare Interventions: Should Anesthetists be Worried?

Harriette Beard, Anavi Prakash, Amit Prakash

ABSTRACT

Recent innovations in the field of anesthesia may improve the safety of sedation outside the anesthetic room. These include developing clear guidelines for assessing and selecting suitable patients for sedation and new pharmacological sedative agents.

Procedural sedation carries multiple risks, and how these are mitigated is vital to the safe execution of a sedation service.[1] These complications are naturally more difficult for physicians not airway-trained or less experienced with sedation than an anesthetist.

As the complexities associated with sedation increase, so must the anesthetist's foresight to manage them and the departments undertaking such a service.

Keywords: Sedation; Capnography; Recovery

KEY POINTS

- Anesthetists need to lead clinical management of procedural sedation outside the operating room.
- Procedural sedation carries multiple risks, and how these are mitigated is vital to the safe execution of a sedation service.[1] These complications are naturally more difficult for physicians not airway-trained or less experienced with sedation than an anesthetist.
- Safety in interventional sedation can be improved by developing clear guidelines for pre-assessment, adequate patient selection, application of appropriate monitoring, especially using capnography, and developing criteria for recovery and discharge.
- Anesthetic departments should endeavor to institute a multidisciplinary sedation committee to discourage silo practice, promote interdepartmental learning and oversee clinical governance.

INTRODUCTION

Procedural sedation safely administers short-acting sedative or dissociative agents, with or without analgesics, to reduce discomfort, apprehension, and potentially unpleasant memories while minimizing cardiorespiratory depression in patients during diagnostic and therapeutic procedures. These effects are distinct from general anesthesia, which provides a state of total unconsciousness, and analgesia alone, which delivers a reduction in or insensibility to pain, not necessarily with a decrease in or a loss of consciousness. Worryingly, closed claims data for all sedation providers have identified that severe adverse events and patient harm related to procedural sedation do occur, even in the hands of experienced anesthesiologists.[2]

Anesthesiologists are experts and well-trained in airway and hemodynamic management. The nonanesthetic sedation provider (NAS) will rarely be formally trained in advanced airway skills, and their experience of the complexities of sedation and sedatives is likely to be limited. Curriculum-based training with a demonstration of competency in procedural sedation has been recommended as an essential component of anesthesia training programs.[3] There is a drive toward having an element of sedation training in the form of a module for all specialties who undertake procedural sedation.

We propose to show the reader a framework for planning and preparation of a safe platform for the anesthetic department supporting the expanding field of nonanesthesia-delivered sedation practice.

■ SEDATION OUTSIDE THE OPERATING ROOM

Multiple specialties use sedation for healthcare interventions (HCIs), and new procedures and areas are being added as the interventional field expands **(Box 1)**. It is important to note that some of these procedures are undertaken in nonhospital environments and sometimes in mobile units, e.g., dental sedation. In addition, multiple procedures within these areas have a shared airway (endoscopic procedures, dental procedures) or a limitation

BOX 1: Departments and specialties utilizing NORS (nonoperating room sedation), showing the specialties taking on sedation for healthcare interventions (HCIs).

- Emergency department
- Dental
- Endoscopy*
- Cardiology*
- Burns/plastics/cosmetic procedures
- Radiology*
- Urology
- Ophthalmology
- Bronchoscopy
- Gynecology
- Dermatology

* Indicates those more commonly practicing sedation[5]

in accessing the airway rapidly in case of an emergency. A combination of inadequately trained operators and limited access to the patient could have disastrous outcomes for patients.

Given the above, multiple organizations, including the AoMRC (Academy of Medical Royal Colleges)[3] and AAGBI (Association of Anaesthetists of Great Britain and Ireland),[4] recommend that anesthesiologists have an overview of sedation practice for HCIs and ideally lead such protocol in the hospital set-up. The role should entail supporting sedation practice in nonanesthetic areas by ensuring adequate guidelines and safety measures are in place to prevent adverse events. This is best approached via the formulation of a sedation committee, which has multidisciplinary representation, to develop a hospital-specific governance structure that reviews safety-related incidences and sedation complications **(Table 1)** regularly.

The overarching principle in NORS (nonoperating room sedation) practice should be safety, and to achieve this, one should consider the following:
- Location
- Patient selection
- Monitoring

TABLE 1: Adverse events associated with sedation of over 1,400 procedures performed.

	Low risk	Moderate risk	High risk	Total
Number (% of procedures with ≥1 event)				
Baseline n = 666				
Total adverse events	132 (19.8%)	4 (0.6%)	11 (1.7%)	147 (22.1%)
Respiratory	106 (15.9%)	–	10 (1.5%)	
Cardiac	26 (3.9%)	–	1 (0.2%)	
Outcomes	–	4 (0.6%)	0	
Intervention				
Predefined	0	12	1	
Open text	56	0	2	
All	56 (8.4%)	12 (1.8%)	3 (0.5%)	
Capnography n = 735				
Total adverse events	82 (11.2%)	1 (0.1%)	10 (1.4%)	93 (12.7%)
Respiratory	77 (10.5%)	–	7 (1.0%)	
Cardiac	5 (0.7%)	–	2 (0.3%)	
Outcomes	–	1 (0.1%)	1 (0.1%)	
Intervention				
Predefined	0	6	1	
Open text	44	0	0	
All	44 (6.0%)	6 (0.8%)	1 (0.1%)	

Source: Modified from Corbett G et al.[10]

- Pharmacology
- Recovery.

Location

Multiple specialties use sedation for HCIs, and new procedures and areas are being added as the interventional field expands (*see* **Box 1**).

Nonoperating room sedation is undertaken in dedicated suites within the hospital, out-of-hospital locations, and mobile units. The majority of these locations are fixed and, therefore, unchangeable, but they can be made safer by a standardized set-up. In addition, multiple procedures within these areas have a shared airway (endoscopic procedures, dental procedures) or a limitation in accessing the airway rapidly in case of an emergency.

Emergency equipment and drugs should be immediately available so that, if required, they may be utilized by either the sedation team if trained to do so or, ultimately, the anesthetic and critical care teams that are assigned to support in such emergencies. Continuous high-flow oxygen supply with paraphernalia to ensure effective delivery, standardized monitoring **(Figs. 1A to C)**, airway management equipment, and a trolley equipped to move into resuscitation position should be available. This is particularly relevant to interventional radiology and cardiac intervention suites. At least

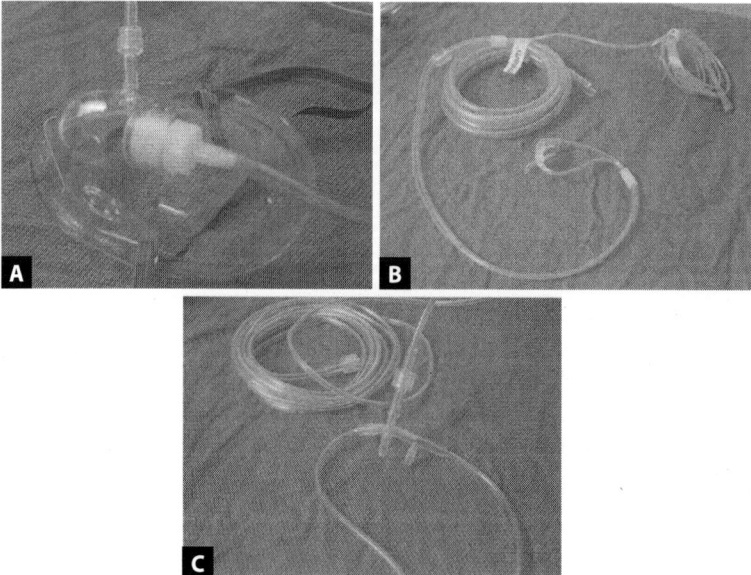

Figs. 1A to C: Oxygen delivery devices with end-tidal carbon dioxide (CO_2) monitoring; (A) a simple facemask with a capnography sidestream line; (B and C) the cannula with the addition of sidestream capnography; this allows simultaneous oxygen delivery and analysis of CO_2.
Source: Reproduced with permission from A Prakash, Clinical Medicine. 2016, vol. 16, No 2:161-3.

one named individual with advanced and/or intermediate life support qualifications should be present.[2] The location must be equipped to suitably monitor and manage a range of complications,[6] which are as follows:
- Respiratory (hypoxemia/apnea)
- Hemodynamic instability (hyper- or hypotension/cardiac arrhythmias)
- Hemorrhage
- Human factors associated with the area itself (lighting/temperature/noise/radiation/distance from support).

Postprocedural sedation, a dedicated recovery should be allocated to continue monitoring the patient until they are ready for discharge to the ward.

■ PATIENT SELECTION

Once the patients are deemed suitable for NORS, they must be counseled effectively to optimize their expectations. Appropriate counseling improves patients' experience while undergoing a HCI.

Several guidelines exist to ensure suitable patient selection for sedation. Each hospital should develop policies and guidelines, and consideration must be given to extremes of age, ASA (American Society of Anesthesiologists) 3 or 4, increasing frailty index, previous anesthetic complications, and anatomical or physiological compromise. Special attention must be paid to airway assessment, considering patients may need bag–mask ventilation far more commonly than endotracheal intubation. Hence, patients with beards or those who are obese or edentulous would also be at risk. Personnel undertaking sedation should endeavor to attain continuos professional development (CPD) in airway management.

Apart from a comprehensive assessment of the cardiorespiratory system, units must develop starvation periods specific to the intervention. The 2- or 6-hour rule for fluids/solids is reasonable in most clinical settings.[7] Ideally, this is the same as anesthesia—although specialties need specific guidance; for instance, standard fasting would not be suitable for a colonoscopy under sedation, as the operator would need to see peristaltic movement.

Gastric point-of-care ultrasound (POCUS) may play a role in trained hands, especially related to nonelective NORS.

One should bear in mind that deeper sedation is akin to general anesthesia, and when these planes are required, stricter fasting may be necessary, given the aspiration risk.

■ MONITORING

Various bodies have set out minimal monitoring standards for anesthesiology [AAGBI, RCOA (Royal College of Anaesthetists), ASA, AoRMC, ESGE (European Society of Gastrointestinal Endoscopy)]. However, there needs to be more consensus on minimal standards for sedation. This is partly due to the length of procedures and the awareness of monitoring techniques, e.g., capnography. Adequate monitoring facilitates early recognition of complications, and units must develop monitoring criteria for moderate sedation as a minimum.

Until 2019, the suggested monitoring for a patient undergoing NORS included pulse oximetry, noninvasive blood pressure (NIBP) monitoring for all, and additional electrocardiogram (ECG) monitoring in those with a cardiac history. The AOMRC in 2021 has recommended end-tidal capnography for all procedures anticipated to be greater than 30 minutes (reference to 2021 update on AOMRC document from 2021).[8]

Applying capnography as a monitor has challenges; its use in sedation is just about being recognized. The reasons for slower uptake are multifactorial. The adage in anesthesia - "No trace = Wrong place[9] to" warn the anesthetist of the possibility of esophageal intubation has apparent flaws concerning sedation, as endotracheal intubation is never undertaken for procedural sedation. In addition, such monitoring requires resources (monitors, disposables), and an understanding of the capnography physiology, and trace followed by continuous education. The equipment for such monitoring is readily available and with integrated capnography lines (*see* **Figs. 1A to C**).

At Cambridge University Hospital, we set out to question the application of capnography to confirm if the recommendation from societies is applicable.[10] We undertook a prospective quality improvement initiative in four clinical services (gastroenterology, cardiology, bronchoscopy, and interventional radiology). We reviewed the adverse events associated with baseline, i.e., interventions without capnography use, to those after introducing capnography. The introduction of capnography has resulted in a significant (43.2%, $p \leq 0.05$) relative risk reduction in adverse events observed during procedural observation (*see* **Table 1**). Also, the multivariate linear regression suggested the use of capnography specifically to be a significant predictor of reduction in procedural sedation-related adverse events. Apart from confirming the recommendation for the benefit of capnography, the study highlighted the challenges in introducing new technology in these areas as it requires an education program and ongoing support. Since the project, the clinicians have reported that the abortion rate for procedures has decreased. They now have more confidence in carrying on with the procedure due to the safety net of additional monitoring.

Adequate monitoring is essential for sedated patients undergoing HCIs.

Apart from minimal monitoring, namely, ECG, NIBP, and peripheral oxygen saturation (SpO_2), units must strive to introduce capnography to improve outcomes. In the future, applying depth of anesthesia monitoring processed electroencephalogram (EEG), bispectral index, and entropy should allow clinicians to monitor for adequate levels of conscious sedation more closely.[11]

PHARMACOLOGY

The pharmacology of anesthetic and sedative agents is paramount to the anesthetic training curriculum, and this complements the daily practice of using such drugs. The sedation practitioner should clearly understand and appreciate the formulation, pharmacokinetics, pharmacodynamics, interactions, and side effects of the drugs being used.

Numerous drugs are available on the market, and the anesthetists are conversant with those that can cross over from sedation to anesthetic, including but not limited to propofol, remifentanil, dexmetomidine, and remimazolam.

The anesthetist is often comfortable with infusion technology and can apply this to sedation; guided and repetitive training is necessary as there is a narrower margin for error compared to bolus administration. Non-anesthetists, however, commonly use combinations of an opioid and midazolam unless trained with other sedatives such as ketamine.

The relaxation and analgesia levels must be considered when selecting the ideal sedative recipe for the patient and procedure. Significant risks associated with sedatives have been highlighted, and therefore, training with specific application to the pharmacodynamics and pharmacokinetics remains necessary, in particular timings of dose conversion from oral to intravenous, the effects of synergism and potentiation of agents, and available reversal and antagonistic agents.

The common routes for sedation include oral, intravenous, and inhalational, and a skilled practitioner will be able to titrate the sedatives to an adequate state of conscious sedation and no further. A single agent is preferable with more predictable pharmacokinetics than a combination of a sedative cocktail. Multiagent sedatives may have an inconsistent onset/offset and time-to-peak effect, quickly altering the ability to titrate and widen the margin for error. However, with that being said, in some instances, there are clear benefits to adding an opiate for analgesia or muscle relaxation.

Midazolam is a benzodiazepine commonly used sedative agent either as the sole agent or in combination with an opioid. It has a rapid onset, and its elimination half-life is between 1 and 3 hours. Its peak effect occurs between 12 and 15 minutes and it is suitable for short procedures. It can be given as slow, repeated boluses (10–100 µg/kg) to a suggested maximum of 5 mg or continuous intravenous infusion (30–100 µg/kg/h). It, however, will suppress the sympathetic nervous system, depress airway reflexes, and blunt the hypercapnic and hypoxic respiratory drive.

The availability and use of lower-strength midazolam (1 mg/mL) are advised, and caution be exercised over the higher-strength formulation. And, although the benzodiazepine antidote, flumazenil, is available (and should be readily so in areas of benzodiazepine use), its regular use and reliance are not advised. Flumazenil itself is not without side effects, including hypertension, vomiting, and dysrhythmias. The application and use of such an agent should be audited against best practices.

Remimazolam is a new contender to benzodiazepine, which presents as a powder that must be reconstituted before injection. It has improved pharmacokinetics compared to midazolam, with a markedly enhanced patient recovery following its quicker offset. However, data and research are still ongoing, and there seems to be insufficient experience in anesthetic practice of its usage.

Analgesic agents commonly used for sedation include morphine and fentanyl and can have a complementary effect with benzodiazepine. The opioid morphine is a widely used adjunct used with midazolam. In a healthy adult, 0.1 mg/kg of morphine given 10–15 minutes before benzodiazepine can help with analgesia, anxiolysis, and sedation. The extremes of age present dosing challenges, given the reduced distribution volume in older people and decreased hepatic clearance in the neonate. Morphine's use complicates nausea and vomiting, bradycardia, hypotension, and, through the action of histamine release, causing itching and bronchospasm. Those who depend on morphine may have built a tolerance to its effect.

Fentanyl, a synthetic phenylpiperidine derivative, is 100 times more potent than morphine. It has a high lipid solubility and extensive distribution. As this is an opioid, it has strong analgesic properties. It results in a dose-dependent respiratory depression that can be more marked in older people. Its rapid onset (2–3 minutes) and offset (30 minutes) are advantageous for sedation, but dosing should not exceed 0.5 µg/kg in a healthy adult. It is a potent respiratory depressant, with its effects being exacerbated by further sedative agents.

With several drugs and combinations available to achieve sedation for procedural sedation, the following still hold: (1) analgesia should proceed with sedation, (2) drugs must be titrated up to a maximum predetermined end dose, and (3) caution must be exercised when considering drugs and dosing the elderly and frail.

■ RECOVERY AND DISCHARGE

Patients do not require the standard postanesthetic care unit (PACU) after sedation. They can move directly from the procedure room to phase 2 of recovery—a medical process unique to anesthetic care. Therefore, recovery step-down and discharge planning can begin at an earlier stage than recovery from general anesthesia. However, a designated area for recovery is vital for identifying postprocedure and post-sedation adverse events. Poor or absent recovery facilities have been identified as a risk factor for complications with NORS.[12] The NAS would need to mirror the close relationship between anesthetists and the recovery team. By appreciating factors that affect recovery, we can design a space and implement a protocol that supports the patient and the recovery team in the postsedation period. Remembering, the first 30 minutes following a procedure is associated with the highest incidence of complications.[13]

Most sedation procedures are day cases; hence, discharge criteria for day care would be applicable. In brief, a pain-free patient who has passed urine, has eaten and drank, returned to baseline consciousness, and has a responsible adult to accompany them for the following 24 hours is suitable for discharge. Supporting a nurse-led discharge can facilitate the efficiency of a sedation service. Clear parameters must be set for this cohort of patients, and therefore, standards must be met to trigger discharge. Two formal scoring systems used after HCIs under sedation are the modified PADSS (Post Anaesthetic Discharge Scoring System) and the modified Aldrete Score.[12] Through these assessments, discharge is achievable once a set score is reached and allows a streamlined process that is economically efficient. Organizational policy for discharge must be clear and agreeable between team members, and training is vital to ensure that the assessments can be followed.

Discharge information must be verbal and written at the point of leaving recovery—a unique area and time for both the patient and clinician. Thus, the clinician must appreciate the variation of mentation and physiology compared to the ward discharge.

■ TRAINING

The Academy of Royal Medical College in the UK recommends sedation practitioners undertake a minimum of 12 hours of CPD per 5 years to maintain accreditation.

Anesthetists should work with specialties to plan regular education activities about sedation training. A single point of contact in the form of a consultant anesthetist can allow direct communication channels to be open. This sedation lead can then oversee training and ensure the regulation of sedation providers in the hospital. The training can be in courses, online modules, or simulation training.

Online learning modules have been designed to supplement the hands-on experience of learning and provide learning ladders for competency base of education into the background of sedation and sedatives. More recently, high-fidelity simulation has allowed clinicians to experience complications in a nonthreatening environment to expedite learning. Simulation now plays an essential role in many specialty-specific accredited training programs, highlighting the limitations of the environment and the human factors working with team members.

GOVERNANCE

A well-structured governance process for sedation practice will allow continuous learning from areas practicing sedation and enable departments to provide the best care for the patient undergoing HCI. Audit activity is vital for assessing and upholding quality standards across hospitals. This would ensure directed training suitable for multidisciplinary teams practicing sedation.

Modular training on sedation for the specialties undertaking sedation for HCIs is becoming increasingly formalized. Representation in such colleges should be encouraged to help formulate curricula for such activities. Across Europe, centers are developing courses with strict regulations, curricula, and assessments to ensure training is standardized. This is a measurable way of overseeing sedation-related education, but one that comes at a cost and is often outsourced.

A no-blame culture is critical to adopt to allow teams to talk openly about the challenges of NAS and NORS. The AOMRC recommends formulating a sedation committee within hospitals to develop a platform for the governance of sedation.

CONCLUSION

With any evolution of the medical field, elements of uncertainty will be unveiled. The concerns of moving from anesthesiology-lead sedation to specialty lead sedation are a form of "scope creep",[14] therefore, governance issues will no longer be answerable to a singular specialty.

We should aspire to have an efficient service, prioritizing patient safety and satisfaction, and as previously highlighted, monitoring is paramount to achieving this. Sedation is not exempt from morbidity and mortality.

The challenges of specialty-led sedation should spur creativity and excellence in training to create a long-term goal of independent sedationists with anesthetic support. We strive to create a service that is answerable to the rigor of anesthetic governance while creating a safe and supportive community of NASPs (nonanesthesia sedation providers).

REFERENCES

1. Hinkelbein J, Schmitz J, Lamperti M, Fuchs-Buder T. Procedural sedation outside the operating room. Curr Opin Anaesthesiol. 2020;33(4):533-8.
2. Guidance for provision of Anesthesia services (GPAS) for sedation services. Chapter 19. RCoA 2016.
3. South West Anaesthetic Research Matrix (SWARM). Sedation practice in six acute hospitals - a snapshot survey. Anaesthesia. 2015;70(4):407-15.
4. Academy of Medical Royal Colleges. (2013). Safe sedation practice for healthcare procedures: standards and guidance. [online] Available from: https://www.aomrc.org.uk/wp-content/uploads/2016/05/Safe_Sedation_Practice_1213.pdf [Last accessed September, 2023].

5. American Society of Anesthesiologists Task Force on Sedation and Analgesia by Non-Anesthesiologists. Practice guidelines for sedation and analgesia by non-anesthesiologists. Anesthesiology. 2002;96:1004-7.
6. Youn AM, Ko YK, Kim YH. Anesthesia and sedation outside of the operating room. Korean J Anesthesiol. 2015;68(4):323-31.
7. Green SM, Leroy PL, Roback MG, Irwin MG, Andolfatto G, Babl FE, et al. An international multidisciplinary consensus statement on fasting before procedural sedation in adults and children. Anaesthesia. 2020;75:374-85.
8. Academy of Medical Royal Colleges. (2021). Safe sedation practice for healthcare procedures: An update. [online] Available from: https://www.aomrc.org.uk/reports-guidance/safe-sedation-practice-for-healthcare-procedures-an-update/ [Last accessed September, 2023].
9. Royal College of Anaesthetists, Difficult Airway Society. Capnography: No Trace = Wrong Place. [online] Available from: https://rcoa.ac.uk/safety-standards-quality/guidance-resources/capnography-no-trace-wrong-place [Last accessed September, 2023].
10. Corbett G, Pugh P, Herre J, See TC, de Monteverde-Robb D, Torrejon Torres R, et al. Service Evaluation of the Impact of Capnography on the Safety of Procedural Sedation. Front Med (Lausanne). 2022;9:867536. Erratum in: Front Med (Lausanne). 2022;9:999862.
11. Miner JR, Biros MH, Seigel T, Ross K. The utility of the bispectral index in procedural sedation with propofol in the emergency department. Acad Emerg Med. 2005;12(3):190-6.
12. Amornyotin S, Chalayonnavin W, Kongphlay S. Recovery pattern and home-readiness after ambulatory gastrointestinal endoscopy. J Med Assoc Thai. 2007;90(11):2352-8.
13. Yamaguchi D, Morisaki T, Sakata Y. Mizuta Y, Nagatsuma G, Inoue S, et al. Usefulness of discharge standards in outpatients undergoing sedative endoscopy: a propensity score-matched study of the modified post-anesthetic discharge scoring system and the modified Aldrete score. BMC Gastroenterol. 2022;22:445.
14. Davidson JE, Bloomberg D, Burnell L. Scope creep: when nursing practice moves beyond traditional boundaries: an evidence-based example using procedural sedation. Crit Care Nurs Q. 2007;30(3):219-32.

CHAPTER 10

Space: The New Frontier for Nonoperating Room Anesthesia

Shagun Bhatia Shah, Rajiv Chawla, Uma Hariharan

ABSTRACT

Space travel and long-term space missions are set to be the future norm, with a definite boom in the coming years. In addition to the National Aeronautics and Space Administration (NASA), commercial space companies (Blue Origin, SpaceX, and Virgin Galactic) have commenced planning and preparations for the long-distance and long-duration space exploration missions to inner solar planets. Besides the absence of gravity (weightlessness), radiation and light are the two main stressors in the space. For comprehensive risk assessment and its mitigation, knowledge of these hazards and the physiological and psychological risks to the human health they pose is quintessential. Besides logistic issues in space, the dilemma of the first-aid versus definitive treatment, surgical challenges associated with open surgery, and the prospect of minimally invasive surgery in space have been discussed. The spectrum of expected anesthetic services in space and anesthetic challenges such as closed-loop environment and effects of microgravity on volatile anesthetic vaporizers, neuromuscular blocking agents, intravenous (IV) fluids and medications, gastroesophageal reflux, endotracheal (ET) intubation, total intravenous anesthesia, neuraxial block, and regional anesthesia hazards have been detailed. Challenges involving cardiopulmonary resuscitation (CPR) in space, the role of telemedicine, and imaging technology are other important topics touched upon.

Keywords: Anesthesia in microgravity; Nonoperating room anesthesia; Space stressors

■ KEY POINTS

- Space travel and long-term space missions are expected to witness a boom.
- Absence of gravity (weightlessness), radiation, and light are the three main stressors in space.
- Space motion sickness, fluid shift toward the upper body, space anemia, bone demineralization, disuse atrophy of muscles, cardiac deconditioning,

disorientation, immune deficits, acute radiation sickness, and increased risk of cancer, infertility, and cataracts are the common pathophysiological changes observed in astronauts
- Airway obstruction, hemopneumothorax, and bleeding are a critical focus for space trauma planning
- Anesthetic challenges include a closed-loop environment (prone to anesthetic vapor contamination, posing a fire hazard), altered physiological responses, autonomic dysfunction, gastroparesis, skeletal muscle disuse atrophy (hyperkalemia), compromised hepatorenal function, inability to measure the weight of drugs or calculate the dose based on per kilogram body weight (since everything is weightless) and limited availability of equipment, drugs, and expertise.
- The ET intubation success rate in a microgravity environment is 8.7 times less than that in the major operation theater because the patient would float if not restrained by his hands and feet being tied to some support, the anesthetist himself would be floating, the laryngoscope and endotracheal tube (ETT) would be weightless, suction would be manual, the vision would be hampered due to safety goggles, larynx may be edematous due to fluid redistribution, assistants would be limited. You cannot call for help in a "cannot ventilate, cannot intubate" situation.

INTRODUCTION

Space travel and long-term space missions will be the future norm, with a definite boom in the coming years. In addition to the National Aeronautics and Space Administration (NASA), commercial space companies (Blue Origin, SpaceX and Virgin Galactic) have commenced planning and preparations for long-distance, long-duration space exploration missions to inner solar planets (Mars) by the 2030s. The concept of space tourism has placed space travel at the confluence of business, hospitality, medicine, and technology.[1] Commercial suborbital spaceflights shall soon transfer passengers from London to Sydney in 2 hours instead of 22 hours.[2] Acceleration from 0 to 28,000 km/s in <9 minutes takes its toll on the human body, howsoever well adapted, well trained, and physically fit an astronaut is. The microgravity space environment interacts with the human body and the standard medical equipment strangely. Space travel manipulates human cells, cardiac contractions, and hemodynamics, thereby regulating the blood pressure. Developing safety concepts for emergencies and airway management in outer space will be challenging.

Aerospace medicine is evolving as a pivotal subfield of medical science to promote the safety and performance of the crew members exposed to the stressors of the space flight. This must be accomplished bearing in mind an inherent conflict of interest between loss of crew (individual risk) and loss of mission of the expedition (risk to the organization) with an acceptance of the residual risk. The surgery in space is not expected to be extensive, but securing an airway is a bare minimum qualification required of a crew medical officer (CMO). An anesthesiologist is adept in managing a difficult airway and well-versed in simple suturing. Aerospace medicine is thus crafted for the anesthesiologist! Considerable overlap and synergy between aerospace medicine, anesthesia, and hyperbaric medicine have led to the core training in anesthesia becoming one of the entry pathways to space medicine in the UK.[3] Space medicine has emerged as a new site for nonoperating room anesthesia (NORA).

STRESSORS IN THE SPACE MILIEU

Overlapping relationships between the earth, aircraft flights, and space milieu in terms of various stressors are depicted in the stacked Venn diagram here **(Fig. 1)**.

Besides the absence of gravity (weightlessness), radiation and light are the two main stressors in the space, and these are highly magnified due to the absence of any intervening atmosphere. For comprehensive risk assessment and its mitigation, knowledge of these hazards and the physiological and psychological risks to the human health they pose is quintessential.

PATHOPHYSIOLOGICAL EFFECTS ON THE HUMAN BODY

- *Weightlessness:* In spaceflights, weightlessness is the root cause of a multitude of health problems (cardiopulmonary, otovestibular, ophthalmic, musculoskeletal, cognitive, and perceptual) **(Fig. 2)**

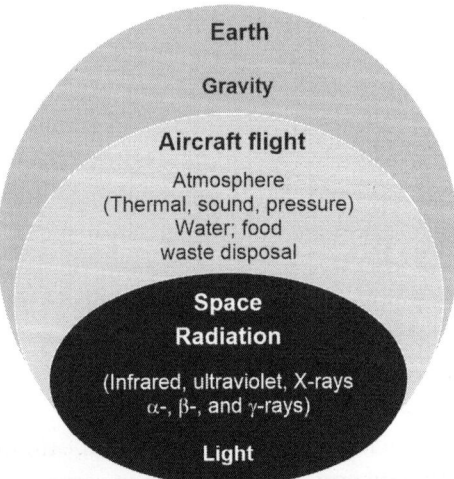

Fig. 1: Stacked Venn diagram comparing stressors on earth, aircraft flights, and space.

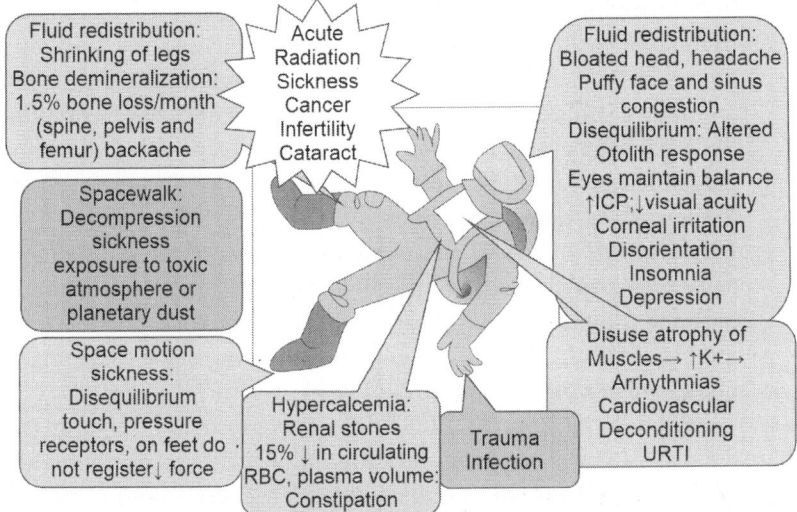

Fig. 2: Color-coded pathophysiological effects of space travel. (ICP: intracranial pressure; RBC: red blood cells; URTI: upper respiratory tract infection)

Note:
Light black: Effects of weightlessness
White: Effects of radiation
Dark black: Miscellaneous effects

- *Space motion sickness (SMS) and disequilibrium:* 75% of the first-time fliers and 50% of the veterans experience SMS caused by extreme fluid shifts and sensory conflicts. Otoliths of the internal ear respond differently to the motion, and the eyes become the prime pathway to the sense motion. Touch and pressure receptors on the feet do not register any downward force. Promethazine is the drug of choice.[4]
- *Fluid redistribution:* The fluid shift toward the upper body is associated with increased renal oxygen transport. This shrinks the legs, causes head and sinus congestion, and makes the face edematous and puffy.[4] Headaches are common. Raised intracranial pressure, reduced visual acuity, and corneal irritation may result.
- *Space anemia:* Astronauts have an estimated 15% decrease in circulating red blood cells and plasma on orbit, the equivalent of class I hemorrhage. Inhibition of erythropoiesis in space, secondary to the increase in kidney tissue oxygen partial pressure (an acute plethora of blood surrounds central organs) and hemolysis suggested by the measured increase in ferritin (+35 to 46%) are the causative factors.[4,5]
- *Bone demineralization:* This does not plateau, and deadaptation continues relentlessly as long as weightlessness persists. Disuse atrophy of weight-bearing bones and muscles occurs. The difference

in bone density compared to preflight is reported to be: Skull +2.2%; thorax/upper limbs −0.7%; lumbar spine/pelvis −6.2%; and lower limbs −5.4%. An average 1.5% monthly bone loss from the spine, pelvis, and femur commonly results in the backache and disk herniation.[6] Renal calculi may result due to hypercalcemia. Nutrient supplements, graded exercise, and bisphosphonates can counter osteoporosis due to space flight-induced bone loss.[1]

- *Disuse atrophy:* Loss of muscle mass and resultant hyperkalemia can cause arrhythmia.[4] Monitoring musculoskeletal deconditioning in space using biomarkers that are accurate and easy to measure to indicate critical musculoskeletal deconditioning before reaching the point of no return is required.[7]
- *Cardiac deconditioning:* Heart rate initially increases, and then decreases while the blood pressure initially decreases, then either continues to decrease or remain constant. Central venous pressure paradoxically remains constant or decreases. Although, the blood volume decreases, there is an increase in intracellular fluid. Cardiac systolic function is preserved while the diastolic function is reduced. Systemic vascular resistance decreases moderately (14%) to massively (39%). After an initial increase in cardiac output, it may either decrease (17–20%) or drastically increase (41%). Baroreflex function is depressed (50%). Aerobic capacity—VO_2 max (22%) and red blood cell mass 10% are reduced. The endothelial function displays deficient vasoconstriction.[8]
- *Disorientation:* Changed sensory input confuses the brain causing occasional disorientation
- *Immune deficits:* Microgravity stress-induced activation of the hypothalamic-pituitary-adrenal and the sympathetic-adrenal-medullary axes produces cortisol and dehydroepiandrosterone (DHEA), which deranges regulation of cellular immunity causing reactivation of latent viruses (Epstein–Barr virus, varicella-zoster virus, and *Cytomegalovirus*). This risk of shedding live, infectious viruses during spaceflight is not mitigated by isolation/quarantine of astronauts before spaceflight, and responses to viral reactivation can be asymptomatic, debilitating, or even life-threatening.[9] Preflight vaccination, polyclonal immunoglobulin, interleukin-2, and adequate exercise and nutrition can counter viral reactivation.
- *Miscellaneous:* Constipation, upper respiratory tract, and urinary tract infections are common. Increased virulence and proliferation of microorganisms in microgravity can produce antibiotic-resistant bacterial infections.[10]
- *Radiation:* Higher doses of radiation cause acute radiation sickness and potentially increase the risk of cancer, infertility, and cataracts.[11] Inventing

radioprotectants against galactic solid cosmic radiation is challenging since lead space suits would be forbiddingly heavy.
- *Isolation and mental health:* Psychological well-being is a vital element in the adaptation of the crew to the occupational demands. Isolation, a closed environment, and distance from the Earth affect the mental health. It is like being locked in a minivan for days and months together. Isolation and chronic stress result in immunodepression, sleep, mood disturbances, and decreased cognitive performance.[12,13] Modafinil, a drug for narcolepsy, sleep apnea, and shift duty-induced daytime sleepiness, has been recently approved for fatigue and circadian rhythm disturbances in astronauts in isolated, confined, and extreme (ICE) environments.[14]

LOGISTIC ISSUES
No Space in Space
Logistical considerations in weight, volume, power, and Crew Medical Officer training constitute a severe limitation of the space medicine community. In monetary terms, the cost of placing 1 kg of any material, e.g., a bottle of colloid and a bottle of crystalloid, into the earth's orbit is 22,000 USD.[8,15] Also, the space inside a spaceship is very limited. Hence, the mass and volume of any medical equipment and drugs need to be minimized. The inventory must comprise drugs with a long shelf-life at the room temperature. No wonder the demand for a physician on board SKYLAB, the first NASA space mission (1973), was rejected, however a small medical kit was provided with training for two crew members to suture cuts, extract teeth, physically examine, and report about fellow crew members. Each mission includes a crew medical officer with 80 hours of training and not necessarily a biomedical background. This has to change for an advanced medical care in the space milieu.

Pharmacological Adjuncts
In the face of the nonavailability of blood products in space, pharmacologic adjuncts (trauma cocktail) such as vasopressin and antifibrinolytics such as aprotinin, tranexamic acid, and recombinant factor VIIa have a potentially significant role.[16] A typical medical kit should include antiallergy medication, antibiotics, analgesics, antipyretics, antiemetics, stimulants, cardiovascular, ophthalmic, otic medication, laxatives, and hypnotics.

THE DAMAGE CONTROL PHILOSOPHY
Damage control (DC) philosophy entails completing only the *most necessary components* of surgery using the most straightforward *techniques*. Emergency open exploratory surgery in space may require a hypovolemic or septic shock to arrive at a specific diagnosis. Four decades back, a committee of trauma surgeons, space physicians, and biomedical engineers pinpointed

the competence to perform laparotomy as the minimum benchmark for the surgical capability to save lives before terrestrial transfer. Damage control resolves problems stemming from a poor physiologic reserve of a patient or resource constraints of a space setting.[17] The principal axiom of DC is compression packing of bleeding solid organs and leaving the abdomen unsutured. Incising the anterior abdominal wall to access the peritoneal cavity quickly is a simple technique of converting noncompressible exsanguination into a directly compressible visceral hemorrhage. Nonphysicians have reportedly performed DC successfully, although psychologically daunted by it.[15] While DC is an attractive option for a significant trauma in low earth orbits (international space station) from where evacuation to earth takes 24 hours, leaving the abdomen open for >72 hours (as required in deeper space missions) can lead to a fatal infection.

SURGICAL CONSIDERATIONS

Surgery should be restricted to the bare minimum essential procedures per the DC policy. Prophylactic prelaunch surgery on earth to prevent in-flight emergencies like acute appendicitis/cholecystitis in astronauts is being considered, as is preventive hysterectomy in menstruating female astronauts.[18,19]

First Aid versus Definitive Treatment

Links in the chain of care of critically injured astronauts include emergency extraterrestrial first-aid at the point of injury, stabilization for space evacuation, space transport (challenges of ascent, entry, and landing), terrestrial landing-site resuscitation and treatment, and terrestrial transportation to the site of definitive treatment.[15] Although imparting definitive medical treatment in space would avert transportation-related dangers, it would exponentially increase capability requirements.

Surgical Challenges in Space

Improved surgical methods like magnetizing surgical tools to stick to surfaces in zero gravity are underway. During open surgery, the intestines would float around the operation site, obscuring the surgical field. Circulating air in the enclosed cabin could put astronauts at risk of infection. Blood-repelling surgical tools and surgical bubbles might be a solution. National Aeronautics and Space Administration has analyzed a closed system consisting of a surgical clear plastic overhead canopy with integrated arm ports. Mechanical restraints, sterile techniques, hemostasis, postoperative care, wound healing, and endothelial leaks are some surgical challenges.[19]

The patient does not lie on an operating table (OT) but will float in space. Once the abdomen is opened, the intubating crew medical officer must secure the floating patient's head between his/her knees to keep the head stationary during laryngoscopy and endotracheal (ET) intubation. Two other crew members hold the patient's ankle/wrist with one hand and the railing/support bar in the spacecraft with the other hand to restrain the patient during anesthetic induction throughout surgery and reversal.[20] Instrument restraints comprise magnetic pads and Velcro for fixing supplies, flypaper area for suture ends, Styrofoam Blocks for sharps, and pockets for biohazardous waste.[19] Operating personnel may be restrained to a waist-level table, horizontal foot bar, and floor-level pellets.

Minimally Invasive Surgery

Minimally invasive surgery (MIS) for traumatic injury has been proven feasible in weightlessness during parabolic flight and as an extrapolation in space.[21] Reducing postoperative morbidity, safeguarding the spacecraft cabin environment from floating patient tissue and the patient from the environmental particulates, maintaining normothermia, and facilitating blood salvage and autotransfusion are attractive potential benefits. The abdominal cavity in weightlessness changes from a flattened oval to a rounded shape creating larger operating space.[15,22] Potential techniques to reduce the skill level required for performing minimally invasive surgery (MIS) include simulated hand-assisted laparoscopy in parabolic flight and telementoring nonsurgeons to perform simple laparoscopic drainage procedures utilizing minilaparoscopes.[15] On the flip side, healthy astronauts have diminished blood volumes and cardiac deconditioning, and serious concerns exist that septicemic or hypovolemic astronauts may not tolerate the physiologic stresses of laparoscopy.[23]

Euthanasia

In the face of complex life-threatening injuries, euthanasia requires multispecialty discussion with all stakeholders to reach a consensus.

■ ANESTHETIC CONSIDERATIONS

Spectrum of Expected Anesthetic Services in Space

Astronauts being amongst the fittest bracket of the human population and screened extensively for comorbidities, traumatic injury would expectedly be the most typical medical emergency in the long-distance space flights. Considering the product of probable incidence and degree of adverse impact on mission and crew health, the highest level of concern has been accorded to trauma by NASA. Resource constraints in the space environs compel medical care to focus on the conditions with the highest probability of occurrence and those with the most significant impact on the crew and mission (the red risks). A 5 × 5 matrix of likelihood (frequency) versus consequence (severity of impact) was created by NASA based on Monte Carlo and engineering analysis of previous space missions for medical risk-analysis [Integrated Medical Model (IMM) a probabilistic risk assessment (PRA) Monte-Carlo simulation tool).[24] The higher the risk, the higher the need for reliable systems, backups, and fault tolerance.[25]

High probability-high impact risks for a mission to the red planet are (1) space radiation health effects of cancer, cardiovascular disease, and cognitive decrements; (2) neuro-ocular syndrome, (3) behavioral health and performance decrements; and (4) inadequate food and nutrition.[26] Recognizing that there are at least three disabling injuries for every traumatic death on earth,[27] all of which would have catastrophic implications in space, and given the risks and isolation inherent in long-duration space flight, a broadly-trained surgically capable emergency/critical care specialist (read anesthesiologist) with critical thinking, decision-making, information processing capabilities, and creativity, to problem-solve and improvise even in hitherto unseen medical scenarios will be required onboard any spaceship.[15] If this anesthetist cum surgeon cum critical care specialist himself/herself turns sick, injured, disabled, or dies, a backup nonphysician trained to treat the most common emergencies should be available.[28]

Airway obstruction, hemopneumothorax, and bleeding are critical focuses for space trauma planning. Securing an adequate airway (ET intubation, laryngeal mask placement, and tracheostomy) is a critical first step in any resuscitation and has been successfully undertaken in parabolic flights.[29] Correct endotracheal tube (ETT) positioning can be sonographically confirmed either remotely or automatically.[30]

Pneumothorax comprises the most common intrathoracic severe injury resulting from blunt trauma. Mortality is preventable using simple interventions like decompression with both needle and tube thoracotomies for tension pneumothorax, as demonstrated in parabolic flights.[31] Detection of hemopneumothorax poses a more significant challenge than treatment. Being a pleural-based disease, pneumothorax is highly amenable to sonographic detection, both in weightlessness and terrestrially. Unfortunately, ultrasound is a very user-dependent tool in which nonanesthesiologist CMOs are unlikely to be proficient and require specialized training for autonomous or remotely guided ultrasonographic evaluations.[32] Extravehicular activity (EVA) may produce hypobaric stresses, aggravating pneumothorax.[33]

Hemorrhage would require the administration of constant pressure infusions of degassed colloids or crystalloids, a feasibility already confirmed by parabolic flight experience.[34] Capability for the onboard generation of medical-grade fluids from processed drinking water would be a boon for severe injuries or burns that would quickly deplete onboard crystalloid stores.[8]

Arresting hemorrhage is much more crucial than fluid administration, considering that fluid overload dilutes clotting factors, exacerbates bleeding, and induces hypothermia.[35] External or compressible hemorrhage is the most accessible source of bleeding to arrest. Tourniquets are essential in buying valuable time while other resources are activated.[36] Tissue sealant bandages, employing fibrin glue-like ingredients, result in significantly reduced blood loss compared to standard packing gauze.[15] New-generation prehospital hemostatics act by two primary mechanisms, i.e., (1) clotting factor activators and (2) adhesive agents. Clotting factor activators like kaolin (QuikClot) initiates the coagulation cascade's intrinsic pathway. Adhesive agents like shellfish shell derived Chitin (Celox and HemCon); form a physical barrier by surface bonding of red blood cells to form an adhesive plug.[37]

Cavitary hemorrhage not amenable to external compression would constitute 76% of all the deaths.[15] Sites of massive internal hemorrhage may be intrapleural, intraperitoneal, and/or retroperitoneal. Both parabolic flight and true space studies suggest that ultrasound can accurately detect thoracic and abdominal blood.

Penetrating micrometeorite injuries may occur during EVA, e.g., construction activity on Moon/Mars surface. The resultant breach of the space suit would cause either a flash fire or explosive decompression to the vacuum of space with zero chances of survival.[38] Crush-type/blunt injuries are more likely because although objects are weightless in space, they retain mass and can therefore generate significant forces (mass × acceleration).[39] The Moon (1/6 G) and Mars (1/3 G) have lower gravitational pull as compared to Earth (G). Mass can appear deceptively light here with the inadvertent acceleration of objects. Helmets and toughened torso space suits may mitigate the occurrence and severity of severe thoracoabdominal injuries at the cost of chronic musculoskeletal strain and over-use injuries.[35] They fail to protect limb injuries. Compound long-bone fractures would be disastrous for a mission, however in true weightlessness; bony integrity might not be required for ambulation. Immobilization could be obtained using simple air or thermoplastic casts/splints.[15] The absence of mechanical, gravitational loading may compromise fractured bone healing rate and quality due to decreased callus volume and angiogenesis. Limited intramembranous ossification instead of the traditional endochondral ossification healing pathway makes malunion/disunion of fractures common in the space. Movement of unfixed bones may compound the risk of fat emboli.[40] Regrettably, previously healthy astronauts might suffer permanent disability without advanced bony fixation techniques and gravitational loading.

Anesthetic Challenges in the Remotest of Remote Locations: Space

Anesthetics challenges include a closed environment (prone to anesthetic vapor contamination posing a fire hazard), altered physiological responses, autonomic dysfunction, gastroparesis, skeletal muscle disuse atrophy (hyperkalemia), compromised hepatorenal function, inability to measure the weight of drugs or calculate the dose based on per kilogram body weight since everything is weightless and limited availability of equipment and drugs.

Closed-Loop Environment

The environment of a spacecraft is tightly sealed. The oxygen administered to the patient cannot be vented into space as it would be too wasteful. An anesthetic gas leak may contaminate the closed-loop environment.[8,21] Low-flow anesthesia with closed circuits and efficient scavenging systems for volatile anesthetics may be used if gaseous anesthetics are unavoidable. The concentrated material from scavenging systems can be dumped overboard. The intravenous drugs should not reach the other crew members via the water reclamation system or by contaminating the spaceship atmosphere. Oxygen from respiratory support equipment may invite a fire hazard if dumped into the cabin atmosphere.

Volatile anesthetic vaporizers: These depend on the gravity-induced separation of gases and fluids and hence malfunction in microgravity.[21]

Neuromuscular blocking agents: Bedridden patients are at risk of succinylcholine-induced hyperkalemia-initiated cardiovascular collapse. Such a theoretical risk is evident in microgravity conditions where astronauts experience disuse atrophy of muscles with neuromuscular junctions exhibiting changes akin to bedridden patients.[8,21]

Intravenous fluids and medications: Fluids and gases do not separate based on different densities in a zero-gravity environment. In an ampoule or a vial containing liquid drug, or an intravenous fluid bag/bottle, only foam/froth will exist in space. This makes infusion/transfusion of intravenous fluids technically very difficult in microgravity milieu, and special bubble-filter incorporated syringes have been designed. These convection and buoyancy issues must be catered to. Medications should be chemically stable, thermally robust, radiation resistant, possess a long shelf-life, undergo rapid metabolism to pharmacologically inactive products, and preferably exist in powdered form.[21] Injectable drugs need to be stored in prefilled syringes.[41] Cardiovascular, hormonal, electrolyte, and immunoglobulin levels changes, accompanied by a reduction in microsomal P-450 and its dependent enzymes, alter drugs' pharmacokinetics and pharmacodynamics in space, necessitating dose alterations.[42]

Intravenous access: Vascular access might be difficult to obtain in a medical contingency. An intraosseous access kit has been integrated into the International Space Station medical gear.[8]

Gastroesophageal reflux: Space motion sickness in most of the crew, gastroparesis, and gastroesophageal reflux are evidenced during and postflight. All patients would need a rapid sequence intubation with Sellick's and cuffed ETT but without succinylcholine and preferably rocuronium as a muscle relaxant to facilitate ET intubation to avert the heightened risk of aspiration in these patients.[8,21]

■ GENERAL ANESTHESIA

Medical evacuation is not an option in airway emergencies.

Endotracheal Intubation

The ET intubation success rate in a microgravity environment is 8.7 times less than in the major operation theater. This is because the patient would float if not restrained by his hands and feet being tied to some support, the anesthetist himself would be floating, the laryngoscope and ETT would be weightless, suction would be manual, vision would be hampered due to safety goggles (like wearing a PPE-kit in the COVID-19 era), larynx may be edematous due to fluid redistribution, assistants would be limited or none and you cannot call for help in a "cannot ventilate cannot intubate" situation **(Table 1)**. One hand cannot stabilize the head-neck and also direct the ETT toward the glottic opening simultaneously since anesthesiologists exert a force of about 40 N, lasting for about 10-20 seconds during direct laryngoscopy (sufficient for a 70 kg human to move about 0.3 m in 1 second in microgravity).[43] Using restraint will stabilize the head and neck so that the hand not holding the laryngoscope can direct the ETT toward the glottic opening. Clutching the head of an unrestrained patient between the anesthetist's knees may provide a quick, stable, although slightly distant, glottic view **(Fig. 3)**.[43] Introducing a supraglottic airway device, preferably a cuffless one like I-gel, would be easier, quicker, safer, and less bulky than the ET intubation assembly.[44] Simulated microgravity prolonged time to initial ventilation by 3.3 seconds for the laryngeal mask, 3.9 seconds for the laryngeal tube, 19.9 seconds for I-gel, and 43.1 seconds for ET intubation, versus similar attempts in normal gravity.[45] To prevent hypoxia, preoxygenate the patient and perform video laryngoscope-guided intubation. In a recent study under simulated microgravity environs, 1/25 direct laryngoscopy attempts by experts against 12/20 attempts by novices failed. In contrast, 1/20 attempts at videolaryngoscope-guided intubation by experts against 5/25 attempts by novices failed.[46]

Astronauts are prone to cardiovascular collapse owing to hypovolemia (10-15% reduced vascular volume), altered baroreflex, and systemic vascular resistance. Clinical assessment of fluid status and prophylactic low-dose vasopressors may be employed to prevent alpine hemodynamic changes. The drug of choice for sedation, induction, and maintenance is ketamine

TABLE 1: Indications, challenges, and solutions to airway management in space.

Indications	Challenges	Solutions
Airway obstruction: • Edema • Anaphylaxis • Laryngospasm • Bronchospasm	Physiological: • Airway edema due to fluid shift • Cardiac deconditioning • Gastroesophageal reflux • Hyperkalemia	• LMA • I-gel • Videolaryngoscope • RSI
Aspiration of foreign body: • Food crumbs • Medication	Technical: • Lack of space • Lack of equipment • Lack of drugs • Restraints required • Vascular access	• Restraints • Clutching the head of an unrestrained patient between the anesthetist's knees
Burns or smoke inhalation	Human: • Lack of skills • Lack of assistance • Hampered vision • Psychological effect on other crewmembers	• Ketamine for induction • Rocuronium as relaxant • Sugammadex for reversal in case of failed intubation
Coma/GCS <8	Degassing of IV fluids and drugs	Intraosseous access kit
GA		• Chemically stable, thermally robust radiation resistant • Long shelf-life • Rapid metabolism to pharmacologically inactive products • Exist in powdered form
Hypoxic cardiopulmonary arrest		Prophylactic low dose vasopressors

(GA: general anesthesia; GCS: Glasgow Coma Scale; IV: intravenous; LMA: laryngeal mask airway; RSI: rapid sequence intubation)

(cardiovascular stability; airway reflexes maintained; less respiratory depression than other IV anesthetics/opioids analgesics at equipotent doses; powdered form exists).[41] Rocuronium is the neuromuscular blocking agent of choice (quick onset, no hyperkalemia-induced arrhythmias unlike succinylcholine, amenable to emergency reversal with sugammadex).

Total Intravenous Anesthesia

Total intravenous anesthesia (TIVA) may avert the need for ET intubation and volatile anesthetics and seems the preferred method for administering general anesthesia (GA) in microgravity environments.[8,21,47]

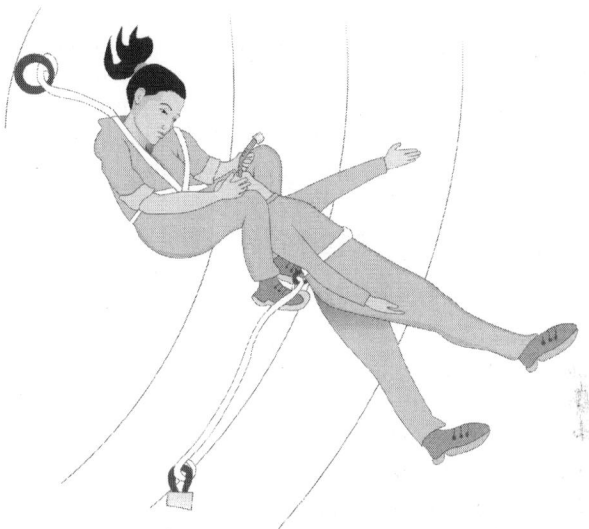

Fig. 3: Endotracheal intubation in the space milieu.

TABLE 2: Comparative analysis of indications, pros, and cons of various modes of anesthesia.

	Indications	Pros	Cons
Conscious sedation	Quick painful procedures	• Technically easy • No apnea • No intubation	• Limited types of surgery • Airway not secured
GA	Invasive head or torso surgery	• Technically easy • All types of surgery possible	• Dangerous (difficult airway, overdose, and hemodynamic instability) • Equipment intensive
RA	Peripheral/limb surgery	• Safe • All four limbs • Less equipment required	• Technically difficult • Steep learning curve • Early skill fade • Spinal not possible • Long block onset time • Compartment syndrome • LA toxicity and allergy
Local infiltration	Limited surgery	• Safe • Hardly any equipment required	• Limited types of surgery • LA toxicity and allergy • Painful

(GA: general anesthesia; LA: local anesthetic; RA: regional anesthesia)

Neuraxial Block and Regional Anesthesia

Local and regional anesthesia may seem more attractive than GA in space, but they have problems **(Table 2)**. The on-board anesthetist may encounter a difficult or failed spinal. Autonomic dysfunction, cardiovascular deconditioning and disruption of central modulation of baroreceptor reflexes, and contracted intravascular volume during and after spaceflight are responsible for exaggerated hypotension and cardiovascular collapse following subarachnoid block. Isobaric local anesthetic agents are suitable (as against conventional hyperbaric ones), but technical expertise is required.[8,21,48] Epidural anesthesia and peripheral nerve blocks are better suited if expertise is available and sterility can be maintained.

CARDIOPULMONARY RESUSCITATION IN SPACE

Chest Compression Techniques

To perform external chest compressions in microgravity, a prerequisite is to be an acrobat. At least three methods have been described to perform chest compressions in space. During cardiopulmonary resuscitation (CPR), the intensivist sits atop the patient's abdomen with legs wrapped along either side of the patient's torso; toes firmly clasped beneath the patient to provide a firm supporting surface on which to perform CPR. The left leg is placed over the patient's right shoulder, while the right leg is placed under the patient's left shoulder. This is the Evetts–Russomano (ER) method. In the second technique (handstand/HS method), the patient is pinned against a spaceship's walls in a plantigrade position. The intensivist assumes the supine position, places his/her legs on one wall of the spaceship, arms stretched out, and both hands on the patient's chest on the opposite wall. The chest compressions are performed by extension and flexion of the hip and knees of the intensivist. The third is the "reverse bearhug (RBH)" method. The patient is placed in the prone position, and the intensivist assumes an identical horizontal position parallel to and above the patient. The intensivist wraps his arms around the patient with his hands on his chest. Arm flexion movements are used to provide chest compressions. On simulators, the HS method gave the best depth of chest compressions, while ER and RBH methods gave the best rate of compressions.[49,50] A video demonstration is available at https://www.innovaspace.org/blog/extraterrestrial-cpr-and-its-simulations-on-earth-air-water.

Defibrillate with Care

When a shock is being applied on the Earth, everybody is supposed to stand clear to avoid electrocution, but other crew members are floating around unpredictably in space, and astronaut chairs could be conductive. Hence, special defibrillators that do not interfere with the electronics of the space station or produce sparks are required.

TELEMEDICINE TECHNOLOGY

Even if information travels at the speed of light, it will take at least 40 minutes to receive an answer from the Earth in response to questions if on a spaceflight to Mars. Anesthesia is a branch of rapid sequence events, and as we all know, even 3 minutes of loss of oxygen supply to the brain can be disastrous and result in irreversible coma. Onboard information systems with data on essential drugs, doses, and emergency algorithms must be available as a backup.

■ IMAGING TECHNIQUES

Currently, radiography, computed tomography (CT), and magnetic resonance (MR) imaging facilities still need to be improved (limited space for large imaging structures, difficulties in interpretation due to microgravity). Only ultrasound is available in space, fueling a series of innovative investigations into newer sonographic techniques to aid the critically injured in space.[51-53]

The terrestrial healthcare industry may reap benefits from this. The Butterfly iQ portable ultrasound probe can be linked directly to a smartphone through cloud computing, allowing physicians/specialists to analyze remote ultrasound images promptly. Future development of a photocathode-based X-ray source may make this possible.[54]

■ AEROSPACE MEDICINE SIEVE

Aerospace medicine sieve is divided into clinical, human performance, and human systems engineering.[4]

Nonclinical Skills

Nonclinical skills may prove to be immensely valuable in managing events with the heaviest potential impact on missions such as sudden cardiac arrest, smoke inhalation, toxic exposure, seizures, and penetrating eye injuries and contribute to healthcare safety. Personnel skills (team coordination, communication, leadership, and logistics) and technical skills (troubleshooting equipment, use of safety equipment, and orientation) are valuable nonclinical skills.[28]

Career Opportunities in Aerospace Medicine

Combining the broad spectrum of medical and aviation sciences, an array of sectors offers lucrative job prospects postcompletion of a degree in Aerospace Medicine.[55]
- NASA
- Federal Aviation Administration
- National Transport and Safety Board
- Airline Medical Department
- Airline Medical Clinic
- Aerospace Manufacturing
- Commercial Spaceflight Operations
- Military.

FUTURE DIRECTIONS
Designing Clinical Trials
Suspended animation techniques could freeze and forward all the significant pathology to the final landing on the Earth. Hydrogen sulfide is a specific, reversible inhibitor of oxidative phosphorylation that has been shown to reduce the metabolism of mice by 90% after 6 hours sans behavioral or functional complications on reversal. Profound hypothermia using extracorporeal circulation has successfully kept severely injured dogs pulseless for 2 hours before returning them to the normal function via resuscitation.[56,57-59] These preliminary results in animal research studies could pave the way for future clinical trials.

Three Dimensional Printer, the Game Changer
The three-dimensional (3D) printer operates by a process called *additive manufacturing*. It involves heating a relatively low-temperature plastic filament and extruding it layer-by-layer to construct the part defined in the design file sent to the 3D printer. In a Zero-G technology demonstration on a space station, 3D printing successfully produced the first object, a printhead faceplate engraved with the names of the collaborating organizations: NASA and Made in Space, Inc. The ultimate dream is a printer printing another 3D printer. The 3D printer is a transformative moment in space research, securing replacement tools and parts for the space station crew with reduced reliance on supply missions from the Earth.[60]

Artificial Intelligence and Robotic Interventions
Telesurgery and telementoring would encounter hurdles like 8–40 minutes round-trip electronic delays.[15] Consequently, any space robot would require guidance from an experienced surgeon or be autonomous with image guidance. Completely robotic autonomous ultrasound-guided central venous access to monitor hemodynamic changes and administer vasopressors and irritant drugs is on the anvil and may prove beneficial before anesthetizing patients in space.[15] A similar robotic device for interventional angiographic embolization of arterial bleeders that are surgically inaccessible is much needed. The "trauma pod" shall be used whenever timely deployment of proper medical personnel is unavailable, and the patient cannot be evacuated quickly to an appropriate medical facility. The platform shall secure the airway, insert an intravenous or intraosseous line, perform hemostasis, manipulate damaged tissue, and position monitoring devices.[61] The 22 kg RAVEN surgical robot (Bio Robotics Lab. University of Washington, Seattle, WA) operates on principles of the DaVinci System (544.3 kg patient-side cart only), has two articulated arms, is easily assembled, and works on the long-distance remote control.[62] Robonaut 2 (a collaborative effort of NASA

Johnson Space Center and General Motors and Oceaneering) is a versatile humanoid surgical robot adept in telemedicine and medical management in autonomous and teleoperation mode.[63]

CONCLUSION

Limited skillsets, lack of support, and limited drug and equipment availability in a stressful, constrained environment can be physically and mentally challenging. Till such time an image-guided autonomous robot is invented, validated, and perfected, a broadly trained, flexible, surgically able, critical care specialist (anesthesiologist) with innate capabilities to solve problem and quickly improvise appropriate solutions would be an apt medical officer in space, the final frontier for NORA.

REFERENCES

1. Krittanawong C, Singh NK, Scheuring RA, Urquieta E, Bershad EM, Macaulay TR, et al. Human Health during Space Travel: State-of-the-Art Review. Cells. 2022;12(1):40.
2. Boyd M. (2023). London to Sydney to take just two hours as new passenger flight will go via space. [online] Available from: https://www.mirror.co.uk/travel/australia-new-zealand/london-sydney-take-just-two-29981475 [Last accessed September, 2023].
3. Smith TG, Buckey JC Jr. Anaesthetists and aerospace medicine in a new era of human spaceflight. Anaesthesia. 2022;77(4):384-8.
4. Hodkinson PD, Anderton RA, Posselt BN, Fong KJ. An overview of space medicine. Br J Anaesth. 2017;119(suppl_1):i143-53.
5. Smith SM. Red blood cell and iron metabolism during space flight. Nutrition. 2002;18(10):864-6.
6. Stavnichuk M, Mikolajewicz N, Corlett T, Morris M, Komarova SV. A systematic review and meta-analysis of bone loss in space travelers. NPJ Microgravity. 2020;6(1):13.
7. Liphardt AM, Fernandez-Gonzalo R, Albracht K, Rittweger J, Vico L. Musculoskeletal research in human space flight-unmet needs for the success of crewed deep space exploration. NPJ Microgravity. 2023;9(1):9.
8. Komorowski M, Fleming S, Kirkpatrick AW. Fundamentals of anesthesiology for spaceflight. J Cardiothoracic Vasc Anesth. 2016;30(3):781-90.
9. Mehta SK, Laudenslager ML, Stowe RP, Crucian BE, Feiveson AH, Sams CF, et al. Latent virus reactivation in astronauts on the international space station. NPJ Microgravity. 2017;3:11.
10. Campbell MR, Johnston SL 3rd, Marshburn T, Kane J, Lugg D. Nonoperative treatment of suspected appendicitis in remote medical care environments: Implications for future spaceflight medical care. J Am Coll Surg. 2004;198(5):822-30.
11. Friedberg W, Darden E. Health aspects of radiation exposure on a simulated mission to Mars. In: Simopulos ES. The Natural Radiation Environment VII: VIIth Int. Symp. On the NRE. Elsevier, Amsterdam 2005: 894-901.

12. Rai B, Foing BH, Kaur J. Working hours, sleep, salivary cortisol, fatigue and neuro-behavior during Mars analog mission: Five crews study. Neurosci Lett. 2012;516(2):177-81.
13. Palinkas LA, Suedfeld P. Psychosocial issues in isolated and confined extreme environments. Neurosci Biobehav Rev. 2021;126:413-29.
14. Wu B, Wang Y, Wu X, Liu D, Xu D, Wang F. On-orbit sleep problems of astronauts and countermeasures. Mil Med Res. 2018;5(1):17.
15. Kirkpatrick AW, Ball CG, Campbell M, Williams DR, Parazynski SE, Mattox KL, et al. Severe traumatic injury during long duration spaceflight: Light years beyond ATLS. J Trauma Manag Outcomes. 2009;3:4.
16. Kirkpatrick AW, Dulchavsky SA, Boulanger BR, Campbell MR, Hamilton DR, Dawson DL, et al. Extraterrestrial resuscitation of hemorrhagic shock: fluids. J Trauma. 2001;50(1):162-8.
17. Mattox KL. Introduction, background, and future projections of damage control surgery. Surg Clin N Amer. 1997;77(4):753-9.
18. Urban R. (2023). [online] Available from: https://spaceimpulse.com/2023/04/10/medical-emergencies-in-space/ [Last accessed September, 2023].
19. Ball CG, Kirkpatrick AW, Williams DR, Jones JA, Polk JD, Vanderploeg JM, et al. Prophylactic surgery prior to extended-duration space flight: Is the benefit worth the risk? Can J Surg. 2012;55(2):125-31.
20. Campbell MR, Williams DR, Buckey JC Jr, Kirkpatrick AW. Animal surgery during spaceflight on the Neurolab Shuttle mission. Aviat Space Environ Med. 2005;76(6):589-93.
21. Norfleet WT. Anesthetic concerns of spaceflight. Anesthesiology. 2000;92(5):1219-22.
22. Panesar SS, Ashkan K. Surgery in space. J British Surg. 2018;105(10):1234-43.
23. Kirkpatrick AW, Keaney M, Hemmelgarn B, Zhang J, Ball CG, Groleau M, et al. Intra-abdominal pressure effects on porcine thoracic compliance in weightlessness: implications for physiologic tolerance of laparoscopic surgery in space. Critical Care Med. 2009;37(2):591-7.
24. Pantalone D, Faini GS, Cialdai F, Sereni E, Bacci S, Bani D, et al. Robot-assisted surgery in space: pros and cons. A review from the surgeon's point of view. NPJ Microgravity. 2021;7(1):56.
25. Antonsen EL, Myers JG, Boley L, Arellano J, Kerstman E, Kadwa B, et al. Estimating medical risk in human spaceflight. NPJ Microgravity. 2022;8(1):8.
26. Patel ZS, Brunstetter TJ, Tarver WJ, Whitmire AM, Zwart SR, Smith SM, et al. Red risks for a journey to the red planet: The highest priority human health risks for a mission to Mars. NPJ Microgravity. 2020;6(1):33.
27. American College of Surgeons Committee. (2004). Trauma Advanced Trauma Life Support for Doctors Chicago. [online] Available from: https://www.facs.org/quality-programs/trauma/education/advanced-trauma-life-support/?page=1 [Last accessed September, 2023].
28. Komorowski M, Fleming S, Mawkin M, Hinkelbein J. Anaesthesia in austere environments: literature review and considerations for future space exploration missions. NPJ Microgravity. 2018;4(1):5.
29. Campbell MR, Billica RD, Johnston SL 3rd, Muller SM. Performance of advanced trauma life support procedures in microgravity. Aviat Space Environ Med. 2002;73(9):907-12.

30. Chun R, Kirkpatrick AW, Sirois M, Sargasyn AE, Melton S, Hamilton DR, et al. Where's the tube? Evaluation of hand-held ultrasound in confirming endotracheal tube placement. Prehosp Disaster Med. 2004;19(4):366-9.
31. Barton ED, Epperson M, Hoyt DB, Fortlage D, Rosen P. Prehospital needle aspiration and tube thoracostomy in trauma victims: a six-year experience with aeromedical crews. J Emerg Med. 1995;13(2):155-63.
32. Kirkpatrick AW, Hamilton DR, Nicolaou S, Sargsyan AE, Campbell MR, Feiveson A, et al. Focused assessment with sonography for trauma in weightlessness: a feasibility study. J Am Coll Surg. 2003;196(6):833-44.
33. Summers RL, Johnston SL, Marshburn TH, Williams DR. Emergencies in space. Ann Emerg Med. 2005;46(2):177-84.
34. Campbell MR. A review of surgical care in space. J Am Coll Surg. 2002;194(6):802-12.
35. Kirkpatrick AW, Campbell MR, Jones JS, Broderick T, Ball CG, McBeth PB, et al. Extraterrestrial hemorrhage control: Terrestrial developments in technique, technology, and philosophy with applicability to traumatic hemorrhage control during long-duration spaceflight. J Am Coll Surg. 2005;200(1):64-76.
36. Navein J, Coupland R, Dunn R. The tourniquet controversy. J Trauma. 2003;54 (5 Suppl):S219-20.
37. Welch M, Barratt J, Peters A, Wright C. Systematic review of prehospital haemostatic dressings. BMJ Mil Health. 2020;166(3):194-200.
38. Kirkpatrick AW, Campbell MR, Novinkov OL, Goncharov IB, Kovachevich IV. Blunt trauma and operative care in microgravity: a review of microgravity physiology and surgical investigations with implications for critical care and operative treatment in space. J Am Coll Surg. 1997;184(5):441-53.
39. McCuaig KE, Houtchens BA. Management of trauma and emergency surgery in space. J Trauma. 1992;33(4):615-25.
40. Gadomski BC, Lerner ZF, Browning RC, Easley JT, Palmer RH, Puttlitz CM. Computational characterization of fracture healing under reduced gravity loading conditions. J Orthop Res. 2016;34(7):1206-15.
41. Komorowski M, Watkins SD, Lebuffe G, Clark JB. Potential anesthesia protocols for space exploration missions. Aviat Space Environ Med. 2013;84(3):226-33.
42. Graebe A, Schuck EL, Lensing P, Putcha L, Derendorf H. Physiological, pharmacokinetic, and pharmacodynamic changes in space. J Clin Pharmacol. 2004;44(8):837-53.
43. Keller C, Brimacombe J, Giampalmo M, Kleinsasser A, Loeckinger A, Giampalmo G, et al. Airway management during spaceflight: a comparison of four airway devices in simulated microgravity. Anesthesiology. 2000;92(5):1237-41.
44. Hinkelbein J, Ahlbäck A, Antwerber C, Dauth L, DuCanto J, Fleischhammer E, et al. Using supraglottic airways by paramedics for airway management in analogue microgravity increases speed and success of ventilation. Sci Rep. 2021;11(1):9286.
45. Warnecke T, Dauth L, Ahlbäck A, DuCanto J, Fleischhammer E, Glatz C, et al. Time to ventilation and success rate of airway devices in microgravity: a randomized crossover manikin-trial using an underwater setting. Acta Anaesthesiol Scand. 2021;65(5):681-7.
46. Starck C, Thierry S, Bernard CI, Morineau T, Jaulin F, Chapelain P, et al. Tracheal intubation in microgravity: a simulation study comparing direct laryngoscopy and videolaryngoscopy. Br J Anaesth. 2020;125(1):e47-53.

47. Drudi L, Ball CG, Kirkpatrick AW, Saary J, Grenon SM. Surgery in Space: Where are we at now? Acta Astronaut. 2012;79:61-6.
48. Reddy P. Challenges to Airway Management in Space. Special Considerations in Human Airway Management. In: Shallik NA (Ed). England: Intechopen Limited; 2021.
49. Rehnberg L, Ashcroft A, Baers JH, Campos F, Cardoso RB, Velho R, et al. Three methods of manual external chest compressions during microgravity simulation. Aviat Space Environ Med. 2014;85(7):687-93.
50. Rehnberg L, Russomano T, Falcao F, Campos F, Everts SN. Evaluation of a novel basic life support method in simulated microgravity. Aviat Space Environ Med. 2011;82(2):104-10.
51. Chiao L, Sharipov S, Sargsyan AE, Melton S, Hamilton DR, McFarlin K, et al. Ocular examination for trauma; Clinical ultrasound aboard the International Space Station. J Trauma. 2005;58(5):885-9.
52. Kirkpatrick AW, Nicolaou S, Rowan K, Liu D, Cunningham J, Sargsyan AE, et al. Thoracic sonography for pneumothorax: the clinical evaluation of an operational space medicine spin-off. Acta Astronautica. 2005;56(9-12):831-8.
53. Sargsyan AE, Hamilton DR, Jones JA, Melton S, Whitson PA, Kirkpatrick AW, et al. FAST at MACH 20: clinical ultrasound aboard the International Space Station. J Trauma. 2005;58(1):35-9.
54. Han JS, Lee SH, Go H, Kim SJ, Noh JH, Lee CJ. High-Performance Cold Cathode X-ray Tubes Using a Carbon Nanotube Field Electron Emitter. ACS Nano. 2022;16(7):10231-41.
55. Leverage Edu. (2023). Career in Aerospace Medicine. [online] https://leverageedu.com/blog/aerospace-medicine/ [Last accessed September, 2023].
56. Behringer W, Safar P, Wu X, Kentner R, Radovsky A, Kochanek PM, et al. Survival without brain damage after clinical death of 60-120 mins in dogs using suspended animation by profound hypothermia. Crit Care Med. 2003;31(5):1523-31.
57. Letsou GV, Breznock EM, Whitehair J, Kurtz RS, Jacobs R, Leavitt ML, et al. Resuscitating hypothermic dogs after 2 hours of circulatory arrest below 6 degrees C. J Trauma. 2003;54(5 Suppl):S177-82.
58. Tisherman SA. Suspended animation for resuscitation from exsanguinating hemorrhage. Crit Care Med. 2004;32(2 Suppl):S46-50.
59. Blackstone E, Morrison M, Roth MB. H2S induces a suspended animation-like state in mice. Science. 2005;308(5721):518.
60. Wright T. (2015). Space Station ER. [online] Available from: https://www.airspacemag.com/space/space-station-er-180956246/ [Last accessed September, 2023].
61. Garcia P, Rosen J, Kapoor C, Noakes M, Elbert G, Treat M, et al. Trauma Pod: a semi-automated telerobotic surgical system. Int J Med Robot. 2009;5(2):136-46.
62. Takács Á, Jordán S, Nagy DÁ, Tar JK, Rudas IJ, Haidegger T. Surgical robotics— Born in space. IEEE 10th Jubilee International Symposium on Applied Computational Intelligence and Informatics, Timisoara. Romania: Institute of Electrical and Electronics Engineers; 2015. pp. 547-51.
63. Pantalos G, Broderick T, Raj A, Morimoto T, Kernagis D, Clark J, et al. (2019). Minimally Invasive Expeditionary Surgical Care Using Human-Inspired Robots. [online] Available from: https://ntrs.nasa.gov/search.jsp?R=20190030296 [Last accessed September, 2023].

Premedication in Pediatric Anesthesia

Dave Barrett, Shireen Edmends

ABSTRACT

Premedication is a longstanding practice in pediatric anesthesia. Evolving from routine antisialagogue administration to combat secretions into practices reducing anxiety, improving mask acceptance, and cannulation. Familiarization, parent presence, distraction, and simple analgesia should be utilized as often as practicable. If sedation is desired, opioids and chloral hydrate can be premedication agents, but the side effects limit their use. The most used agents in current practice are clonidine and midazolam, each with side effect profiles. Ketamine appears slightly more efficacious than midazolam but must be dose adjusted depending on the administration. Dexmedetomidine is becoming more commonly used, where available, owing to its considerable efficacy and a more favorable hemodynamic profile over clonidine. Overall, each child requires a tailored approach, and understanding pharmacokinetics, pharmacodynamics, and efficacy of the available premedication agents in children aids this endeavor.

Keywords: Premedication; Pediatric; Anesthesia; Sedation; Anxiolysis

KEY POINTS

- Familiarization, distraction, and parent presence should be used whenever possible.
- A low threshold should be given to utilizing simple analgesia.
- The dose and administration should be tailored to each child if sedatives are used.
- The oral route, while masking foul taste, is preferential for premedication.
- Clonidine and midazolam are the most commonly used agents at present.
- Dexmedetomidine is proving to be an ideal agent with minimal adverse effects.
- Diamorphine and chloral hydrate are falling out of favor for premedication.
- Melatonin may prove helpful with evolving literature on efficacious dosing.

INTRODUCTION

Premedication in children undergoing general anesthesia for various procedures has been ongoing for nearly a century. Its uses for anxiolysis, sedation, and/or analgesia are widespread. Early use of antisialagogues to prevent excessive secretions in the airway was every day with the use of older anesthetic agents such as ethyl chloride and ether. More recently, newer sedative drugs have given us a wider choice of drugs to tailor to the individual patient. This review will discuss the various strategies and nonparenteral drugs used globally for premedication in children. Premedication in neonates will not be discussed as techniques, pharmacokinetics, and pharmacodynamics are vastly different in this highly specialized field.

PSYCHOLOGICAL FACTORS

Children presenting for anesthesia and surgery are often distressed and anxious. Whether this is more than in previous generations can be debated, but there is undoubtedly more acknowledgment and openness about anxiety and stress in older children and parents.

Play therapy is one of the most valuable tools in preparing a child for anesthesia and surgery. Methods of distraction and familiarization can reduce the requirement for pharmacological intervention,[1,2] but often needs considerable time and effort, which is difficult to achieve on a fast-turnover list. More recently, the introduction of electronic devices and age-appropriate applications are as effective as oral premedication.[2,3] Children and their parents can develop post-traumatic stress reactions following surgery.[4] Minimizing any anxiety during their perioperative journey is crucial.

EXTRINSIC FACTORS

Prehospital preparation, including information booklets, videos, or hospital tours, can help reduce preoperative anxiety and requirements for anxiolysis. The theater environment, with minimal extraneous noise and well-trained and informed staff, can all contribute to smoothing the induction of anesthesia.[5]

CHOOSING THE IDEAL AGENT

The route of administration can be challenging in pediatric patients. Many patients are needle-phobic, and venous access is only sometimes obtained before general anesthesia. This reduces options for parenteral administration routes for premedication drugs. The oral route is preferred due to the ease of administration and comfort of the patient. Due to the availability of the different concentrations of drugs and the use of combinations of drugs, large volumes of liquid can potentially be given; however, there is little risk of pulmonary aspiration in the elective population.[6] Other routes of administration include rectal, buccal, and intranasal, although these routes can pose difficulties when faced with an uncooperative child. Discussion with the nursing staff and carers is a key to successfully administering premedication. The choice of agent will depend on other comorbidities, e.g., hypovolemia, cardiac abnormalities, obesity, and obstructive sleep apnea. It may be influenced by previous experience on the part of the child or the parent. Many drugs will have additional benefits such as a reduction in postoperative delirium, reduction in anesthetic requirements, reduction in vomiting, and prolongation of analgesic effects of other drugs. There is also an observed calming effect when a familiar taste (e.g., paracetamol syrup) is associated with improved mood and general well-being, as parents commonly administer it at home (personal communication). As several drugs given orally are unavailable as elixirs or syrups, masking their taste by adding small volumes of fruit cordial (or added to paracetamol syrup) can encourage consumption by the patient. The intranasal route requires proximity to the patient and can irritate the nasal mucosa, which can be impractical and may limit cooperation on future occasions.

■ DISCUSSION OF COMMON AGENTS

Paracetamol

A commonly available agent proposed to be nonspecifically inhibiting cyclooxygenase (COX) enzymes centrally causing its analgesic and antipyretic actions.[7] Paracetamol has an excellent oral bioavailability of 80%, a large volume of distribution, is metabolized by the liver enzyme cytochrome p450 family 2 subfamily E member 1 (CYP2E1), and is predominantly eliminated by the kidneys.[8] The hepatotoxic intermediate metabolite, N-acetyl-p-benzoquinone imine, is produced in small quantities at regular therapeutic doses but is rapidly metabolized by hepatic glutathione with normal liver function.[8] While limited evidence exists, the authors can share anecdotal evidence that loading doses of paracetamol in children can have a slight sedative/relaxation effect, making it an invaluable premedication agent irrespective of its well-established analgesic actions. Peak serum concentrations can be reached within 60 minutes orally but over 2 hours rectally with variable bioavailability, making oral administration the preferred choice in this context.[9]

Ibuprofen

Another commonly available agent that reversibly and nonselectively inhibits cyclooxygenase 1 (COX1) and two enzymes to cause analgesia and antipyretic actions.[8] Ibuprofen has an oral bioavailability of 80% and a volume of distribution of 0.1-0.3 L/kg (reducing with age).[10] The onset of ibuprofen varies depending on the formulation used, with the suspension formulation quickest at 30 minutes and tablets slowest at up to 1.5 hours, making suspension the ideal formulation for premedication.[11] The inactive R isomer of the racemic mixture is slowly converted to the active S isomer, which then undergoes hepatic oxidation.[7] The elimination of ibuprofen is predominantly through the kidneys.[8] Consideration must be given to the nonsteroidal anti-inflammatory drugs (NSAIDs) risk of gastrointestinal events, which appears to be a lower incidence in children than in adults and is generally conservatively managed.[12] Similarly, NSAID-induced asthma or bronchospasm is a risk but incidence is less than that of the adult population, and cardiac events associated with COX inhibition have not been recorded in children.[12] Overall, the authors feel that ibuprofen is a safe and valuable addition to paracetamol for premedication in children before anesthesia.

Midazolam

A commonly available benzodiazepine that activates the α-subunit of postsynaptic γ-aminobutyric acid sub-type A receptor ($GABA_A$) receptors to promote chloride influx and neuronal membrane hyperpolarization resulting in sedation and amnesia.[8] Midazolam can be delivered orally, buccally, and intranasally as premedication with an oral bioavailability approaching 40% and intranasal and buccal between 60 and 80%, respectively.[13] Oral midazolam has an onset within 30 minutes, buccal and intranasal within 10 minutes (prolongs with age).[14] It has a volume of distribution of about 1.2 L/kg. It is predominantly metabolized via hydroxylation into an active compound via the same CYP enzyme as alfentanil, prolonging the duration of both if used together.[8] Oral administration with grapefruit juice can be catastrophic due to its ability to inhibit CYP enzymes, thereby reducing first-pass metabolism and increasing plasma concentrations of midazolam by >50%.[15] Midazolam's clearance is approximately 20 times that of diazepam (6-10 mL/kg/min), and alongside its rapid redistribution, constitutes a much shorter duration of action with an elimination half-life of only 1-4 hours (shortened with age and lengthened with oral administration).[16] Delivery of intranasal midazolam can cause nasal burning and pain, and as such, consideration should be given to anesthetizing the nares with lidocaine before utilization.[17] Midazolam often provides ideal conditions for anesthesia induction as a premedication. However, it has been linked to higher rates of emergence agitation, hiccups, and respiratory depression compared to other premedication agents such as dexmedetomidine.[18]

Clonidine

An often-available α-adrenergic agonist with selectivity for α-2:α-1 of approximately 200:1, thereby reducing sympathetic outflow, increasing endogenous opiate release, and modulating descending inhibition.[8] Clonidine can be delivered orally in tablet form or suspension, rectally, or intranasally using intravenous preparation or formulated drops.[19] It has an oral and rectal bioavailability of almost 100% in adults, but the evidence is developing that it is closer to 55% in children with a volume of distribution around 2 L/kg.[8,20] Approximately 50% is metabolized in the liver to inactive metabolites, and the remainder is excreted renally as active metabolites, warranting dose reduction in renal impairment.[8] The time to peak effect orally is ~60 minutes, intranasally ~30 minutes, and rectally ~50 minutes, with an elimination half-life of about 6 hours in children, increasing with age.[21] The adverse effects of hypotension and bradycardia commonly associated with clonidine as a sole agent have limited incidence and clinical significance at routine premedication doses in children,[22] but subsequent use of sedative-hypnotics on induction can precipitate profoundly low heart rates and blood pressure. As such, it is generally best practice also to administer atropine at the time of premedication.[23] Clonidine has improved mask acceptance with reduced postoperative nausea and vomiting, postoperative shivering, and postoperative agitation compared to other premedication agents such as benzodiazepines, thereby making it an invaluable premedication agent where available.[24]

Dexmedetomidine

A newer, promising, highly selective α-2 adrenergic receptor agonist with variable but often limited availability produces similar sedation and analgesia to clonidine with a more favorable adverse effect profile following its better selectivity (eight times more selective than clonidine).[8] Limited evidence supports oral dexmedetomidine (1-4 µg/kg), likely secondary to its poor oral bioavailability of only 15%.[25] Fortunately, intranasal and buccal administration confers greater bioavailability of 65 and 80%, respectively, becoming much more practicable as a premedication agent.[26,27] Dexmedetomidine has a highly variable volume of distribution depending on the patient's age but averages around 2.2 L/kg in children.[28] Dexmedetomidine is metabolized hepatically with no known toxic or active metabolites and is predominantly excreted renally.[28] Anxiolysis onset is around 10 minutes intranasally and buccally (increasing with age), with sedation seen after 30-60 minutes and overall duration of action of fewer than 2 hours following a single dose.[29] As a novel agent, the literature is beginning to explore multimodal premedication strategies, including dose-reduced dexmedetomidine and ketamine, with promising additive effects for improved mask tolerance, cannulation success, and reduced parental separation anxiety.[30] Furthermore, the comparatively long duration of action of dexmedetomidine can be considered helpful in the proper context, with postoperative rousable sedation often observed in the recovery room, thereby also providing anxiolysis in this foreign environment.[31] Overall, dexmedetomidine, if available, is a valuable and promising premedication agent with similar efficacy to benzodiazepines, reduced incidence of hemodynamic compromise compared to clonidine, and reduced rates of postoperative agitation and pain compared to benzodiazepines.[28]

Ketamine

A powerful sedative analgesic and amnesic working as a noncompetitive N-methyl-D-aspartate (NMDA) receptor antagonist, more commonly delivered in the intravenous and intramuscular route for sedation and induction of anesthesia.[8] The parenteral formulation can be delivered orally in juice, rectally, and intranasally as a premedication agent with bioavailabilities of ~15–30% for oral and rectal delivery, and ~45% for nasal delivery using an atomizer and splitting the dose between nostrils.[32] Onset is seen around 45 minutes rectally, 20–30 minutes orally, and 15 minutes intranasally, with an analgesic duration of approximately 60 minutes and sedation of approximately 45 minutes.[33,34] The overall volume of distribution of ketamine is between 2.1 and 3.1 L/kg (increases with age) with very low protein binding of only 10–30%.[35] Ketamine is metabolized hepatically, with the first stage an active metabolite, norketamine—this has a potency of ~25% compared to the parent—and subsequent stages producing inactive compounds predominantly excreted renally.[35] The commonly cited emergence agitation seen in adults is much less prevalent in children. As such, concomitant benzodiazepines are generally not needed.[36] Of importance, ketamine causes hypersalivation and does not suppress laryngeal reflexes, so if used as a sole premedication and induction agent can contribute to laryngospasm if airway or pharyngeal manipulation takes place.[37] Furthermore, despite of being a sympathomimetic, ordinarily increasing heart rate and blood pressure, ketamine is a direct myocardial depressant, so in situations of high sympathetic activity or heart failure, the administration of ketamine can still cause dose-dependent hypotension.[32] Overall, ketamine is more efficacious than midazolam as a premedication agent in terms of sedation and overall procedure accomplishment, with success rates approaching that of dexmedetomidine.[34,38]

Morphine

A naturally occurring predominantly mu (μ)-opioid receptor agonist with some kappa (κ) and delta (δ) activity causing the closure of presynaptic neuronal calcium channels and the opening of postsynaptic potassium channels, thereby hyperpolarizing nerves and reducing neurotransmitter release, providing analgesia and sedation.[8] Morphine can be delivered orally in tablet or suspension form with a bioavailability of 15–33%, an onset of around 30 minutes, and a dose-dependent duration of around 2–5 hours.[39] Rectal administration has unpredictable kinetics in children, significantly increasing the risk of severe adverse events, including death with prolonged use.[40] Morphine has a poor lipid solubility and a bimodal volume of distribution of 2–5 L/kg with higher values observed in very young and older children.[41] Morphine is metabolized principally hepatically into the likely neurotoxic compound morphine-3-glucuronide and highly active compound morphine-6-glucuronide; both are predominantly excreted renally, prompting avoidance with renal impairment.[42] Morphine as a premedication agent appears to be falling out of favor in current practice, with a paucity of recent literature mentioning its use.[43,44] This reluctance is likely due to the prevalence of adverse effects such as respiratory depression (particularly in children with sleep apnea), nausea and vomiting, urinary retention, pruritus, and hemodynamic changes on induction, combined with its prolonged duration of action delaying discharge.[43,44] Furthermore, the histamine release associated with morphine can be compounded with other drugs prone to do the same, which can significantly increase the risk of bronchospasm.[45] However, morphine may prove beneficial as a premedication agent with appropriately selected patient populations in resource-limited settings where other agents are not as readily available.

Diamorphine

Diamorphine (i.e., diacetylmorphine or heroin) is an inactive prodrug that is rapidly converted into the active compound 6-monoacetylmorphine by plasma and liver esterases and then slowly converted into morphine, exerting the same effects and side effects as morphine above.[46] Diamorphine has very poor and unpredictable oral bioavailability and undergoes some enterohepatic circulation, prompting intranasal as the preferred method of administration with a respective bioavailability of approximately 50%.[46] Diamorphine is far more lipid soluble, constituting a faster onset of action of approximately 5 minutes and relative equianalgesic potency of approximately 200% compared to morphine.[46] Ultimately, pharmacokinetic and pharmacodynamic data on diamorphine in children are scarce in the literature, and dosing is mainly based on adult or historical data.[47] Diamorphine has all the prospective side effects of morphine, with a greater propensity for euphoria. As such, limited studies have compared its efficacy in the premedication space in the recent literature, focusing more on neonatal withdrawals, acute pain, and palliative care.[47] The beneficial properties of diamorphine could make it a reasonable premedication agent in high-turnover surgical lists while noting its prominent adverse effects.

Fentanyl

Fentanyl is a potent synthetic, predominantly μ-opioid receptor agonist culminating in similar effects to morphine with less histamine release.[8] On ingestion, fentanyl is heavily ionized and therefore somewhat trapped in the stomach, then made slowly available for absorption in the small bowel but undergoes significant first-pass metabolism conferring very poor and unpredictable oral bioavailability of ~30%.[48] Fortunately, buccal administration with lozenge formulations and nasal administration using parenteral formulation has 70 and 90% bioavailabilities, respectively, with an intranasal onset of action within 10 minutes owing to its very high-lipid solubility of approximately 600 times that of morphine,[48] however, the duration of fentanyl is dose-dependent, approximating 2-4 hours, and is mainly secondary to redistribution with a highly variable volume of distribution between 5 and 15 L/kg owing to dose, age (younger patient = higher distribution), and body habitus (higher adiposity = higher distribution).[48,49] Fentanyl is metabolized hepatically via N-dealkylation to norfentanyl and further hydroxylated to inactivate metabolites and predominantly excreted renally (~75%) with <10% as an unchanged drug.[8] Preoperative anxiolysis in children is typically seen around 10 minutes, sedation at approximately 20 minutes, and limited postoperative sedation is observed depending on the length of the procedure.[31]

Furthermore, fentanyl has shown similar efficacy to dexmedetomidine and superiority to midazolam regarding mask acceptance, parental separation anxiety, and cannulation success.[31] Dosages for larger children may require dual nares administration alongside higher concentration formulations to reduce the amount of liquid administered and consequential unpredictable pharmacokinetics following ingestion. Buccal administration with lozenge formulations, while showing higher acceptance levels, can occasionally cause higher rates of over-sedation and desaturation, likely secondary to complex titration and less predictable absorption, thereby falling out of favor as a premedication formulation.[50,51] Irrespective of more predictable pharmacokinetics, intranasal fentanyl is still at risk of causing oversedation and respiratory depression in specific patient populations. Outside of bradycardia and chest wall rigidity seen at very high doses, fentanyl is generally hemodynamically stable except the hypovolemic patient, and care must be taken on induction with the additive effect of sedative-hypnotic agents.[8] Overall, fentanyl is a beneficial, widely available agent with favorable side effect profiles and efficacy in the premedication space when used intranasally.

Chloral Hydrate

Chloral hydrate is a previously widely used prodrug converted hepatically via hepatic alcohol dehydrogenase into its active component trichloroethanol to exert its sedative effects via a largely unknown mechanism.[52] Chloral hydrate has unpredictable rectal absorption but is readily absorbed orally, with a bioavailability approaching 95%.[53] Following oral administration, the onset of sedation begins around 15-30 minutes, with a duration of action of up to 2 hours.[54] Chloral hydrates active components are further hepatically glucuronidated, prompting avoidance in liver disease, and its metabolites are primarily excreted renally.[55] The rare adverse effects of rapid comatose state or malignant cardiac dysrhythmias in higher doses are less prevalent in children under the age of 4 years; irrespective of this, it should be known that chloral hydrate has a narrow therapeutic index and should be dosed with caution as numerous reports of death have been recorded following dosing error.[56]

Furthermore, the sedation involved with higher doses of 75-100 mg/kg can cause respiratory depression, desaturation, and airway obstruction; however, lower doses can still do the same.[57] Its use remains somewhat common to facilitate diagnostic investigations, however it has been removed from circulation in some countries due to concerns for carcinogenicity and the mounting case reports of unintentional fatal overdoses.[57] Other prominent side effects of chloral hydrate at regular doses include nausea, vomiting, agitation, gastric irritation, and unpleasant taste, which can be masked by mixing with juice.[52] Recent literature comparing chloral hydrate's efficacy as a premedication agent is limited, but in facilitating diagnostic investigations, comparisons show that it provides similar onset, with more profound and more prolonged sedation (at doses of 75 mg/kg) compared to midazolam (0.5 mg/kg).[58] Overall, with careful, appropriate dosing and observation, chloral hydrate can prove helpful as a premedication agent, recognizing that the effects of induction agents are likely additive.

Melatonin

Melatonin is the primary hormone secreted from the pineal gland. It acts by activating ML1 and ML2 receptors which regulate circadian rhythms such as sleep-awake, neuroendocrine rhythms, and body temperature cycles. Following oral administration, peak concentration arises within 60 minutes. Bioavailability is 10-56%, rapidly metabolized primarily in the liver and secondarily in the kidney.[59] Ingestion of melatonin induces fatigue and sleepiness; and is used therapeutically in sleep disorders, psychiatric disorders, and cancer.[59] Melatonin's anxiolytic properties for premedication in adults, and its usefulness in children with autism spectrum disorder (ASD), make it a promising drug for premedication in children. Melatonin appears to produce reduced sedation and less emergence delirium compared to midazolam.[60] Several studies have shown variable results using melatonin for preoperative anxiolysis using dose ranges from 0.05 to 0.75 mg/kg.[60-62] This may be a dose-dependent effect, and we await further studies to determine the most efficacious dose in what could potentially be a very useful agent with minimal side effects.

TABLE 1: Pharmacological overview of common agents.

Agent	Mechanism of action	Sedation	Analgesia	Route	Common dose	Admin time	Important considerations
Paracetamol	Likely central nonspecific COX inhibition	+/−	++	• Oral • Rectal	• Oral loading 15–30 mg/kg • Maximum 90 mg/kg/day	Oral ~30 minutes prior	• Caution in hepatic dysfunction • Rectal absorption slower and less predictable
Ibuprofen	Reversible nonspecific COX inhibition	+/−	++	Oral	• Oral loading 10 mg/kg • Maximum 30–40 mg/kg/day	Oral ~30 minutes prior	• Caution with history of GI bleeding or reactive airways • Tablet absorption slower than suspension
Midazolam	Postsynaptic GABA$_A$ activation	+++	−	• Oral • Buccal • Nasal	• Oral 0.2–0.5 mg/kg • Buccal and nasal 0.1–0.2 mg/kg	• Oral ~30 minutes prior • Buccal and nasal ~15 minutes prior	• Oral is slower onset and longer lasting • Do not mix midazolam with grapefruit juice • Respiratory depression, hiccups, nasal irritation, and emergence agitation are prominent side effects
Clonidine	Alpha-adrenergic agonist and predominantly α-2	++	+	• Oral • Rectal • Nasal	Nasal, oral, and rectal 2–4 µg/kg	• Nasal ~30 minutes prior • Rectal and oral ~45 minutes prior	Consider coadministration of nasal atropine at 20 µg/kg or oral at 30–40 µg/kg to mitigate bradycardia and hypotension on induction

Contd...

Contd...

Agent	Mechanism of action	Sedation	Analgesia	Route	Common dose	Admin time	Important considerations
Dexmedetomidine	Highly selective α-2 adrenergic agonist	++	+	• Nasal • Buccal	Nasal and buccal 1–2 μg/kg	~45 minutes prior	• Note unpredictable and poor oral bioavailability • Note dose-dependent duration of action
Ketamine	Noncompetitive NMDA receptor antagonist that blocks glutamate	++	+++	• Nasal • Oral • Rectal	• Nasal 3–5 mg/kg • Oral and rectal 4–6 mg/kg	Nasal ~15 minutes prior Oral ~30 minutes prior Rectal ~45 minutes prior	• Note risk of laryngospasm if sole anesthetic agent—consider antisialagogue • Note still a risk of hypotension in maximally stimulated or heart failure patients
Morphine	Natural predominantly Mu opioid receptor agonist	++	++	Oral	Oral 0.1–0.3 mg/kg	~30 minutes prior	• Note the significant risk of respiratory depression • Avoid use in renal dysfunction and obstructive sleep apnea • Avoid concomitant use of agents prone to cause histamine release
Diamorphine	Prodrug converted into 6-monoacetylmorphine and morphine	++	++	Nasal	Nasal 0.05–0.1 mg/kg	Nasal 5–10 minutes prior	• Note significant risk of respiratory depression • Avoid use in renal dysfunction and obstructive sleep apnea • Avoid concomitant use of agents prone to cause histamine release

Contd...

Contd...

Agent	Mechanism of action	Sedation	Analgesia	Route	Common dose	Admin time	Important considerations
Fentanyl	Synthetic predominantly Mu opioid receptor agonist	++	++	• Nasal • Buccal	Nasal and buccal 1–1.5 µg/kg	Nasal and buccal 10–20 minutes prior	Intranasal use of parenteral formulation is preferred due to higher risks of oversedation and respiratory depression when administering buccal lozenges
Chloral hydrate	Unknown mechanism	+++	-	Oral	Oral 25–75 mg/kg	Oral 15–20 minutes prior	• Avoid use in children over 3 years old and those with liver disease • The lowest dose possible should be utilized under close monitoring to avoid the well-documented severe adverse events of oversedation or dysrhythmia
Melatonin	ML1 and ML2 receptor activation	+/-	-	Oral	Oral 0.25–0.75 mg/kg	45–60 minutes prior	Care with hepatic impairment (limited data). Potential wide-dose range

(COX: cyclooxygenase; GABA$_A$: γ-aminobutyric acid type A; GI: gastrointestinal; NMDA: N-methyl-D-aspartate)

CONCLUSION

Creating the optimum environment to improve parental separation, mask acceptance, and cannulation should involve a holistic and multifaceted approach. Familiarization techniques can be logistically complicated but should not be underestimated and may prove more efficient than other measures in the foreseeably anxious or combative child. Parental presence can be helpful, and distraction is a powerful augmenting tool. If pharmacological premedication is desired, paracetamol, and ibuprofen are invaluable owing to familiar flavors, analgesia, and possibly providing a calming effect; and can be combined with other agents. There are several other drugs to choose from **(Table 1)**. If using sedative agents, consideration of patient risk factors, route of administration, and resources available is essential so that the appropriate agent, at the appropriate dose, can be administered promptly with the least risk of side effects. Children having repeat procedures and obese children present extra complexities, and combinations of drugs may be beneficial.[5]

The sedative agents most commonly utilized include clonidine and midazolam, both with associated risks as described earlier. Dexmedetomidine is a valuable agent, often providing optimum conditions in theater and the recovery room with fewer side effects but a slower onset of action. For opioids, morphine—although commonly available, has an unfavorable adverse effect profile compared to other agents. Fentanyl seems to be the most efficacious of the opioids for premedication owing to its synthetic nature, high lipid solubility, fast redistribution, and fewer adverse effects. However, fentanyl should be administered intranasally for safer and more predictable outcomes, which may be problematic in some children. Diamorphine has limited evidence to support its use as a premedication agent, and chloral hydrate has similar efficacy to midazolam yet has a narrow therapeutic window and developing concerns for carcinogenicity. The predictable bioavailability and consequent methods of administration of ketamine make it useful in an array of situations if dose adjusted, particularly if potent analgesia is also desired. Melatonin may be an effective premedicant, but the evidence is currently conflicting.

Whichever therapeutic options are chosen, having a firm understanding of the pharmacokinetics and pharmacodynamics of the agents available will improve the chances of a seamless anesthetic with the potentially anxious or combative child.

REFERENCES

1. Yahya AL-Sagarat A, Al-Oran HM, Obeidat H, Hamlan AM, Moxham L. Preparing the family and children for surgery. Crit Care Nurs Q. 2017;40(2):99-107.
2. Marechal C, Berthiller J, Tosetti S, Cogniat B, Desombres H, Bouvet L, et al. Children and parental anxiolysis in paediatric ambulatory surgery: a randomized controlled study comparing 0.3 mg kg^{-1} midazolam to tablet computer based interactive distraction. Br J Anaesth. 2017;118(2):247-53.

3. Manyande A, Cyna AM, Yip P, Chooi C, Middleton P. Non-pharmacological interventions for assisting the induction of anaesthesia in children (Review). Cochrane Database Syst Rev. 2015;7(3):CD0006447.
4. Turgoose DP, Kerr S, De Coppi P, Blackburn S, Wilkinson S, Rooney N, et al. prevalence of traumatic psychological stress reactions in children and parents following paediatric surgery: a systematic review and meta-analysis. BMJ Paediatr Open. 2021;5(1):e001147.
5. Heikal S, Stuart G. Anxiolytic premedication for children. BJA Educ. 2020;20(7):220-5.
6. Andersson H, Zarén B, Frykholm P. Low incidence of pulmonary aspiration in children allowed intake of clear fluids until called to the operating suite. Pediatr Anesth. 2015;25(8):770-7.
7. Przybyła GW, Szychowski KA, Gmiński J. Paracetamol—An old drug with new mechanisms of action. Clin Exp Pharmacol Physiol. 2021;48(1):3-19.
8. Peck T, Harris B. Pharmacology for Anaesthesia and Intensive Care, 5th edition. United Kingdom: Cambridge University Press; 2021.
9. Hahn T, Henneberg S, Holm-Knudsen R, Eriksen K, Rasmussen S, Rasmussen M. Pharmacokinetics of rectal paracetamol after repeated dosing in children. Br J Anaesth. 2000;85(4):512-9.
10. Mehlisch D, Sykes J. Ibuprofen blood plasma levels and onset of analgesia. Int J Clin Prac. 2013;67(178):3-8.
11. Scott CS, Retsch-Bogart GZ, Kustra RP, Graham KM, Glasscock BJ, Smith PC. The pharmacokinetics of ibuprofen suspension, chewable tablets, and tablets in children with cystic fibrosis. J Pediatr. 1999;134(1):58-63.
12. Kanabar DJ. A clinical and safety review of paracetamol and ibuprofen in children. Inflammopharmacology. 2017;25(1):1-9.
13. Bagheri M. The Use of Midazolam in Paediatric Dentistry: A Review of the Literature. Razavi Int J Med. 2014;2(3):1-6.
14. Lee-Kim SJ, Fadavi S, Punwani I, Koerber A. Nasal versus oral midazolam sedation for pediatric dental patients. J Dent Child (Chic). 2004;71(2):126-30.
15. Goho C. Oral midazolam-grapefruit juice drug interaction. Pediatr Dent. 2001;23(4):365-6.
16. Al-Rakaf H, Bello L, Turkustani A, Adenubi J. Intra-nasal midazolam in conscious sedation of young paediatric dental patients. Int J Paediatr Dent. 2001;11(1):33-40.
17. Chiaretti A, Barone G, Rigante D, Ruggiero A, Pierri F, Barbi E, et al. Intranasal lidocaine and midazolam for procedural sedation in children. Arch Dis Child. 2011;96(2):160-3.
18. Sheta SA, Al-Sarheed MA, Abdelhalim AA. Intranasal dexmedetomidine vs midazolam for premedication in children undergoing complete dental rehabilitation: a double-blinded randomized controlled trial. Pediatr Anesth. 2014;24(2):181-9.
19. Hanning SM, Orlu Gul M, Toni I, Neubert A, Tuleu C. A mini-review of non-parenteral clonidine preparations for paediatric sedation. J Pharm Pharmacol. 2017;69(4):398-405.
20. Larsson P, Nordlinder A, Bergendahl HTG, Lönnqvist P-A, Eksborg S, Almenrader N, et al. Oral bioavailability of clonidine in children. Pediatr Anesth. 2011;21(3):335-40.

21. Xie HG, Cao YJ, Gauda EB, Agthe AG, Hendrix CW, Lee H. Clonidine clearance matures rapidly during the early postnatal period: a population pharmacokinetic analysis in newborns with neonatal abstinence syndrome. J Clin Pharmacol. 2011;51(4):502-11.
22. Nishina K, Mikawa K, Shiga M, Obara H. Clonidine in paediatric anaesthesia. Pediatr Anesth. 1999;9(3):187-202.
23. Mitra S, Kazal S, Anand LK. Intranasal clonidine vs. midazolam as premedication in children: a randomized controlled trial. Indian Pediatr. 2014;51(2):113-8.
24. Bergendahl H, Lönnqvist PA, Eksborg S. Clonidine in paediatric anaesthesia: review of the literature and comparison with benzodiazepines for premedication. Acta Anaesthesiol Scand. 2006;50(2):135-43.
25. Mahmoud M, Mason K. Dexmedetomidine: review, update, and future considerations of paediatric perioperative and periprocedural applications and limitations. Br J Anaesth. 2015;115(2):171-82.
26. Anttila M, Penttilä J, Helminen A, Vuorilehto L, Scheinin H. Bioavailability of dexmedetomidine after extravascular doses in healthy subjects. Br J Clin Pharmacol. 2003;56(6):691-3.
27. Iirola T, Vilo S, Manner T, Aantaa R, Lahtinen M, Scheinin M, et al. Bioavailability of dexmedetomidine after intranasal administration. Eur J Clin Pharmacol. 2011;67(8):825-31.
28. Potts AL, Anderson BJ, Warman GR, Lerman J, Diaz SM, Vilo S. Dexmedetomidine pharmacokinetics in pediatric intensive care—a pooled analysis. Pediatr Anesth. 2009;19(11):1119-29.
29. Yuen VM, Hui TW, Irwin M, Yao TJ, Wong G, Yuen M. Optimal timing for the administration of intranasal dexmedetomidine for premedication in children. Anaesthesia. 2010;65(9):922-9.
30. Qiao H, Xie Z, Jia J. Pediatric premedication: a double-blind randomized trial of dexmedetomidine or ketamine alone versus a combination of dexmedetomidine and ketamine. BMC Anesthesiol. 2017;17(1):1-7.
31. Chatrath V, Kumar R, Sachdeva U, Thakur M. Intranasal fentanyl, midazolam and dexmedetomidine as premedication in pediatric patients. Anesth Essays Res. 2018;12(3):748-53.
32. Peltoniemi MA, Hagelberg NM, Olkkola KT, Saari TI. Ketamine: A Review of Clinical Pharmacokinetics and Pharmacodynamics in Anesthesia and Pain Therapy. Clin Pharmacokinet. 2016;55(9):1059-77.
33. Turhanoğlu S, Kararmaz A, Özyilmaz M, Kaya S, Tok D. Effects of different doses of oral ketamine for premedication of children. Eur J Anesthesiol. 2003;20(1):56-60.
34. Bahetwar S, Pandey R, Saksena A, Girish C. A comparative evaluation of intranasal midazolam, ketamine and their combination for sedation of young uncooperative pediatric dental patients: a triple blind randomized crossover trial. J Clin Pediatr Dent. 2011;35(4):415-20.
35. Mion G, Villevieille T. Ketamine pharmacology: an update (pharmacodynamics and molecular aspects, recent findings). CNS Neurosci Ther. 2013;19(6):370-80.
36. Ng KT, Sarode D, Lai YS, Teoh WY, Wang CY. The effect of ketamine on emergence agitation in children: A systematic review and meta-analysis. Pediatr Anesth. 2019;29(12):1163-72.

37. Green SM, Roback MG, Krauss B, Brown L, McGlone RG, Agrawal D, et al. Emergency Department Ketamine Meta-Analysis Study Group. Predictors of airway and respiratory adverse events with ketamine sedation in the emergency department: an individual-patient data meta-analysis of 8,282 children. Ann Emerg Med. 2009;54(2):158-68.e1-4.
38. Natarajan SM, Pandey RK, Saksena AK, Kumar R, Chandra G. A comparative evaluation of intranasal dexmedetomidine, midazolam and ketamine for their sedative and analgesic properties: a triple blind randomized study. J Clin Pediatr Dent. 2014;38(3):255-61.
39. Dawes JM, Cooke EM, Hannam JA, Brand KA, Winton P, Jimenez-Mendez R, et al. Oral morphine dosing predictions based on single dose in healthy children undergoing surgery. Pediatr Anesth. 2017;27(1):28-36.
40. Gourlay G, Boas R. Fatal outcome with use of rectal morphine for postoperative pain control in an infant. BMJ. 1992;304(6829):766-7.
41. Hunt A, Joel S, Dick G, Goldman A. Population pharmacokinetics of oral morphine and its glucuronides in children receiving morphine as immediate-release liquid or sustained-release tablets for cancer pain. J Pediatr. 1999;135(1):47-55.
42. Lugo RA, Kern SE. Clinical pharmacokinetics of morphine. J Pain Palliat Care Pharmacother. 2002;16(4):5-18.
43. Strauss L. Premedication in paediatrics. South Afr J Anaesth Analg. 2021;27(6):131-5.
44. Strom S. Preoperative evaluation, premedication, and induction of anesthesia in infants and children. Curr Opin Anaesthesiol. 2012;25(3):321-5.
45. Parameswara G. Anesthetic concerns in patients with hyper-reactive airways. Karnataka Anaesth J. 2015;1(1):8-16.
46. Gastine S, Morse JD, Leung MTY, Wong ICK, Howard RF, Harrop E, et al. Diamorphine pharmacokinetics and conversion factor estimates for intranasal diamorphine in paediatric breakthrough pain: systematic review. BMJ Support Palliat Care. 2022:bmjspcare-2021-003461.
47. Morse JD, Anderson BJ, Gastine S, Wong IC, Standing JF. Pharmacokinetic modeling and simulation to understand diamorphine dose-response in neonates, children, and adolescents. Pediatr Anesth. 2022;32(6):716-26.
48. Lötsch J, Walter C, Parnham MJ, Oertel BG, Geisslinger G. Pharmacokinetics of non-intravenous formulations of fentanyl. Clin Pharmacokinet. 2013;52(1):23-36.
49. Katz R, Kelly W. Pharmacokinetics of continuous infusions of fentanyl in critically ill children. Crit Care Med. 1993;21(7):995-1000.
50. Sengupta S, Bhattacharya P, Nag DS, Sahay N. Search for the ideal route of premedication in children. far from over? Indian J Anaesth. 2022;66(Suppl 4):S188-92.
51. Moore PA, Cuddy MA, Magera JA, Caputo A, Chen AH, Wilkinson LA. Oral transmucosal fentanyl pretreatment for outpatient general anesthesia. Anesth Prog. 2000;47(2):29-34.
52. Ashrafi MR, Mohammadi M, Tafarroji J, Shabanian R, Salamati P, Zamani GR. Melatonin versus chloral hydrate for recording sleep EEG. Eur J Paediatr Neurol. 2010;14(3):235-8.
53. Zimmermann T, Wehling M, Schulz H. The relative bioavailability and pharmacokinetics of chloral hydrate and its metabolites. Arzneimittelforschung. 1998;48(1):5-12.

54. Olson DM, Sheehan MG, Thompson W, Hall PT, Hahn J. Sedation of children for electroencephalograms. Pediatrics. 2001;108(1):163-5.
55. Nandini DM. Premedication and induction of anaesthesia in paediatric patients. Indian J Anaesth. 2019;63(9):713-20.
56. Grissinger M. Chloral hydrate: Is it still being used? Are there safer alternatives? PT. 2019;44(8):444-5.
57. Krauss B, Green SM. Procedural sedation and analgesia in children. Lancet. 2006;367(9512):766-80.
58. Wheeler DS, Jensen RA, Poss WB. A randomized, blinded comparison of chloral hydrate and midazolam sedation in children undergoing echocardiography. Clin Pediatr (Phila). 2001;40(7):381-7.
59. Tordjman S, Chokron S, Delorme R, Charrier A, Bellisant E, Jaafari N, et al. Melatonin: Pharmacology, Functions and Therapeutic benefits. Curr Neuropharmacol. 2017;15(3):434-43.
60. Mellor K, Papaioannou D, Thomason A, Bolt R, Evans C, Wilson M, et al. Melatonin for pre-medication in children: a systematic review. BMC Pediatr. 2022;22:107.
61. Kain ZN, MacLaren JE, Herrmann L, Mayes L, Rosenbaum A, Hata J, et al. Preoperative melatonin and its effects on induction and emergence in children undergoing anesthesia and surgery. Anesthesiology. 2009;111(1):44-9.
62. Kurdi MS, Muthukalai SP. A comparison of the effect of two doses of oral melatonin with oral midazolam and placebo on pre-operative anxiety, cognition and psychomotor function in children: a randomised double-blind study. Indian J Anaesth. 2016;60(10):744-50.

12

Anesthesia for Robotic Surgeries in Children

Neerja Bhardwaj, Ravi P Kanojia

ABSTRACT

Robot-assisted laparoscopic surgery in children, including infants and neonates, is rapidly gaining interest as it improves the surgeon's three-dimensional (3D) view making the surgery easier. An anesthesiologist should know the anesthetic challenges in a child undergoing robotic surgery. These may be related to the positioning of the patient, limited access to the airway and intravenous (IV) lines, pressure injury of nerves and tissues, and the possibility of hypothermia. In addition, knowledge of the physiological changes produced by pneumoperitoneum (PnP) and its impact on the various organ systems is also essential. The lung ventilatory strategies required to maintain oxygenation and avoid hypercarbia and atelectasis include delivery of a tidal volume of 6–7 mL/kg, positive end-expiratory pressure (PEEP) of 5 mm Hg, and peak airway pressure limited to 25 cmH$_2$O with a higher respiratory rate. Postoperative pain management is essential to anesthesia care and may be achieved by a multimodal approach, including nerve blocks.

Keywords: Pediatric anesthesia; Robot-assisted surgery; Laparoscopic surgery; Minimally invasive surgery; Anesthesia management; Postoperative pain; Complications

KEY POINTS

- The popularity of robotically performed, minimally invasive surgery has significantly increased in pediatric patients.
- Knowledge of the pathophysiological effects of PnP on various organ systems and the potential complications which can occur is essential to provide safe anesthesia during robot-assisted surgery in infants and children.
- Anesthetic management for pediatric robotic surgery focuses on close physiological monitoring, optimum ventilation strategies, careful positioning, stabilization, and protection of the patient from potential injury related to the moving robot arms and equipment.
- Pain management should be multimodal and should consider multiple sources of pain: incisional, diffuse abdominal and shoulder, and visceral pain.

INTRODUCTION

The last 10–15 years have seen an exponential rise in the use of minimally invasive approaches to surgery in children owing to the many advantages seen with this approach **(Box 1)**. However, more expensive and complex, robot-assisted surgery is an extension of laparoscopic surgery. It was conceptualized with the primary aim of improving the surgical quality as well as accessibility for the complex surgical procedures which would be otherwise difficult and require open surgery. This has led to the introduction of the robot in all surgical fields, including pediatric surgery. With the inclusion of robots in the pediatric surgeon's armamentarium, various authors have published their experience of robotic surgery, mainly for urological procedures such as pyeloplasty, nephrectomy, ureteric implantation, and gastrointestinal surgery, including cholecystectomy, choledochal cyst excision, and Kasai's portoenterostomy.[1,2] In addition to these procedures, the authors have experience managing neonates undergoing repair of tracheoesophageal fistula and congenital diaphragmatic hernia using a robot. Robotic surgery in neonates and infants is challenging owing to the reduced anatomical working space, which limits the movement of robotic instruments.

There is a need for consensus guidelines on the type of patients and the procedures for robotic surgery in children. The Italian Society of Pediatric and Neonatal Anesthesia and Intensive Care (SARNePI) and the Italian Society of Pediatric Surgery (SICP) published a joint consensus statement for managing children undergoing robot-assisted surgery.[3] With the increasing use of robotic surgery in infants and children, it is crucial for pediatric anesthesiologists to understand the basics of the robotic system as well as its impact on anesthesia management. This includes the challenges of the positioning of the patient, limited airway and intravenous (IV) access, long duration of the procedure, and the possibility of hypothermia, and understanding the physiological changes produced by pneumoperitoneum (PnP) to provide safe and effective perioperative anesthesia. This review aims to inform readers about anesthesia management principles for a safe perioperative outcome in children undergoing robot-assisted surgery.

BOX 1: Advantages of laparoscopic surgery.

- Smaller scars
- Better healing
- Decreased blood loss
- Less need for postoperative analgesia
- Lower postoperative respiratory and wound complications
- Earlier ambulation
- Decreased length of stay in hospital

THE ROBOTIC SYSTEM

The robotic system provides improved surgical field visibility using three-dimensional (3D) imaging systems and instrument movement by creating 7° of motion mimicking the wrist's movement, thereby producing better control of fine movements and preventing hand tremors through a computer scaling system. There are several robotic systems available for commercial use currently; however, the Da Vinci system by Intuitive Surgical (Sunnyvale, CA, USA) is one of the first and most widely adopted robotic systems worldwide. The Da Vinci system has three major components which are: (1) the vision cart, (2) a master console, and (3) a movable robotic tower **(Fig. 1)** housed around the patient during a procedure.

The patient cart is the mobile part with four robotic arms for endoscopic instruments. This is docked over the patient during the procedure **(Fig. 2)**. This is the most significant part that fully covers the patient. In most cases, the patient cart is placed on the side of the table so that the head and foot end of the patient are free for any access. The anesthetist has to double-check the cart's position concerning the airway and the IV infusion lines once the

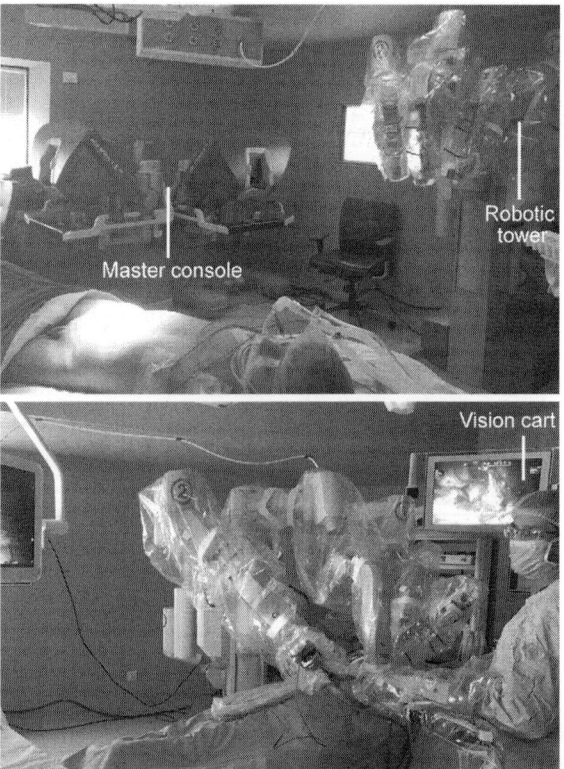

Fig. 1: Da Vinci surgical robot with the components.

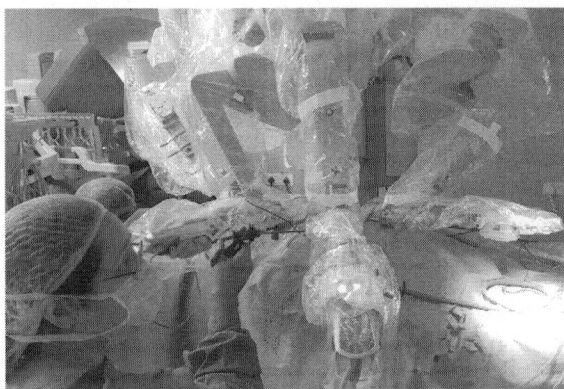

Fig. 2: The robotic system after docking.

four arms are finally docked. This can be a significant concern in pediatric patients and should be actively discussed with the surgeon.

The surgeon's console is at a distance from the operation table, housed within the same room, and should be in direct line of sight of the surgeon so that he can view the patient at all times. The console gives a 3D inside view of the surgical field and is used to maneuver the surgical instruments docked inside the patient. Most robotic systems have a dual console, the second console used for assistance and teaching.

The vision cart is the video tower that houses the display, insufflator, energy sources, and central computer. This is also housed away from the patient, and the surgical assistant and the anesthetist use the screen to see the procedure and synchronize with the surgeon.

Concerns of Robotic System

Safety during a robotic procedure is a top priority, as much hardware surrounds the patient. Apart from the problems related to the robotic arms docked on the patient, there are other concerns regarding the access to the airway, infusion lines, and extremes of the position that are part of any minimally invasive surgery.

Positioning of Patient and Access after Docking

For nearly all types of minimal access surgery, the patient is placed supine with the operative site aligned with the principles of the Trendelenburg position. The patient is in a head-up position for upper abdominal procedures involving the stomach, liver, and spleen. On the other hand, for pelvic procedures, there is a head low position. The robotic system is docked so that the main cart is on the side of the operation table, and the arm's pillar housing is rotatable to align with the operative site. The arms are often in the way and can obstruct access to the airway. There is a minor play in the arm adjustment to move it away from such an inappropriate position. This is something that the anesthetist has to actively see while the surgeon is docking the robot, checking for access to the patient from various sides.

Preventing Pressure Injuries due to the Robot

The robotic arms, once docked, will be angulating and leaning over the patient's body, and there is a fair chance that one of the arms is putting pressure on the face or chest. This is to be actively seen by the surgical assistant on the patient's side, who checks and keeps soft padding over the pressure areas. The assistant must alert the console surgeon if the robotic arms have undue movement, which might hit the patient's body parts.

Emergency Conversion during Surgery

An emergency conversion to an open surgical approach may be required mainly because of the blood loss or any major vascular injury. The procedures related to hepatobiliary systems are very prone to emergency conversions. In such a case, the robot must be rapidly undocked by the assistant surgeon on the patient's side and the scrub nurse until the lead surgeon can join to open up the patient. In such cases, the anesthetist must be ready with the protocol for massive transfusion and volume replacement products to maintain hemodynamic stability.

■ LAPAROSCOPIC SURGERY

Laparoscopic surgery involves the introduction of carbon dioxide gas into the abdomen to improve the visibility of the surgical field and thereby help the surgeon operate through small incisions. Carbon dioxide is the most commonly used gas for PnP as it meets nearly all the criteria of an ideal gas for insufflation **(Box 2)**.[4] The drawback of carbon dioxide is that it is absorbed intravascularly across the peritoneum. Air, oxygen, and nitrous oxide all support combustion, so they are not preferred. Helium is a good gas but is expensive, and if intravascular embolization occurs, its relative insolubility can lead to severe cardiovascular collapse.

BOX 2: Characteristics of an ideal gas for pneumoperitoneum.

Properties:
- It should not support combustion
- It should have limited systemic absorption
- If absorbed, it should have limited systemic effects
- It should be rapidly excreted
- It should be highly soluble in blood
- It should have limited physiological effects if intravascular embolism occurs

Physiological Effects of Pneumoperitoneum

Pneumoperitoneum induces pathophysiological changes in various organ systems via physical pressure and due to systemic absorption of carbon dioxide (CO_2). The absolute amount of intra-abdominal pressure (IAP) and the length of time this pressure is applied affect the extent of the pressure applied.

Physiological Effects due to Increased Intra-abdominal Pressure

Cardiovascular System

At IAP levels above 15 mm Hg, venous return decreases mainly because of a decrease in preload and an increase in afterload by compression of the inferior vena cava and the surrounding collateral vessels.[5] This leads to a fall in the cardiac output (CO) and hypotension, followed by an increase in the systemic vascular resistance (SVR) and arterial blood pressure in healthy patients with normal cardiovascular function. The aforementioned changes can reopen the antenatal shunts (transiently or permanently) in small children, therefore laparoscopic surgery may be challenging in neonates and infants with congenital.[6] Even at IAP levels <15 mm Hg, there is a "squeezing" out of blood from the splanchnic venous bed, increasing the venous return and thereby producing an increase in CO. The CO may also increase because of sympathetically-mediated peripheral vasoconstriction.[7]

Impact on Children

Neonates and infants below 3 months of age have a relatively fixed CO and cannot increase contractility because of the immature myocardial fibers. They can increase the CO only by an increase in the heart rate. These cardiovascular effects can be magnified by patient's positioning and the extent of the rise in IAP. A head-up position during laparoscopy as for a cholecystectomy can increase venous pooling, thereby reducing venous return and CO followed by hypotension in a hypovolemic child; whereas a head-down position, as is done for pelvic procedures, can cause an increase in venous return and preload with an increase in the central venous pressure (CVP), pulmonary capillary wedge pressure (PCWP), and mean arterial pressure.[8] Children have a high resting vagal tone, and a rapid PnP or insertion of trocars causes stimulation of the peritoneum, provoking bradycardia or asystole.[9]

Respiratory System

The increased IAP causes splinting and a cephalad shift of the diaphragm, leading to decreased functional residual capacity (FRC), lung compliance, and increased atelectasis. It also causes an increase in airway resistance, ventilation–perfusion (V/Q) mismatch with preferential ventilation of nondependent regions, and an increased possibility of bronchial mainstem intubation. The aforementioned changes result in the risk of developing hypoxia, hypercarbia, changes in ventilatory pressure, and risk of barotrauma during intermittent positive pressure ventilation (IPPV).[10] The Trendelenburg position worsens these effects, and the effect is less with the reverse Trendelenburg position.[11]

The difference between alveolar and intrapleural pressure is called transpulmonary pressure (Ptp). It leads to lung parenchymal injury with an increased risk of acute lung injury and respiratory distress syndrome as the Ptp increases. Pneumoperitoneum increases the external and intrapleural pressure, but PtP decreases so that one can safely increase the ventilator pressures proportional to the pressure provided.[4]

Impact on Children

The oxygen consumption in infants is higher (6–8 mL/kg/min) than in adults (2–3 mL/kg/min), making them more prone to hypoxia. There are increased chances of atelectasis in children because of their lower FRC making them prone to hypercarbia.[12] In otherwise healthy children, the impact of these respiratory changes is minimal and can be offset by changing the ventilatory parameters; however, hypoxia and hypercarbia may not be tolerated in children with respiratory diseases. In rare situations, an inadvertent venous rupture can lead to CO_2 emboli which can enter the arterial circulation via intrapulmonary shunting or a patent foramen ovale leading to hemodynamic collapse.[13]

Central Nervous System

Hypercarbia, increased SVR, head-down positioning, and elevated IAP develop whenever there is an increased intracranial pressure and a decrease in cerebral perfusion pressure. The creation of PnP causes an increase in the middle cerebral artery blood flow velocity even if CO_2 reactivity is normal in younger children.[14] Preterm infants may be at risk for intraventricular hemorrhage in these situations.[15]

Renal System

The PnP causes an increase in renovascular resistance and decreases flow through the renal vein by compression of the renal parenchyma and vessels. It also causes increased release of antidiuretic hormone, activating the renin-angiotensin system.[16] Patients may develop oliguria during the laparoscopic surgery, which may continue for many hours postoperatively.[17]

Gastrointestinal System

Pneumoperitoneum can lead to a decrease in splanchnic circulation and, therefore, a decrease in hepatic blood flow and bowel perfusion.[18] In contrast, hypercarbia can lead to splanchnic vasodilatation, causing no significant effect on blood flow.[19]

Ophthalmic System

Pneumoperitoneum and Trendelenburg position can increase the intraocular pressure (IOP), which may last 45–60 minutes after surgery in adults.[20] In adults, a steep Trendelenburg position may lead to a rare but severe complication like blindness, especially if the surgery is prolonged, however there is no evidence that this blindness can occur in children.[21] This is important in children with glaucoma, where the increase in IOP can be magnified, leading to vision loss.

Other Effects

An increase in IAP can increase static venous blood flow increasing the chances of deep vein thrombosis, especially during lengthy procedures. It has been shown that laparoscopy causes reduced release of acute stress mediators (glucose, leucocyte, and C-reactive protein) and interleukin compared to laparotomy and a decrease in plasma concentration of catecholamine, cortisol, insulin, epinephrine, prolactin, and growth hormones.[8]

Physiological Effects due to Increased Carbon Dioxide Absorption

The effect of systemic CO_2 absorption on the body depends on the amount of CO_2 which diffuses. The amount of CO_2 that diffuses across the peritoneum and into the bloodstream depends on the Fick's law [Vgas α A/t.D (P1–P2)].[4] According to this law, the gas diffusion across a membrane is proportional to the area of the membrane in contact with the gas (A), the difference in partial pressure of the gas across the membrane (P1–P2), and a diffusion constant (D). The diffusion is, therefore, proportional to the solubility of the gas and inversely proportional to the square root of the molecular weight and the thickness of the membrane.

If the surgical procedure continues for >1 hour, it results in hypercarbia because of increased CO_2 absorption. This hypercarbia stimulates the sympathetic system causing an increase in pulse rate, systemic blood pressure, and sensitization of the myocardium to the arrhythmogenic effects of catecholamines while using volatile anesthetic agents.[22] This requires increased minute ventilation to restore the end-tidal carbon dioxide ($ETCO_2$) to the baseline. For about 10 minutes after deflation of the abdomen, CO_2 decreases, leading to a difference between the arterial and end-tidal CO_2 (0.33–8.8 mm Hg). Hypercarbia is magnified in children mainly because of an increased ratio of peritoneal surface area to mass, less peritoneal thickness, smaller muscle bulk, and less distance between vessels and the serous surface. Even an IAP of <10 mm Hg causes CO_2 absorption.[23]

Which Patients should be Selected for Robotic Surgery?

There are no specific parameters to select patients for robotic surgery in children. The expert consensus from Italian Society of Pediatric and Neonatal Anesthesia and Intensive Care (SARNePI) and Italian Societies of Pediatric Surgery (SICP) was that robotic surgery is highly costly and should be performed mainly in complex pediatric reconstructive procedures such as pyeloplasty, fundoplication, and choledochal cyst removal.[3] Its use in patients <1 year or weighing <10 kg is challenging. However, based on the surgeon's experience, robotic surgery can also be performed in patients with lower weight or age. In general, any procedure which can be done by laparoscopic approach can also be done by robotic surgery. The patient's physical size is essential, as the robotic system requires a minimum distance of 8–10 cm between two adjacent ports. If this can be achieved on a patient, then the surgical procedure is feasible by the robot. Enhanced Recovery After Surgery (ERAS®) protocols may be adopted for all the robotic surgical procedures for economic sustainability.[24]

■ PREREQUISITES FOR ROBOTIC PROCEDURES

Two IV lines with long extensions are placed in the upper limb before the surgical robot is docked because securing another IV line will be difficult in an emergency. Intravenous access in the upper limb is desirable to avoid the slow onset of the effect of drugs given in the lower limb owing to increased IAP. In addition, one of these IV lines can be used to measure intraoperative electrolytes or hematocrit in the event of bleeding. Infusion lines should be of extra length and have no kinking or obstruction. The injection ports on IV lines should be easy to access. It is preferable to keep one arm free for access if needed by the anesthetist. Attention should be paid to the fixation of the IV, arterial, and central venous access lines to avoid damage to the vessel wall. Malfunction, erosion, inflammation, thrombosis, occlusion, and exit-site infections are also possible.

Placing a nasogastric tube is essential for decompressing the stomach to prevent obscuring the surgeon's surgical view and prevent gastric injury while introducing the trocars. It also lowers the risk of regurgitation, which increased IAP may cause. Urinary catheter placement is required for the measurement of urine output, for fluid management during surgery, and to avoid bladder injury during trocar placement.

Positioning of the patient during robotic surgery is aimed at optimizing the visibility of the surgical field view, giving access to the patient to the anesthesiologist, and at the same time, minimizing the development of compression injuries. Considering the above factors, the position should be established in consultation between the surgeon and the anesthesiologist. Patients are either supine or in a lateral decubitus position for robotic surgery.

For facilitating surgical visualization, the bed is tilted laterally. Patients should be secured firmly to the operating table, preferably with the mattress to avoid slipping, and soft pillows, a foam ring, or padding should protect the patient's head and pressure points. It should be ensured that moving robotic arms do not touch the patient. One should protect the eyes and aids to prevent nerve injuries (e.g., heel and elbow pads, cotton padding, and pillows).

PREOPERATIVE ASSESSMENT AND INVESTIGATIONS

During the preoperative assessment, one should identify any underlying medical condition likely to impact anesthesia management by history and physical examination and stratify the risk. *Congenital anomalies* involving the cardiovascular, respiratory, and central nervous systems should be diagnosed and investigated because they may get aggravated by PnP and surgery. IAP and CO_2 absorption impact the cardiorespiratory changes and could influence the development and severity of hypoxia and pulmonary hypoperfusion. Minimally invasive surgery is thus avoided in pediatric patients with congenital heart disease (CHD);[25] however, studies about these issues in children of <5 years of age with CHD have not shown any harmful effect if the IAP is kept between 8 and 12 mm Hg.[6] However, in children with severe heart disease, transesophageal echocardiography monitoring is essential, and a pediatric cardiac anesthetist should perform presurgical evaluation and be available during perioperative management. In children with glaucoma, IOP should be stabilized before robotic surgery.[26]

Based on the clinical state of the child, laboratory investigations are performed. Blood loss during robotic laparoscopic procedures is usually minimal. However, there is always a possibility of damage to blood vessels, so blood should be readily available. A preoperative hemoglobin value, renal function tests in case of kidney disease, liver function tests for liver dysfunction, and electrocardiography (ECG) and echocardiography (ECHO) in children with cardiac disease may be required as a baseline.

Preoperative Preparation

The child should fast before surgery based on the 6-4-2/1 rule. Drinking clear fluids up to 1–2 hours prior is recommended, as it has been shown to improve perioperative outcomes. It is also one of the essential components of ERAS® protocol.[24]

Premedication is not required in the neonatal population but would be required in children >1 year of age to allay anxiety. The most frequently used agent is midazolam, administered orally or by IV, depending on the availability of vascular access. However, α-adrenergic antagonists such as clonidine and dexmedetomidine may also be utilized for premedication. Children with airway reactivity may require high-flow nebulization of a bronchodilator and an anticholinergic; aspiration prophylaxis with histamine type 2 (H_2)-antagonists and motility agents may be required in children with gastric distension/delayed gastric emptying; some may like to give an anticholinergic agent, to blunt cholinergic-mediated airway reactivity and prevent bradycardia during laparoscopy. The intravascular volume should be checked in neonates coming for surgery.

MONITORING

Monitoring is routine, including electrocardiography, heart rate, noninvasive blood pressure (NIBP), oxygen saturation (SpO_2) both pre- and postductal, especially in neonates and infants, $ETCO_2$, temperature, urine output and inspired and expired concentration of oxygen, air, and anesthetic agent. Peak inspiratory pressure (PIP) and exhaled tidal volume should be measured to detect any ventilatory leak pre- and postinsufflation. Bispectral index (BIS) or entropy should be used for easier titration of anesthetic agents for early recovery. Monitoring neuromuscular blockade helps avoid patient movement during surgery, preventing vascular or organ injury.

Invasive blood pressure (IBP) is optional but essential for measuring arterial carbon dioxide partial pressure ($PaCO_2$) as there is a significant gradient between $ETCO_2$ and $PaCO_2$ during PnP and for calculating the base deficit and electrolytes. Central venous access is not mandatory but must be based on specific needs such as administration of hyperosmolar fluids, blood, antibiotics, and vasoactive drugs. Depending on the child's age and the anesthesiologist's expertise, it can be placed under ultrasound guidance via the internal jugular, subclavian, brachiocephalic, or axillary vein.

During anesthesia, children are prone to hypothermia as their body surface area to mass ratio is more and subcutaneous fat is less. This is compounded by introducing cold, nonhumidified CO_2 into the abdominal cavity and prolonged operative time. Hypothermia can be avoided by using a warming mattress, heat humidifier, forced air blankets, warm IV fluids and blood, and warm insufflating gas with flows below 2 L/min are recommended, therefore monitoring the core body temperature of the child is essential.

ANESTHESIA MANAGEMENT

Anesthetic management is not specific to the robotic surgery. Induction can be inhalational or IV, depending on the availability of IV access. A modified rapid sequence induction may be practiced in children undergoing emergency laparoscopy. Cuffed endotracheal tube (ETT) should be utilized for intubation to avoid a decrease in tidal volume (due to increased gas leak around the ETT) caused by a reduction in pulmonary compliance without increasing peak airway pressure and fresh gas flow to keep minute ventilation at adequate levels. The endotracheal tube should be correctly and securely fixed, and arms placed on the side of the body.

A balanced anesthetic technique with controlled ventilation using inhalational agents (isoflurane, desflurane, and sevoflurane), or TIVA (propofol and opioids—fentanyl and remifentanil) and nondepolarizing muscle relaxant (such as atracurium and vecuronium) is preferred. Nitrous oxide is avoided because it causes a decrease in the inspired oxygen concentration (FiO_2) and a probable risk of venous embolism. It may also cause distension of the bowel which will hamper the surgeon's view during laparoscopic surgery as well as causes an increase in the incidence of postoperative nausea and vomiting (PONV).

Controlled ventilation facilitates CO_2 removal and minimizes the FRC reduction caused by an increased IAP and patient positioning. To maintain $ETCO_2$ and counteract the reduction in respiratory compliance and increased resistance, an increase in minute ventilation by 25–30% and an increase in peak inspiratory pressure is required to maintain normocarbia or hypercarbia is limited. Positive end-expiratory pressure (PEEP) counteracts the effects of increased IAP on the lower lung zones and the development of atelectasis, and an increase in FiO_2 is required to maintain the oxygen saturation.

Balanced salt solutions are the preferred IV fluids administered during the surgical procedure following the Holliday-Segar formula or the guidelines made by the Association of the Scientific Medical Societies of Germany.[27] Fluid administration should be guided by maintaining euvolemia and avoiding hypotension and anuria after the institution of PnP. The calculated fluid deficit before surgery is replaced in the first hour, followed by maintenance IV fluids. The advantage of this fluid resuscitation is reducing the incidence of hypotension with the PnP and in urine production throughout the surgery. A background infusion of 10 mL/kg/h of a buffered isotonic polyelectrolyte solution with 1–2% glucose can be established. The infusion regimen can be adjusted based on the duration of surgery, blood loss, acid-base balance, and glucose level.

When the surgical procedure ends, the peritoneum should be completely deflated. The neuromuscular blockade should be reversed using a combination of neostigmine and atropine or glycopyrrolate. Postoperative nausea and vomiting prophylaxis with dexamethasone (0.15–0.2 mg/kg) or ondansetron (0.2 mg/kg) is also recommended.

Pneumoperitoneum and Ventilation Strategies

In pediatric laparoscopies, a moderate-to-low IAP of 6–10 mm Hg (compared to an IAP of 12–15 mm Hg in adults) is recommended as it minimally alters the splanchnic perfusion, thereby causing minimal and transient organ dysfunction.[28] Also, due to decreased compliance of the abdominal wall in children, adequate operating conditions can be achieved at lower levels of IAP.[29] In addition, insufflation pressures of >10 mm Hg cannot increase the workspace in infants, therefore, the pressure produced by the PnP should be maintained as 6-10 mm Hg in children <2 years old, 10-12 mm Hg in 2-10 years old, and 12 mm Hg in >10 years old.[3] The volume of insufflating gas is kept at 0.9 L, and the flow rate is kept below 2 L/min in children compared to 2.5-5 L and 4-5 L/min, respectively in the adults.

Volume-controlled and volume-targeted pressure-controlled ventilation (PCV) can be utilized in children undergoing minimally invasive surgery.[30,31] In a study by Kim et al., the mean airway pressure and dynamic compliance were significantly higher when using pressure-controlled ventilation with 5 cmH$_2$O PEEP compared to volume-controlled ventilation (VCV) with 5 cmH$_2$O. The authors found no differences in other ventilatory parameters and oxygen saturation, so they recommended that VCV and PCV can be safely used in children undergoing laparoscopic procedures.[30]

General anesthesia (GA) leads to a loss of FRC, thereby inducing pulmonary atelectasis. In the pediatric population, the effect of GA on FRC is aggravated due to their compliant chest wall and easily collapsible airways. The creation of PnP in laparoscopic surgeries further increases the shunt fraction and dead space. In the lung-protective ventilation strategy (LPVS), administration of lower TV, sustained PEEP, and the decreased concentration of FiO$_2$ is practiced to avoid lung barotrauma caused by the increased abdominal pressures; however, LPVS leads to a steady decline in FRC and the development of alveolar collapse. The incidence of atelectasis in infants has been reported to exceed 50% within the first minute of induction of GA, and the incidence increases further during laparoscopic surgeries. Various studies have shown that applying a recruitment maneuver/sustained higher positive pressure can help decrease atelectasis in the dependent portions of the lungs.[12,32-35]

■ POSTOPERATIVE MANAGEMENT OF PAIN

Laparoscopic surgery generally causes less postoperative pain than the open surgery. The pain may be due to the incision made for placement of laparoscopic ports and diffuse abdominal and shoulder pain due to the PnP. The cause of shoulder pain may be related to the diaphragm's peritoneal surface getting irritated and desiccating the peritoneum with the insufflated dry CO$_2$ gas. For incisional pain, local anesthetic infiltration into the port site, caudal blockade, nonsteroidal anti-inflammatory drugs (NSAIDs) such as ketorolac, and low doses of opioids can be utilized.[36] Nerve blocks such as transversus abdominis plane (TAP) block, paravertebral block, and erector spinae block can be performed using local anesthetics alone or in combination with additives such as clonidine and dexmedetomidine.[37-39]

■ COMPLICATIONS

The incidence of complications during robotic laparoscopic surgery is relatively low and is related to the surgeon's experience and type of procedure. The possible complications are summarized in **Table 1**.

TABLE 1: Complications associated with robotic laparoscopic surgery.

Cardiovascular	Respiratory	Others
• Hypotension • Hypertension • Arrhythmias	• Pneumothorax • Pneumopericardium • Pneumomediastinum • Subcutaneous emphysema • Gas embolism • Hypoxia • Hypercarbia • Atelectasis • Bronchospasm • Endobronchial intubation	• Hypothermia • Peripheral neuropathy • Plexus injury • Airway, facial, and brain edema • Soft tissue injury • Perioperative visual loss • Vascular, bowel, and bladder injury • Compartment syndrome • Thromboembolism

CONCLUSION

The introduction of robots in the field of pediatric surgery has produced challenges for both the surgeon and the anesthetist. To have a successful surgical outcome, the anesthetist must understand the robot's configuration and the physiological impact it causes. The anesthesia management must focus on the problems caused due to patient positioning, limited airway and IV access, hypothermia, pneumoperitoneum, and ventilation.

REFERENCES

1. Bansal D, Cost NG, DeFoor WR, Reddy PP, Minevich EA, Vanderbrink BA, et al. Infant robotic pyeloplasty: comparison with an open cohort. J Pediatr Urol. 2014;10(2):380-5.
2. Ostlie DJ, Miller KA, Woods RK, Holcomb GW 3rd. Single cannula technique and robotic telescopic assistance in infants and children who require laparoscopic Nissen fundoplication. J Pediatr Surg. 2003;38(1):111-5.
3. Tesoro S, Gamba P, Bertozzi M, Borgogni R, Caramelli F, Cobellis G, et al. Pediatric robotic surgery: issues in management—expert consensus from the Italian Society of Pediatric and Neonatal Anesthesia and Intensive Care (SARNePI) and the Italian Society of Pediatric Surgery (SICP). Surg Endosc. 2022;36(11):7877-97.
4. Lasersohn L. Anaesthetic considerations for paediatric laparoscopy. S Afr J Surg. 2011;49(1):22-6.
5. Atkinson TM, Giraud GD, Togioka BM, Jones DB, Cigarroa JE. Cardiovascular and ventilatory consequences of laparoscopic surgery. Circulation. 2017;135(7):700-10.
6. Kim J, Sun Z, Englum BR, Allori AC, Adibe OO, Rice HE, et al. Laparoscopy is safe in infants and neonates with congenital heart disease: a national study of 3684 patients. J Laparoendosc Adv Surg Tech A. 2016;26(10):836-9.
7. De Waal EE, Kalkman CJ. Haemodynamic changes during low-pressure carbon dioxide pneumoperitoneum in young children. Paediatr Anaesth. 2003;13(1):18-25.
8. O'Leary E, Hubbard K, Tormey W, Cunningham AJ. Laparoscopic cholecystectomy: haemodynamic and neuroendocrine responses after pneumoperitoneum and changes in position. Br J Anaesth. 1996;76(5):640-4.

9. Jung KT, Kim SH, Kim JW, So KY. Bradycardia during laparoscopic surgery due to high flow rate of CO_2 insufflation. Korean J Anesthesiol. 2013;65(3):276-7.
10. Tobias JD. Anaesthesia for minimally invasive surgery in children. Best Pract Res Clin Anaesthesiol. 2002;16(1):115-30.
11. Kalmar AF, Foubert L, Hendrickx JFA, Mottrie A, Absalom A, Mortier EP, et al. Influence of steep Trendelenburg position and CO(2) pneumoperitoneum on cardiovascular, cerebrovascular, and respiratory homeostasis during robotic prostatectomy. Br J Anaesth. 2010;104(4):433-9.
12. Acosta CM, Sara T, Carpinella M, Volpicelli G, Ricci L, Poliotto S, et al. Lung recruitment prevents collapse during laparoscopy in children: a randomised controlled trial. Eur J Anaesthesiol. 2018;35(8):573-80.
13. Lalwani K, Aliason I. Cardiac arrest in the neonate during laparoscopic surgery. Anesth Analg. 2009;109(3):760-2.
14. Kim MS, Bai SJ, Lee JR, Choi YD, Kim YJ, Choi SH. Increase in intracranial pressure during carbon dioxide pneumoperitoneum with steep trendelenburg positioning proven by ultrasonographic measurement of optic nerve sheath diameter. J Endourol. 2014;28(7):801-6.
15. Kamata M, Hakim M, Walia H, Tumin D, Tobias JD. Changes in cerebral and renal oxygenation during laparoscopic pyloromyotomy. J Clin Monit Comput. 2020;34(4):699-703.
16. Dunn MD, McDougall EM. Renal physiology. Laparoscopic considerations. Urol Clin North Am. 2000;27(4):609-14.
17. Gómez Dammeier BH, Karanik E, Glüer S, Jesch NK, Kübler J, Latta K, et al. Anuria during pneumoperitoneum in infants and children: a prospective study. J Pediatr Surg 2005;40(9):1454-8.
18. Kotake Y, Takeda J, Matsumoto M, Tagawa M, Kikuchi H. Subclinical hepatic dysfunction in laparoscopic cholecystectomy and laparoscopic colectomy. Br J Anaesth. 2001;87(5):774-7.
19. Meierhenrich R, Gauss A, Vandenesch P, Georgieff M, Poch B, Schütz W. The effects of intraabdominally insufflated carbon dioxide on hepatic blood flow during laparoscopic surgery assessed by transesophageal echocardiography. Anesth Analg. 2005;100(2):340-7.
20. Karabayirli S, Çimen NK, Muslu B, Tenlik A, Gözdemir M, Sert H, et al. Effect of positive end-expiratory pressure administration on intraocular pressure in laparoscopic cholecystectomy: randomised controlled trial. Eur J Anaesthesiol. 2016;33(9):696-9.
21. Ripa M, Schipa C, Kopsacheilis N, Nomikarios M, Perrotta G, De Rosa C, et al. The impact of steep Trendelenburg position on intraocular pressure. J Clin Med. 2022;11(10):2844.
22. Fitzgerald SD, Andrus CH, Baudendistel LJ, Dahms TE, Kaminski DL. Hypercarbia during carbon dioxide pneumoperitoneum. Am J Surg. 1992;163(1):186-90.
23. Pennant JH. Anesthesia for laparoscopy in the pediatric patient. Anesthesiol Clinics N Am. 2001;19(1):68-88.
24. Shinnick JK, Short HL, Heiss KF, Santore MT, Blakely ML, Raval MV. Enhancing recovery in pediatric surgery: a review of the literature. J Surg Res. 2016;202(1):165-76.
25. Gillory LA, Megison ML, Harmon CM, Chen MK, Anderson S, Chong AJ, et al. Laparoscopic surgery in children with congenital heart disease. J Pediatr Surg. 2012;47(6):1084-8.

26. Astuto M, Minardi C, Uva MG, Gullo A. Intraocular pressure during laparoscopic surgery in paediatric patients. Br J Ophthalmol. 2011;95(2):294-5.
27. Sumpelmann R, Becke K, Brenner S, Breschan C, Eich C, Hohne C. et al. Perioperative intravenous fluid therapy in children: guidelines from the Association of the Scientific Medical Societies in Germany. Pediatr Anesth. 2017;27(1):10-8.
28. Sureka SK, Patidar N, Mittal V, Kapoor R, Srivastava A, Kishore K, et al. Safe and optimal pneumoperitoneal pressure for transperitoneal laparoscopic renal surgery in infant less than 10 kg, looked beyond intraoperative period: a prospective randomized study. J Pediatr Urol. 2016;12(5):281.e1-7.
29. Van Batavia JP, Casale P. Robotic surgery of the kidney and ureter in pediatric patients. Curr Urol Rep. 2013;14(4):373-8.
30. Kim JY, Shin CS, Lee KC, Chang YJ, Kwak HJ. Effect of pressure-versus volume-controlled ventilation on the ventilatory and hemodynamic parameters during laparoscopic appendectomy in children: a prospective, randomized study. J Laparoendosc Adv Surg Tech A. 2011;21(7):655-8.
31. Feldman JM. Optimal ventilation of the anesthetized pediatric patient. Anesth Analg. 2015;120(1):165-75.
32. Cinnella G, Grasso S, Spadaro S, Rauseo M, Mirabella L, Salatto P, et al. Effects of recruitment maneuver and positive end-expiratory pressure on respiratory mechanics and transpulmonary pressure during laparoscopic surgery. Anesthesiology. 2013;118(1):114-22.
33. Kim JY, Shin CS, Kim HS, Jung WS, Kwak HJ. Positive end-expiratory pressure in pressure-controlled ventilation improves ventilatory and oxygenation parameters during laparoscopic cholecystectomy. Surg Endosc. 2010;24(5):1099-103.
34. Acosta CM, Vargas MPL, Oropel F, Valente L, Ricci L, Natal M, et al. Prevention of atelectasis by continuous positive airway pressure in anaesthetised children: A randomised controlled study. Eur J Anaesthesiol. 2021;38(1):41-8.
35. Bhardwaj N, Sarkar S, Yaddanapudi S, Jain D. Effect of two different levels of positive end-expiratory pressure (PEEP) on oxygenation and ventilation during pneumoperitoneum for laparoscopic surgery in children: a randomized controlled study. Saudi J Anaesth. 2022;16(4):430-6.
36. Molinaro F, Krasniqi P, Scolletta S, Giuntini L, Navarra C, Puzzutiello R, et al. Considerations regarding pain management and anesthesiological aspects in pediatric patients undergoing minimally invasive surgery: robotic vs. laparoscopic-thoracoscopic approach. J Robot Surg. 2020;14(3):423-30.
37. Karnik PP, Dave NM, Shah HB, Kulkarni K. Comparison of ultrasound-guided transversus abdominis plane (TAP) block versus local infiltration during paediatric laparoscopic surgeries. Indian J Anaesth. 2019;63(5):356-60.
38. Faasse MA, Lindgren BW, Frainey BT, Marcus CR, Szczodry DM, Glaser AP, et al. Perioperative effects of caudal and transversus abdominis plane (TAP) blocks for children undergoing urologic robot-assisted laparoscopic surgery. J Pediatr Urol. 2015;11(3):121.e1-7.
39. Srinivasan AK, Shrivastava D, Kurzweil RE, Weiss DA, Long CJ, Shukla AR. Port site local anesthetic infiltration Vs single-dose intrathecal opioid injection to control perioperative pain in children undergoing minimal invasive surgery: a comparative analysis. Urology. 2016;97:179-83.

CHAPTER 13

Hepatobiliary Disease and Anesthesia

Tejal Desai, Hesham Youssef, Achal Dhir

ABSTRACT

The liver is a vital organ that performs several essential functions. Liver disease is a multisystem condition with far-reaching consequences. Anesthesia and surgery can cause complications, resulting in significant morbidity and mortality, even in patients with compensated cirrhosis. Patients with liver cirrhosis undergo a surgical procedure in their last 2 years of life. Perioperative mortality is 2–10 times higher in patients with cirrhosis than those without cirrhosis.

A thorough understanding of liver disease pathophysiology is imperative to manage sick patients. Depending on the time interval between the triggering event and the onset of symptoms, liver disease can be classified as acute, acute-on-chronic, or chronic. With the advent of direct antiviral agents, the disease burden of the hepatitis C virus (HCV) is declining. In contrast, alcohol and fatty liver disease remains the most common causes of chronic liver disease. Various scoring systems have been developed for disease severity and to stratify these patients for candidacy for the liver transplantation.

For optimal outcomes, preoperative optimization and safe anesthetic management are essential in patients with liver disease undergoing surgery. This chapter highlights the issues encountered while managing patients with hepatobiliary disease.

Keywords: Hepatobiliary disease; Liver cirrhosis; Portal hypertension; End-stage liver disease; Chronic liver disease

■ KEY POINTS

- Hepato-biliary diseases account for 4% of all the deaths worldwide.
- Preoperative diagnosis, optimization, and perioperative management are vital for patients with liver disease.
- Acute liver failure results in rapid deterioration of liver function, causing encephalopathy and coagulopathy in individuals without preexisting liver disease. Survival rates have changed for the better with liver transplantation.

- Acute-on-chronic liver failure is a severe clinical syndrome due to acute deterioration of chronic liver disease, leading to high short-term death rates. It is managed by treating the underlying etiology and precipitating factors while controlling and treating the complications.
- Chronic liver disease is a continuous hepatic inflammation and destruction, followed by liver parenchyma regeneration and fibrotic band formation termed cirrhosis. Cirrhosis typically has a phase of asymptomatic compensation followed by decompensation and its associated complications.
- Uncompensated cirrhosis may present as jaundice, ascites, encephalopathy, portal hypertensive gastrointestinal bleeding, and the involvement of systemic organs like kidneys, lungs, and portal circulation.
- An understanding of physiological alterations in liver disease is crucial for intraoperative management.

INTRODUCTION

Although the liver constitutes around 2.5% of the body weight, it receives one-fourth of the cardiac output.[1] It performs several vital functions; such as plasma protein synthesis, bile production, gluconeogenesis, drug, and lipid metabolism; and storage of vitamins, minerals, and glucose. It synthesizes procoagulants, anticoagulants, fibrinolytics, and antifibrinolytics, hence playing an essential role in hemostasis.[2] Hepatic function is disrupted due to various disease states, resulting in dysfunction or failure.

Deaths from hepatobiliary diseases account for 4% of all the deaths worldwide, or over 2 million annually.[3] Globally, alcohol is the primary etiology of alcohol-associated hepatitis and cirrhosis and accounts for 60% of the cases in Europe and the Americas[4,5] followed by nonalcoholic fatty liver disease (NAFLD).[3] In patients with cirrhosis, nontransplant surgery and anesthesia can lead to postoperative complications.[6] Preoperative diagnosis, optimization, and perioperative management are vital for patients with liver disease. This chapter focuses on the pathophysiology of liver disease prognosis based on the scoring systems and anesthetic management in acute and chronic liver disease.

ANATOMY AND PHYSIOLOGY

The portal triad encompassing the portal vein, hepatic artery, and bile duct sits at each corner of the hexagonal structure known as the *lobule* (**Fig. 1**).

This lobule, a nonhomogenous unit, has three zones. Blood, rich in oxygen, nutrients, and metabolic products, flows opposite to the flow of bile.[7]
- Zone 1, the periportal area, is highly perfused. It involves glucose, fatty acid, cholesterol, and urea metabolism.
- Zone 3 surrounds the central vein and is responsible for bile acid, glycolysis, and drug metabolism.
- Zone 2 lies between zones 1 and 3.[8]

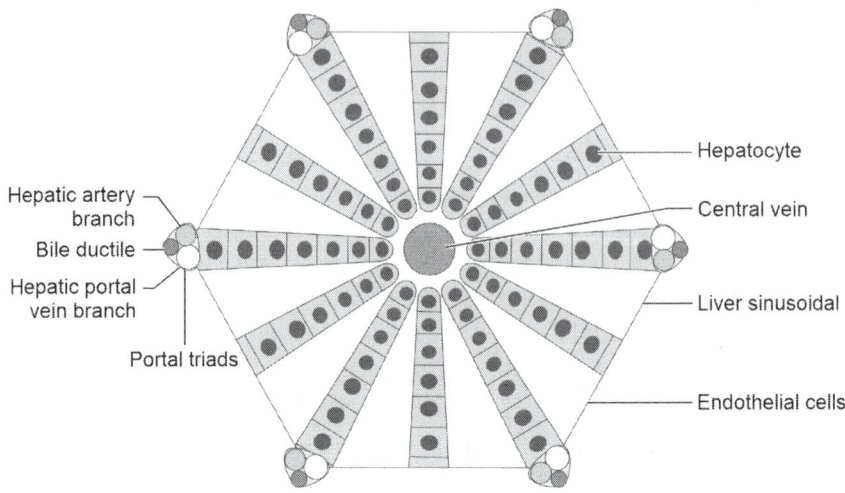

Fig. 1: Hepatic lobule.

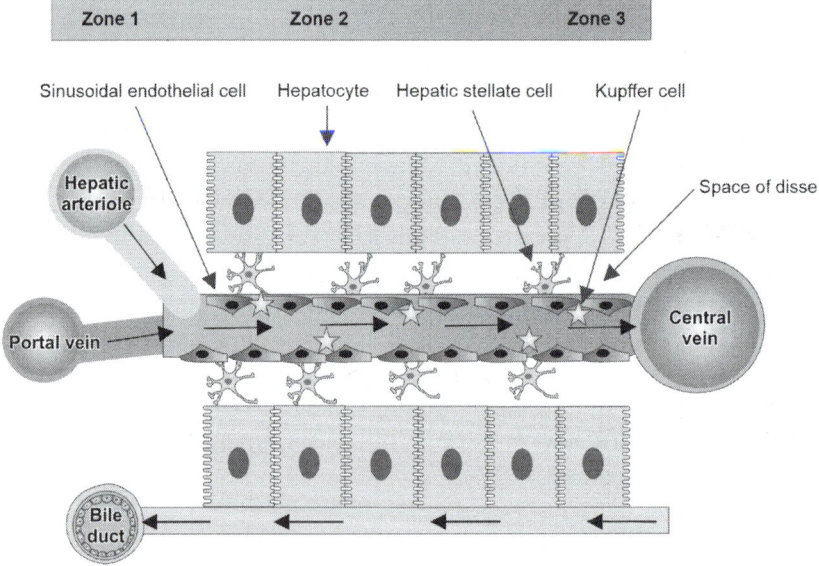

Fig. 2: Schematics of hepatic lobule and three zones.

Sinusoidal channels direct blood flow from the portal triad to the hepatic venules. Kupffer cells (KCs) and specialized liver sinusoidal endothelial cells (LSECs) line the sinusoids.[9] LSECs separate blood from hepatocytes and stellate cells.[10] They are characterized by the fenestrations allowing the exchange of essential nutrients and metabolic by-products **(Fig. 2)**.

Liver sinusoidal endothelial cells ensure a low portal pressure regardless of fluctuations in hepatic flow during digestion.[10] After liver resection surgery, increased blood flow increases the shear stress on hepatocytes. This high shear stress then stimulates the production of nitric oxide and hepatocyte growth factor by the LSECs, leading to liver regeneration.[11] However, extensive resections can lead to very high shear stress due to high blood flow per unit volume of the liver, ultimately causing irreversible damage to the LSECs.[10] Attenutation of this shear stress by procedures that modulate hepatic blood flow such as portosystemic shunts, splenectomy, and splenic artery embolization can prevent postoperative liver failure.[12,13] While LSECs play an essential role in liver regeneration, aberrant LSEC activation can lead to liver fibrosis.[14]

Hepatic stellate cells (HSCs) are present in the subendothelial space and serve many functions, such as hepatic development, regeneration, immune modulation, angiogenesis, and storage of vitamin A.[15] These cells get activated in response to liver injury, and transform into cells with fibrogenic and contractile capacity.[15] Kupffer cells are macrophages present in the liver that reduce endotoxins and improve the host defense system.[16]

LIVER DISEASE

Liver disease can be classified as an acute, chronic, or acute-on-chronic, depending on the time between the onset of symptoms, disease progression, and the triggering events.

Acute Liver Disease

Acute liver failure (ALF) is a rare condition in which rapid deterioration of liver function results in encephalopathy and coagulopathy in individuals without preexisting liver disease. The most widely accepted definition of ALF includes evidence of coagulation abnormality, usually an international normalized ratio (INR) of above 1.5, and any degree of encephalopathy in a patient without preexisting cirrhosis occurring within <26 weeks from the beginning of symptoms.[17] The duration of onset of encephalopathy differs in different geographies and varies between 4 and 24 weeks.[18] Acute liver failure results from massive hepatocellular damage and has a complex course.[19] Its mortality can range from 40 to 50%, depending on the etiology and inappropriate treatment decisions.[19] Survival rates have changed for the better with liver transplantation; however, sudden cerebral herniation due to brain edema can lead to significant early mortality.[20] In most others with ALF, death is due to sepsis and multiorgan failure (MOF).[19] Drug overdose (paracetamol), autoimmune hepatitis, and metabolic diseases are the most common causes in the Western world,[21] viral hepatitis contributes to 90% of the cases in India, with contributions from antitubercular drugs and complementary and alternative therapies as well.[22]

Prognosis of Acute Liver Failure

The goal of prognostication of ALF is to ascertain which patients will benefit from liver transplantation and which are expected to undergo spontaneous recovery. Etiology, age, and severity of encephalopathy are the most important factors for predicting outcomes in ALF. In a prospective study, survival without needing a liver transplant was more than half in patients with ALF due to acetaminophen overdose, hepatitis A, ischemia, or pregnancy, but survival was poor when Budd–Chiari syndrome, Wilson disease, hepatitis B, autoimmune hepatitis, cancer, or an indeterminate cause led to ALF.[23]

Predictive models used in ALF are King's College criteria (KCC), Clichy score, model for end-stage liver disease (MELD) score, chronic liver failure sequential organ failure assessment (CLIF-SOFA), and acute liver failure early dynamic (ALFED) score. CLIF-SOFA may be better than MELD in predicting mortality in ALF.[24]

King's College criteria shows 68% sensitivity, and 82% specificity in predicting outcomes in nonparacetamol-induced ALF.[25] Specificity was most accurate in severe encephalopathy grades and when the criteria were assessed at regular intervals during the clinical trajectory of ALF. The ALFED score is deemed to be an appropriate score in Indian patients.[21] Clichy criteria were derived in 1986 for prognostication in patients with hepatitis B-related ALF but require factor V measurements.[24]

Pathophysiology of Acute Liver Failure

The clinical picture of ALF is either due to the etiology of primary liver injury or secondary to MOF. Secondary MOF shows a sepsis-like view with low systemic vascular resistance, dysfunctional oxygen delivery to the tissues, poor gas exchange, and lactic acidosis. Dysregulation of renovascular and cerebrovascular tone causes functional renal failure and hepatic encephalopathy (HE). Later in the clinical course, an anti-inflammatory response culminates in immunosuppression and the possibility of infection.[26]

Inflammation causes changes in the permeability of the blood–brain barrier (BBB), leading to the buildup of glutamine and activated microglia, and this, in turn causes cerebral edema.[27]

Management of Acute Liver Failure

Detailed management of acute liver failure is beyond the scope of this chapter, and this section will encompass the general management of critically ill patients with ALF in the intensive care unit. N-acetyl cysteine has shown improved outcomes without needing liver transplants in nonparacetamol ALF in patients with lower grades of encephalopathy.[28] Management of lower grades of encephalopathy includes lactulose to lower ammonia levels. More severe grades of encephalopathy will need endotracheal intubation and mechanical ventilation because of the risks of airway obstruction and aspiration.[29] Mild hyperventilation can help regulate end-tidal CO_2 in raised intracranial pressure (ICP) cases. Management of raised ICP includes frequent neurological monitoring and

ICP monitors to guide management with mannitol and hypertonic saline.[30] Short-acting barbiturates may be used in refractory cases as a short-term salvage therapy and hypothermia to a core temperature of 35–36° C.[31,32] Early initiation of continuous venovenous hemofiltration leads to adequate clearance of ammonia.[33] Due to the risk of hypoglycemia in this group of patients, intravenous glucose infusions may be needed. Hypotonic fluids can lead to hyponatremia and worsen cerebral edema, so they must be used judiciously.[31] Coagulopathy may be corrected by vitamin K or fresh frozen plasma (FFP). Vasopressors can help achieve a mean arterial pressure (MAP) of >80 mm Hg and cerebral perfusion pressure of >60 mm Hg.[34] Vasopressin increases cerebral perfusion without increasing ICP and is an excellent agent to add to norepinephrine. **Table 1** depicts the management of ALF patients with raised ICP and cerebral edema.

Acute-on-chronic Liver Failure

Acute-on-chronic liver failure (ACLF) is a severe clinical syndrome due to acute deterioration of chronic liver disease, leading to high short-term death rates. While about half of the ACLF cases have no precipitating cause, sepsis, continued alcohol intake, and relapse of viral hepatitis can lead to clinical deterioration characteristic of ACLF.[35] Prognostic scores can guide treatment strategies to achieve good outcomes for these patients.

Strategies for Managing Acute-on-chronic Liver Failure

Currently, there is no specific treatment for ACLF. Management strategy includes treating the underlying etiology and precipitating factors while preventing, controlling, and treating the complications. Artificial liver support systems and liver transplantation remain viable options. Stem cell therapy appears promising, albeit results of ongoing clinical trials are awaited.[36] Acute-on-chronic liver failure management is summarized in **Table 2**.

Admission of ACLF patients should be considered, preferably in a center performing liver transplants. Close organ-specific monitoring and treatment are required to restrict the development of MOF.

TABLE 1: Management of patients in acute liver failure with cerebral edema.[30]

General measures	Reduce brain volume	Reduce cerebral blood flow
Intubation and ventilation	Continuous renal replacement therapy	Propofol sedation
Head in a neutral position; elevation of the head of the bed to 30°	Hypertonic saline	Hyperventilation
Minimal environmental stimulation	Mannitol	Moderate hypothermia in refractory cases

Chronic Liver Disease/Cirrhosis

When liver function continues to deteriorate for 6 months, it is termed chronic liver disease (CLD). It is a continuous hepatic inflammation and destruction process, followed by liver parenchyma regeneration and fibrotic band formation. These bands surround regenerative nodules, and this is termed *cirrhosis*.

Etiology

Chronic liver disease commonly leads to cirrhosis. **Table 3** summarizes the etiology of CLD/cirrhosis. In the developed world, the most common

TABLE 2: Treatment strategies for managing acute-on-chronic liver failure.

Etiology	Treatment
Viral infections	Antiviral agents
Alcohol hepatitis	• Corticosteroids • Pentoxifylline • N-acetylcysteine
Bacterial and fungal infections	• Antibiotics • Antimicrobials
All etiologies	• Granulocyte-macrophage colony-stimulating factor (G-CSF) • Stem cells • Liver transplantation

TABLE 3: Etiology of chronic liver disease.

Pathology	Examples
Viral	• Hepatitis B • Hepatitis C • Hepatitis D
Toxins	• Alcohol • Drugs
Autoimmune	Autoimmune hepatitis
Cholestatic	• Primary biliary cirrhosis • Primary sclerosing cholangitis
Vascular	• Budd–Chiari syndrome • Sinusoidal obstruction syndrome • Cardiac cirrhosis
Metabolic	• Nonalcoholic steatotic hepatitis (NASH) • Hemochromatosis • Wilson's disease • Alpha-1 antitrypsin deficiency • Cryptogenic cirrhosis

causes are hepatitis C virus (HCV), alcoholic liver disease, and nonalcoholic steatohepatitis (NASH), while hepatitis B virus (HBV) and HCV still dominate in the developing world.[37]

Pathophysiology

Untreated CLD ultimately leads to fibrosis, regenerative nodules, and the development of hepatic cirrhosis. Initially, fibrosis is reversible, but later, it usually becomes irreversible.

Multiple cells play a significant role in the development of liver cirrhosis. Activated HSCs become myofibroblasts and deposit collagen, leading to fibrosis. With chronic alcohol consumption, LSECs lose their fenestrations, causing perisinusoidal fibrosis.[38,39] Kupffer cells release harmful mediators after an insult,[40] and damaged hepatocytes also release inflammatory mediators along with reactive oxygen species that cause liver fibrosis by activating HSCs.[41]

Clinical Manifestations of Chronic Liver Disease

The disease progression in cirrhosis is typically a phase of asymptomatic compensated cirrhosis, followed by decompensated cirrhosis and its associated complications. These include jaundice, ascites, encephalopathy, and portal hypertensive gastrointestinal (GI) bleeding. Spontaneous bacterial peritonitis (SBP) can develop in patients with ascites, precipitating hepatorenal syndrome (HRS). **Box 1** depicts the signs and abnormal tests of CLD.

■ OTHER SYSTEM INVOLVEMENT IN LIVER DISEASE

Renal

Acute kidney injury (AKI) is also one of the most severe complications of cirrhosis, occurring in up to 50% of the hospitalized patients. It has been associated with higher mortality, increasing the severity of AKI. Hepatorenal syndrome is one of the phenotypes of AKI that occurs in patients with advanced cirrhosis and is characterized by decreased kidney blood flow that is unresponsive to volume expansion.

Most AKI in end-stage liver disease (ESLD) is either prerenal (diuresis, low circulating volume, etc.) or acute tubular necrosis due to nephrotoxic agents. About one-third of ARF in ESLD occurs due to true HRS and is more of a diagnosis by exclusion. Precipitating factors include large-volume paracentesis, major variceal bleeding, or SBP. Treatment of HRS includes vasoconstriction with vasopressin or terlipressin, norepinephrine, midodrine, octreotide, and volume expansion with albumin, but sometimes may require renal replacement therapy (RRT). With successful liver

BOX 1: Symptoms, signs, and laboratory tests of chronic liver disease.

- *Portal hypertension:*
  - Ascites
  - Splenomegaly
  - Caput medusae
  - Cruveilhier–Baumgarten murmur—epigastric venous hum
  - Thrombocytopenia
- *Liver dysfunction:*
  - *Hepatocellular damage*:
    - Raised AST and ALT
  - *Cholestasis:*
    - Elevated ALP, GGT, and 5'NT
  - *Synthetic dysfunction:*
    - Jaundice (nonspecific indicator)
    - *Coagulopathy:** Raised PT/INR
    - Low serum albumin
    - Low platelet count
- *Hepatic encephalopathy:*
  - Confusion
  - Asterixis
  - Fetor hepaticus
  - Coma
- *Stigmata of CLD:*
  - Spider telangiectasias
  - Palmar erythema
  - Dupuytren's contractures
  - Gynecomastia
  - Testicular atrophy
  - Loss of chest, axillary, and/or pubic hair
- *Miscellaneous:*
  - Bilateral parotid enlargement

*Refer to Coagulation in Chronic Liver Disease section.
(ALP: alkaline phosphatase; ALT: aspartate transaminase; AST: alanine transaminase; CLD: chronic liver disease; GGT: gamma-glutamyl transferase; INR: international normalizing ratio; 5'NT: 5'nucletidase; PT: prothrombin time)

transplantation, HRS resolves typically. However, some patients may require a kidney transplant, either simultaneous with the liver transplant or later, in the hope of spontaneous kidney recovery.

Circulatory

With the release of several vasodilator substances of different varieties, patients with ESLD are known to have systemic vasodilation leading to hypotension. This induces autonomic stimulation, leading to a hyperdynamic state. Over time, it leads to β-receptor down-regulation, autonomic dysfunction, and inotropic and chronotropic incompetence. Hence, conventional tests (e.g., dobutamine stress echo and radionucleotide scans) to rule out coronary artery disease (CAD) are unreliable in ESLD patients. Though circulation in cirrhosis is hyperdynamic, around half of the patients have some degree of hepatic cardiomyopathy, defined by systolic and diastolic dysfunction and electrophysiological abnormalities like prolongation of QT interval.

Respiratory

Hepatopulmonary syndrome (HPS) is another well-known complication of ESLD. Patients are hypoxic and on oxygen therapy. Type-1 HPS occurs due to massive dilation of pulmonary capillaries with multiple layers of RBCs far away from alveoli, not participating in gas exchange and causing right to the left intrapulmonary shunting. Type-2 HPS is due to actual arteriovenous malformation. Though the results of a liver transplant may not be suitable for HPS, a liver transplant remains the only treatment modality. Portopulmonary hypertension (PoPH) is another serious complication of ESLD. Severe PoPH is considered a contraindication to liver transplant as the right heart may fail, causing congestion and failure of the graft. Regular evaluation of the right heart and pulmonary artery pressures by echocardiography is recommended to diagnose PoPH in the early stages.

Hepatic hydrothorax is an extension of ascites. The fluid leaks through the defects in the diaphragm. Hepatic hydrothorax is another important cause of respiratory compromise in patients with CLD.

Portal Hypertension

The natural progression of cirrhosis is such that 90% of the patients will develop portal hypertension (PHT), which is a precursor of complications that can be fatal.[42] PHT can also exist without cirrhosis, termed *noncirrhotic portal hypertension*.[43] Portal hypertension leads to complications, such as ascites, gastroesophageal varices, hypersplenism, HRS, SBP, HPS, and possibly hepatocellular carcinoma.[44,45]

Classification and Causes of Portal Hypertension

Based on etiology, PHT is grouped into prehepatic, intrahepatic, and posthepatic. However, intrahepatic etiology accounts for over 95% of causes of PHT, and cirrhosis is the primary etiology. Prehepatic causes include portal vein thrombus and neoplasms. Intrahepatic causes are cirrhosis and veno-occlusive disease, and posthepatic has right heart failure, hepatic venous obstruction—Budd-Chiari syndrome, and inferior vena cava obstruction.

Pathophysiology of Portal Hypertension

Factors responsible for developing portal hypertension, particularly in liver cirrhosis are:
- Hyperdynamic circulation with increased cardiac output and splanchnic vasodilatation leads to augmented portal venous flow
- Resistance to centripetal portal venous flow into the liver
- Within the liver, there are anatomical and functional changes in the blood circulation.[46,47]

Due to PHT, portosystemic collateral vessels develop de novo or from preexisting vasculature, leading to complications mentioned earlier.

Diagnosis of Clinically Significant Portal Hypertension

Invasive tools are associated with higher costs and may cause few complications. Hence, efforts have been made to promote noninvasive means.
- *Invasive tools:* Hepatic venous pressure gradient (HVPG) is assessed by balloon catheterization of the hepatic vein to measure portal pressure (PP). Values of HVPG are described as normal (3-5 mm Hg), mild PHT (5-10 mm Hg), and clinically significant portal hypertension (CSPH) (>10 mm Hg). 12 mm Hg is the cut-off value above which there is a higher risk of variceal bleeding, and <12 mm Hg is considered protective (VH).[48]
- *Noninvasive methods for assessing portal hypertension:* The initial investigation of choice is ultrasound in patients to diagnose cirrhosis and/or portal hypertension and thrombosis in the portal and hepatic veins.[49]
- Portosystemic collaterals are one of the most reliable clues for diagnosing portal hypertension.
- Hepatic and splenic stiffness (Normal <2.9 kPa), measured by magnetic resonance elastography (MRE), can make a prediction of severe PHT in asymptomatic or compensated cirrhosis. Values of >20-25 kPa accurately diagnose CSPH in >90% of the cases.[50,51] Limited availability and high cost are the main limitations of MRE.

Management of Portal Hypertension

The aim of managing portal hypertension is to correct and prevent all complications of PHT, including variceal bleeding. Strategies for managing portal hypertension are shown in **Table 4**. Interventional radiological procedures are the mainstay of managing portal hypertension.

Carvedilol, a nonspecific β-blocker (NSBB), decreases portal venous inflow and vascular tone within the liver. It is the preferred NSBB because it dramatically reduces HVPG at low doses.[52,53] Statins, which improve endothelial dysfunction and decrease portal pressure, are a novel, promising treatment.

TABLE 4: Management strategies for portal hypertension.

General therapy	• Maintaining healthy BMI • Abstinence from Alcohol • Moderate aerobic exercise

Pharmacological measures	• *Long-term:* NSBBs *(propranolol, nadolol, and carvedilol—agent of choice)*
	• *Short-term:*
	  – *Somatostatin analogs:* Octreotide
	  – *Vasopressin and analogs:* Terlipressin
	• *Miscellaneous:* Statins

Interventions	• Banding of varices (prevention of upper GI bleed) • TIPS • Surgical portosystemic shunts

(BMI: body mass index; GI: gastrointestinal; NSBBs: nonspecific β-blockers, TIPS: transjugular intrahepatic portosystemic shunt)

Coagulation in Chronic Liver Disease

Due to significant changes in hemodynamics, procoagulant, and anticoagulant mechanisms, coagulation is said to be rebalanced. This can change toward either a procoagulant or anticoagulant process by several factors.[54]

Both procoagulant and anticoagulant factors (antithrombin, protein C, and protein S) are reduced in the broad spectrum of liver pathologies. However, the FVIII and Von Willebrand factor (vWF) levels are raised in cirrhosis and lead to enhanced platelet aggregation.[55] Thrombocytopenia, high nitric oxide concentrations, and prostacyclin reduce platelet function.[55] Splenic sequestration of platelets, combined with reduced synthesis of thrombopoietin by the liver and immune-mediated platelet destruction in sepsis and inflammations, causes thrombocytopenia.[56]

In cirrhosis and ALF, the INR can be raised modestly or remarkably; however, the bleeding risk during invasive procedures may not increase due to increased thrombin generation.[57] In ACLF, due to sepsis and inflammation, coagulation changes from a procoagulant to an anticoagulant state.[58-60]

Excessive transfusion of blood products to normalize INR or aPTT may be harmful, leading to transfusion-related acute lung injury (TRALI) and volume overload.[61,62]

Global coagulation assays [thrombin generation, thromboelastography (TEG), or rotational thromboelastometry (ROTEM)] interpret the interaction between clotting and anticlotting pathways, which assess bleeding risk and guide treatment.

■ SCORING SYSTEMS

Different scoring systems have been developed over the years to assess and stratify the severity of CLD. Most of them were introduced to determine the need for liver transplantation (LT), but they also stratify the severity of CLD. The performance of these scoring systems is diverse in application, and it is still uncertain which system is better. The following are the most used scoring systems for CLD.

Child–Turcotte–Pugh Score

Parameters required for this score are serum bilirubin and albumin concentrations, INR, grade of encephalopathy, and ascites. Patients can then belong to the A, B, or C class. The score predicts postoperative outcomes post-hepatic and other abdominal surgeries.

Advantages include easy availability of parameters and simple bedside calculations. Disadvantages include the subjective nature of ascites and encephalopathy, leading to inter-observer variability. They also change with response to treatment. CTP score excludes renal parameters, which will help prognosticate better as renal dysfunction is often present in this population. Additionally, all variables are given the same weight: 1–3 points, with ceiling effects for bilirubin. This limits accurate, individualized risk assessment.

Model for End-stage Liver Disease Score

The MELD score initially predicted survival outcomes in patients with transjugular intrahepatic portosystemic shunt (TIPS) procedures. However, it now allocates organs to patients awaiting transplantation and predicts the prognosis of patients with cirrhosis.[63,64] It is also an accurate predictor of risk in patients undergoing other surgeries besides liver transplants. Many studies have demonstrated that MELD is now the preferred score over the CTP.[65] The MELD score is logarithmic and calculated using total bilirubin, serum creatinine, and INR.

Hyponatremia is a robust independent predictor of early mortality, and its inclusion improves MELD's accuracy when MELD scores are low.[66-68] Other modifications of MELD include an integrated model for end-stage liver disease (i-MELD), a model for end-stage liver disease to sodium (MESO) index, United Kingdom end-stage liver disease (UKELD) score, updated MELD and MELD XI have been introduced to improve the prognostic accuracy even more in CLD.[69-71]

Mayo Clinic Postoperative Mortality Risk in Patients with Cirrhosis Calculator

This web-based calculator includes patient age, ASA class, and etiology of cirrhosis as its predictive parameters.

VOCAL-Penn Model

Veterans Outcomes and Costs Associated with Liver Disease (VOCAL): The Penn score is one of the newest scores for preoperative risk calculation in patients with cirrhosis for nontransplant surgeries. This online calculator incorporates nine variables: surgical category, emergency indication, fatty liver disease, ASA classification, and obesity, among others. The score predicts the risk of death after surgery at 1-, 3-, and 6-month. It has demonstrated the best risk discrimination, especially for 90-day postoperative mortality, over other scores, and this has been validated in external cohorts.[72,73]

PATIENTS WITH HEPATOBILIARY DISEASE COMING FOR NONHEPATIC SURGERY: PERIOPERATIVE RISKS

Cirrhotic patients, compared to noncirrhotic counterparts, have up to 10 times higher perioperative mortality.[74] The reported in-hospital mortality rates after various nontransplant surgical procedures range from 8.3 to 25% in cirrhotic patients, compared to 1.1% in noncirrhotic patients.[75]

Cardiovascular surgery patients experienced a 31.2% postoperative mortality when their MELD score was above 20. These patients had the highest rates of postoperative bleeding and take-backs for thoracotomy, postoperative respiratory and renal failure, requirements for high-dose catecholamines, and mechanical circulatory assistance.[76]

Cirrhotic patients' most common surgical procedures include hepatic resection for tumors and liver transplantation. However, these patients also frequently require other nonhepatic surgical procedures, cholecystectomy being the commonest.[75] Abdominal surgeries carry higher morbidity and mortality due to increased bleeding from portal hypertension and hepatic ischemia. Upper gastrointestinal surgery in patients with CTP-A and CTP-B cirrhosis has acceptable risks; however, CTP-C patients have a very high risk of developing perioperative complications.[77] In patients with compensated cirrhosis, laparoscopic surgical procedures are considered safer than the open approach.[78]

Elective primary total knee or hip arthroplasties can be safely performed in CTP-A and CTP-B patients.[79] However, cirrhosis is associated with a significantly increased risk of periprosthetic joint infection, transfusion, and frequent need for revision surgery.[80]

PATIENTS WITH HEPATOBILIARY DISEASE PRESENTING FOR NONHEPATIC SURGERY: PREOPERATIVE ASSESSMENT

Patients may have undiagnosed liver disease or fulminant hepatic failure and may present for emergency surgery. Detailed preoperative history and a thorough physical examination, especially stratifying the severity of liver disease, are the essential components of preoperative assessment.

History of blood transfusions, tattoos, illicit drugs, unprotected sex, alcohol consumption, and travel history must be taken. Other vital aspects of history-taking include a family history of liver disease and details of prescription and nonprescription medications.[81]

Details of hepatic decompensation features and whether any treatment was obtained must be ascertained. Decompensated cirrhosis has a much higher risk of precipitating ACLF in the postoperative period, with poor outcomes.[82] Traditional scoring systems should be used to predict outcomes after surgery. Recently published clinical guidelines have an algorithm for stratifying and management of patients undergoing elective surgery.[77]

PREOPERATIVE INVESTIGATIONS

Liver function tests (LFT) can be divided into markers of hepatocellular injury, cholestasis, or synthetic dysfunction. Alanine transaminase and ALT may lack some sensitivity in chronic liver disease but can be markedly elevated in acute hepatitis.[83] For hepatic injury, ALT is more specific than AST, and alcoholic liver disease usually has an AST/ALT ratio >2.

Markers on synthetic dysfunction include bilirubin, albumin, and prothrombin time (PT). Serial measurements are more valuable in assessing disease progression. Total blood count is essential to evaluate the extent of anemia and thrombocytopenia.

During preoperative assessment, major red flags include hypovolemia, coagulopathy, and thrombocytopenia. Electrolyte imbalance should be corrected and infection treated to prevent perioperative encephalopathy. Restricting sedative medications and branched-chain amino acids are helpful.[84] However, in preoperatively hyponatremic patients, rapid correction of sodium, higher than 8 mEq/L in 24 hours, may lead to central pontine myelinolysis.[85]

Prothrombin time and activated partial thromboplastin time (aPTT) only measure the decreased synthesis of procoagulant factors and can be misleading in these patients. In addition, these are performed on plasma rather than whole blood and thus do not reflect factors contributing to clot formation. As per the 7th International Coagulation in Liver Disease Conference, the PT/INR and the aPTT are not helpful and should be avoided for bleeding risk assessment or help blood product transfusion in patients with advanced chronic liver disease (ACLD).[86]

Instead, point-of-care viscoelastic tests (VET) such as TEG and ROTEM can be used. The most helpful VET parameter is the clot stiffness, measured as the maximum clot formation (MCF) in ROTEM or maximum amplitude (MA) in TEG.[87]

Platelet transfusion is recommended with TEG MA of 30–55 mm and EXTEM MCF of 40 mm. FIBTEM MCF of <8 mm indicates cryoprecipitate transfusion.[87] Advanced chronic liver disease patients without hypocoagulability, as measured by VETs, could benefit from regional anesthesia techniques; however, more research needs to be conducted to recommend this.[88] Depending on the invasiveness of planned surgery and clinical condition, ACLD patients need a preoperative echocardiography. A positive contrast echocardiography also aids in diagnosing HPS by demonstrating intrapulmonary vascular dilatation.[89] A chest X-ray or a bedside ultrasound can diagnose large pleural effusions that may need thoracocentesis. Patients with intractable ascites/hydrothorax also benefit from TIPS procedures to reduce PHT.

ANESTHETIC MANAGEMENT OF PATIENTS WITH CHRONIC LIVER DISEASE

General Principles

In cirrhotic patients, anesthesia and surgical stress could cause acute hepatic decompensation, and understanding physiological alterations in liver disease is crucial for intraoperative management.[90]

Typically, ACLD patients have vasodilation in the splanchnic circulation, PHT, and have relative central hypovolemia. Albumin is better than crystalloids and is indicated in patients undergoing large-volume paracentesis. Albumin prevents paracentesis-induced circulatory dysfunction, and 8 g should be given for every liter of ascites drained. Albumin is also indicated in SBP.[91] Fluid overloads should be prevented, and MAP should be maintained to ensure organ perfusion with judicious use of vasopressors and fluids.[92]

Treatment of concomitant HRS includes terlipressin, norepinephrine, midodrine and octreotide, and volume expansion, but sometimes also may need RRT.[93]

Patients with decompensated cirrhosis having ascites are at an increased risk of aspiration under general anesthesia; a rapid sequence induction may be warranted.

Basal atelectasis due to ascites and hepatic hydrothorax may worsen respiratory distress, and patients may not tolerate procedural sedation.

Ascites causes increased intra-abdominal pressure; hence, central venous pressure (CVP) alone can be misleading for assessing volume status. However, central venous access is helpful for quick correction of electrolyte and acid–base status.[94] Dynamic measures of fluid responsiveness should be used to guide fluid therapy. Transesophageal echocardiography may guide fluid and hemodynamic management in some patients, albeit in the absence of large varices. In patients with suspected right ventricular dysfunction and/or pulmonary hypertension, a pulmonary artery catheter (PAC) may be indicated for monitoring and guiding therapy.[91]

Large-bore intravenous access and invasive blood pressure monitoring are indicated when these patients are present for major surgery. Rapid infusers should be available when patients present with massive hemorrhage due to bleeding varices or hypocoagulopathy-related bleeding. For about 10–20 mL/kg of crystalloids should be the first choice of treatment in hypovolemic patients.[91] Patients with hyperchloremic acidosis may benefit from balanced salt solutions like Plasmalyte.[91]

In patients booked for high-risk procedures and with a platelet count of <50,000/L and/or fibrinogen levels under 100 mg/dL, prophylactic transfusion of platelets or fibrinogen concentrate should be considered.[88] Thrombopoietin receptor (TPO-R) agonists, lusutrombopag, or avatrombopag have been approved for high-risk invasive procedures with severe thrombocytopenia.[88] International guidelines recommend VET-guided transfusions and discourage fresh frozen plasma or prothrombin complex concentrate (PCC) for correcting prolonged INR.[95]

Postoperative pain management after major surgery is a significant concern.[88] A low dose of 2–3 g/day of acetaminophen for short term is safe in patients with ACLD. Since nonsteroidal anti-inflammatory drugs (NSAIDs) can precipitate AKI and gastrointestinal bleeding, they should be avoided in ACLD patients. Since these patients may decompensate in the postoperative period, intensive care unit admission is advisable.

Anesthetic Drugs

Metabolism of drugs occurs in the liver via enzyme reactions of the hepatic cytochrome P450 (CYP) system, conjugation to different groups, biliary excretion, and then elimination.[96] Activity of various cytochrome P450 (CYP450) enzymes seems to be different in patients with ACLD. CYP450-mediated reactions seem to be affected more than glucuronidation in mild to moderate cirrhosis; however, in advanced cirrhosis, both functions are significantly reduced.[97]

With lower production of albumin and plasma proteins, the volume of distribution for highly protein-bound substances is higher. Water-soluble drugs also have a higher volume of distribution due to ascites and volume overload.[97] Reduced functional units of hepatocytes with reduced enzymes lead to impaired drug elimination in hepatobiliary disease.[98] With the development of portosystemic shunts, substances also bypass hepatic elimination.[97]

Splanchnic and hepatic circulations are affected by general anesthesia to different levels. Most anesthetics reduce cardiac output and thereby decrease portal blood flow. Hepatic arterial blood flow can be reduced, increased, or no change with anesthesia. Even when hepatic arterial blood flow increases, it is insufficient to compensate for a fall in portal blood flow; anesthesia usually causes decreased total hepatic blood flow.[99]

However, surgical manipulations affect total hepatic blood flow more than current inhalational anesthetic agents. Total blood flow during an anesthetic may decrease by 30–50%.[100] Sevoflurane showed the fewest complications, while desflurane and isoflurane have shown hepatic blood flow to be unaffected.[88]

Propofol is highly protein-bound and has an increased volume of distribution in cirrhotic patients. Although recovery times are slightly longer in ACLD patients, patients awaken at the same plasma concentrations as noncirrhotic patients, probably due to extrahepatic metabolism.[88]

Induction doses of etomidate have a rapid onset and short duration of action, limited by redistribution. Although the metabolism of etomidate occurs in the liver, the clinical effect is unchanged after a single injection.[98]

Thiopental, an ultrashort-acting barbiturate, is exclusively metabolized in the liver. However, the risk of prolonged effects with thiopental is low in cirrhotic patients. Patients may be prone to acute intoxication due to increased unbound fraction of thiopental.[98]

Benzodiazepines are metabolized in the liver. Agents such as diazepam, clonazepam, and midazolam are metabolized via oxidation and have prolonged effects on ACLD. On the other hand, metabolism of lorazepam, oxazepam, and temazepam is via conjugation. These agents do not have active metabolites, and their half-lives are minimally affected in cirrhosis.[88]

The metabolism of opioid medications depends upon liver and renal function. A decrease in drug dosage may be required in patients with coexistent kidney dysfunction such as HRS.[96] Opioids upregulate central mu-opioid receptors and alter gut microbiota. With opioid-induced sluggish intestinal motility, increased intestinal absorption of ammonia and inflammatory mediators can precipitate HE.[101] Long-term and chronic opioid uses are an independent risk of HE.[101] In healthy people, morphine or fentanyl has high hepatic extraction and low bioavailability; however, in cirrhosis, their bioavailability is increased. Their metabolism is slowed by impaired hepatic blood flow. As a single dose, kinetics is unchanged with fentanyl and sufentanil. Liver disease does not affect the bioavailability of methadone and other drugs with low hepatic extraction, but hepatic clearance may be significantly reduced.[96] Clearance of drugs with high biliary excretion is compromised in severe cholestasis. The dose of buprenorphine, which has high biliary clearance, requires reduced dosage or complete avoidance.[96]

The pharmacokinetics of remifentanil are unchanged in ACLD patients; however, patients may be more sensitive to its respiratory depressant effects. However, these effects are of minimal significance due to remifentanil's ultra-short duration of action, being metabolized by nonspecific esterases.[102]

Since hepatobiliary disease is associated with reduced plasma cholinesterase activity, succinylcholine shows prolonged neuromuscular block. With an increased volume of distribution, nondepolarizing neuromuscular blocking agents may have a slow onset of action in cirrhotic patients. Atracurium, cisatracurium, and mivacurium are eliminated via Hofmann's degradation without hepatic involvement and are safe for liver disease. A small dose of vecuronium is terminated by redistribution; however clearance of more significant amounts of vecuronium depends on hepatic clearance, with an increased duration of action in ACLD.[103] A 28% reduction in the clearance of rocuronium and a 55% increase in elimination half-life have been observed.[104] Sugammadex is safe and effective in patients with liver dysfunction for reversing rocuronium.

Even though ESLD alters hepatic extraction, renal excretion, and serum proteins, the net effects of these changes on the drug metabolism and elimination are unpredictable, making general recommendations for the administration of drugs challenging.[105]

CONCLUSION

Liver disease has a broad-spectrum ranging from mild dysfunction to fulminant hepatic failure. The anesthesiologist needs to understand the implications of different manifestations of liver disease in the perioperative environment. Though not perfect, various prognostication scores can guide anesthesiologists in the decision-making regarding care, risks, and futility in patients of hepatobiliary disease presenting for nontransplant surgery. It is important to emphasize that coagulation in advanced liver disease is balanced, and unwarranted use of blood products may lead to bleeding from varices or major thromboses. Drug metabolism and elimination are affected to varying degrees in liver disease, and judicious administration of anesthetic agents must be practiced based on the knowledge of underlying pharmacology. The postoperative period requires vigilant monitoring of patients as they may decompensate during this period.

REFERENCES

1. Eipel C, Abshagen K, Vollmar B. Regulation of hepatic blood flow: the hepatic arterial buffer response revisited. World J Gastroenterol. 2010;16(48):6046-57.
2. In: Wagener G (Ed). Liver Anesthesiology and Critical Care Medicine. Cham: Springer International Publishing; 2018.
3. Devarbhavi H, Asrani SK, Arab JP, Nartey YA, Pose E, Kamath PS. Global burden of liver disease: 2023 update. J Hepatol. 2023;79(2):516-37.
4. Avila MA, Dufour JF, Gerbes AL, Zoulim F, Bataller R, Burra P, et al. Recent advances in alcohol-related liver disease (ALD): summary of a Gut round table meeting. Gut. 2020;69(4):764-80.
5. Stein E, Cruz-Lemini M, Altamirano J, Ndugga N, Couper D, Abraldes JG, et al. Heavy daily alcohol intake at the population level predicts the weight of alcohol in cirrhosis burden worldwide. J Hepatol. 2016;65(5):998-1005.
6. Millwala F, Nguyen GC, Thuluvath PJ. Outcomes of patients with cirrhosis undergoing non-hepatic surgery: Risk assessment and management. World J Gastroenterol. 2007;13(30):4056-63.

7. Nilsson S. Recapitulating the liver niche in vitro. Advances in Stem cells and Their Niches, 1st edition. Amsterdam: Elsevier; 2022. pp. 1-55.
8. Kalra A, Yetiskul E, Wehrle CJ, Tuma F. Physiology, Liver. In: StatPearls. Treasure Island (FL): StatPearls Publishing; 2023.
9. Krishna M. Microscopic anatomy of the liver. Clin Liver Dis (Hoboken). 2013;2(Suppl 1):S4-7.
10. Poisson J, Lemoinne S, Boulanger C, Durand F, Moreau R, Valla D, et al. Liver sinusoidal endothelial cells: Physiology and role in liver diseases. J Hepatol. 2017;66(1):212-27.
11. Schoen JM, Wang HH, Minuk GY, Lautt WW. Shear stress-induced nitric oxide release triggers the liver regeneration cascade. Nitric Oxide. 2001;5(5):453-64.
12. Hanafy AS. Prediction and Prevention of Post-hepatectomy Liver Failure: Where Do We Stand? J Clin Transl Hepatol. 2021;9(3):281-2.
13. Theodoraki K, Vezakis A, Massaras D, Louta A, Arkadopoulos N, Smyrniotis V. Splenic Artery Ligation: An Ontable Bail-Out Strategy for Small-for-Size Remnants after Major Hepatectomy: A Retrospective Study. J Pers Med. 2022;12(10):1687.
14. Lafoz E, Ruart M, Anton A, Oncins A, Hernández-Gea V. The Endothelium as a Driver of Liver Fibrosis and Regeneration. Cells. 2020;9(4):929.
15. Lee Y, Friedman SL. Fibrosis in the liver: acute protection and chronic disease. Prog Mol Biol Transl Sci. 2010;97:151-200.
16. Lautt WW. Hepatic Circulation: Physiology and Pathophysiology. San Rafael (CA): Morgan & Claypool Life Sciences; 2009.
17. Polson J, Lee WM. American Association for the Study of Liver Disease. AASLD position paper: The management of acute liver failure. Hepatology. 2005;41(5):1179-97.
18. Shalimar, Acharya SK. Management in Acute Liver Failure. J Clin Exp Hepatol. 2015;5(Suppl 1):S104-15.
19. Bower WA, Johns M, Margolis HS, Williams IT, Bell BP. Population-based surveillance for acute liver failure. Am J Gastroenterol. 2007;102(11):2459-63.
20. Wang DW, Yin YM, Yao YM. Advances in the management of acute liver failure. World J Gastroenterol. 2013;19(41):7069-77.
21. Acharya SK. Acute Liver Failure: Indian Perspective. Clin Liver Dis (Hoboken). 2021;18(3):143-9.
22. Shalimar, Acharya SK, Lee WM. (2013). Worldwide differences in acute liver failure. [online] Available from: https://www.futuremedicine.com/doi/10.2217/ebo.12.326 [Last accessed October, 2023].
23. Ostapowicz G, Fontana RJ, Schiødt FV, Larson A, Davern TJ, Han SHB, et al. Results of a prospective study of acute liver failure at 17 tertiary care centers in the United States. Ann Intern Med. 2002;137(12):947-54.
24. Goel A, Lalruatsanga D, Himanshu D, Bharti V, Sharma D. Acute Liver Failure Prognostic Criteria: It's Time to Revisit. Cureus. 2023;15(7):e33810.
25. McPhail MJW, Farne H, Senvar N, Wendon JA, Bernal W. Ability of King's College Criteria and Model for End-Stage Liver Disease Scores to Predict Mortality of Patients with Acute Liver Failure: A Meta-analysis. Clinical Gastroenterol Hepatol. 2016;14(4):516-25;quiz e43-5.

26. Chung RT, Stravitz RT, Fontana RJ, Schiodt FV, Mehal WZ, Reddy KR, et al. Pathogenesis of Liver Injury in Acute Liver Failure. Gastroenterology. 2012;143(3):e1-7.
27. Shah NJ, Royer A, John S. Acute Liver Failure. In: StatPearls. Treasure Island (FL): StatPearls Publishing; 2023.
28. Lee WM, Hynan LS, Rossaro L, Fontana RJ, Stravitz RT, Larson AM, et al. Intravenous N-Acetylcysteine Improves Transplant-Free Survival in Early-Stage Non-Acetaminophen Acute Liver Failure. Gastroenterology. 2009;137(3):856-64.e1.
29. Lee WM, Stravitz RT, Larson AM. Introduction to the Revised American Association for the Study of Liver Diseases Position Paper on Acute Liver Failure 2011. Hepatology. 2012;55(3):965-7.
30. Kok B, Karvellas CJ. Management of Cerebral Edema in Acute Liver Failure. Semin Respir Crit Care Med. 2017;38(6):821-9.
31. Bernal W, Wendon J. Acute liver failure. N Engl J Med. 2013;369(26):2525-34.
32. Rabinowich L, Wendon J, Bernal W, Shibolet O. Clinical management of acute liver failure: Results of an international multi-center survey. World J Gastroenterol. 2016;22(33):7595-603.
33. Slack AJ, Auzinger G, Willars C, Dew T, Musto R, Corsilli D, et al. Ammonia clearance with haemofiltration in adults with liver disease. Liver Int. 2014;34(1):42-8.
34. Stravitz RT, Kramer DJ. Management of acute liver failure. Nat Rev Gastroenterol Hepatol. 2009;6(9):542-53.
35. Hernaez R, Solà E, Moreau R, Ginès P. Acute-on-chronic liver failure: an update. Gut. 2017;66(3):541-53.
36. Hoang DM, Pham PT, Bach TQ, Ngo ATL, Nguyen QT, Phan TTK, et al. Stem cell-based therapy for human diseases. Signal Transduct Target Ther. 2022;7(1):272.
37. Sharma B, John S. Hepatic Cirrhosis. In: StatPearls. Treasure Island: StatPearls Publishing; 2023.
38. Braet F, Wisse E. Structural and functional aspects of liver sinusoidal endothelial cell fenestrae: a review. Comp Hepatol. 2002;1(1):1.
39. Deaciuc I, D'Souza N, Fortunato F, Hill D, Sarphie T, McClain C. Alcohol-induced sinusoidal endothelial cell dysfunction in the mouse is associated with exacerbated liver apoptosis and can be reversed by caspase inhibition. Hepatol Res. 2001;19(1):85-97.
40. Kolios G, Valatas V, Kouroumalis E. Role of Kupffer cells in the pathogenesis of liver disease. World J Gastroenterol. 2006;12(46):7413-20.
41. Bataller R, Brenner DA. Liver fibrosis. J Clin Invest. 2005;115(2):209-18.
42. de Franchis R, Primignani M. Natural history of portal hypertension in patients with cirrhosis. Clin Liver Dis. 2001;5(3):645-63.
43. Khanna R, Sarin SK. Non-cirrhotic portal hypertension – diagnosis and management. J Hepatol. 2014;60(2):421-41.
44. Bosch J, García-Pagán JC. Complications of cirrhosis. I. Portal hypertension. J Hepatol. 2000;32(1 Suppl):141-56.
45. Ripoll C, Groszmann R, Garcia-Tsao G, Grace N, Burroughs A, Planas R, et al. Hepatic venous pressure gradient predicts clinical decompensation in patients with compensated cirrhosis. Gastroenterology. 2007;133(2):481-8.
46. Martell M, Coll M, Ezkurdia N, Raurell I, Genescà J. Physiopathology of splanchnic vasodilation in portal hypertension. World J Hepatol. 2010;2(6):208-20.

47. Groszmann RJ, Abraldes JG. Portal hypertension: from bedside to bench. J Clin Gastroenterol. 2005;39(4 Suppl 2):S125-30.
48. Abraldes JG, Villanueva C, Bañares R, Aracil C, Catalina MV, Garci A-Pagán JC, et al. Hepatic venous pressure gradient and prognosis in patients with acute variceal bleeding treated with pharmacologic and endoscopic therapy. J Hepatol. 2008;48(2):229-36.
49. Margini C, Berzigotti A. Portal vein thrombosis: The role of imaging in the clinical setting. Dig Liver Dis. 2017;49(2):113-20.
50. Friedrich-Rust M, Müller C, Winckler A, Kriener S, Herrmann E, Holtmeier J, et al. Assessment of liver fibrosis and steatosis in PBC with FibroScan, MRI, MR-spectroscopy, and serum markers. J Clin Gastroenterol. 2010;44(1):58-65.
51. Lemoine M, Katsahian S, Ziol M, Nahon P, Ganne-Carrie N, Kazemi F, et al. Liver stiffness measurement as a predictive tool of clinically significant portal hypertension in patients with compensated hepatitis C virus or alcohol-related cirrhosis. Aliment Pharmacol Ther. 2008;28(9):1102-10.
52. Villanueva C, Albillos A, Genescà J, Garcia-Pagan JC, Calleja JL, Aracil C, et al. β blockers to prevent decompensation of cirrhosis in patients with clinically significant portal hypertension (PREDESCI): a randomised, double-blind, placebo-controlled, multicentre trial. Lancet. 2019;393(10181):1597-608.
53. Villanueva C, Torres F, Sarin SK, Shah HA, Tripathi D, Brujats A, et al. Carvedilol reduces the risk of decompensation and mortality in patients with compensated cirrhosis in a competing-risk meta-analysis. J Hepatol. 2022;77(4):1014-25.
54. Lisman T, Caldwell SH, Burroughs AK, Northup PG, Senzolo M, Stravitz RT, et al. Hemostasis and thrombosis in patients with liver disease: the ups and downs. J Hepatol. 2010;53(2):362-71.
55. Premkumar M, Saxena P, Rangegowda D, Baweja S, Mirza R, Jain P, et al. Coagulation failure is associated with bleeding events and clinical outcome during systemic inflammatory response and sepsis in acute-on-chronic liver failure: An observational cohort study. Liver Int. 2019;39(4):694-704.
56. Northup PG, Caldwell SH. Coagulation in liver disease: a guide for the clinician. Clin Gastroenterol Hepatol. 2013;11(9):1064-74.
57. Agarwal B, Wright G, Gatt A, Riddell A, Vemala V, Mallett S, et al. Evaluation of coagulation abnormalities in acute liver failure. J Hepatol. 2012;57(4):780-6.
58. Blasi A, Calvo A, Prado V, Reverter E, Reverter JC, Hernández-Tejero M, et al. Coagulation Failure in Patients with Acute-on-Chronic Liver Failure and Decompensated Cirrhosis: Beyond the International Normalized Ratio. Hepatology. 2018;68(6):2325-37.
59. Fisher C, Patel VC, Stoy SH, Singanayagam A, Adelmeijer J, Wendon J, et al. Balanced haemostasis with both hypo- and hyper-coagulable features in critically ill patients with acute-on-chronic-liver failure. J Crit Care. 2018;43:54-60.
60. Bedreli S, Sowa JP, Gerken G, Saner FH, Canbay A. Management of acute-on-chronic liver failure: rotational thromboelastometry may reduce substitution of coagulation factors in liver cirrhosis. Gut. 2016;65(2):357-8.
61. Case JJ, Khan N, Delrahim M, Dizdarevic J, Nichols DJ, Schreiber MA, et al. Association of Massive Transfusion for Resuscitation in Gastrointestinal Bleeding with Transfusion-related Acute Lung Injury. Indian J Crit Care Med. 2017;21(8):506-13.

62. Kumar M, Ahmad J, Maiwall R, Choudhury A, Bajpai M, Mitra LG, et al. Thromboelastography-Guided Blood Component Use in Patients With Cirrhosis With Nonvariceal Bleeding: A Randomized Controlled Trial. Hepatology. 2020;71(1):235-46.
63. Kamath PS, Kim WR; Advanced Liver Disease Study Group. The model for end-stage liver disease (MELD). Hepatology. 2007;45(3):797-805.
64. Malinchoc M, Kamath PS, Gordon FD, Peine CJ, Rank J, ter Borg PC. A model to predict poor survival in patients undergoing transjugular intrahepatic portosystemic shunts. Hepatology. 2000;31(4):864-71.
65. Befeler AS, Palmer DE, Hoffman M, Longo W, Solomon H, Di Bisceglie AM. The safety of intra-abdominal surgery in patients with cirrhosis: model for end-stage liver disease score is superior to Child-Turcotte-Pugh classification in predicting outcome. Arch Surg. 2005;140(7):650-4; discussion 655.
66. Londoño MC, Cárdenas A, Guevara M, Quintó L, de Las Heras D, Navasa M, et al. MELD score and serum sodium in the prediction of survival of patients with cirrhosis awaiting liver transplantation. Gut. 2007;56(9):1283-90.
67. Biggins SW, Rodriguez HJ, Bacchetti P, Bass NM, Roberts JP, Terrault NA. Serum sodium predicts mortality in patients listed for liver transplantation. Hepatology. 2005;41(1):32-9.
68. Biggins SW, Kim WR, Terrault NA, Saab S, Balan V, Schiano T, et al. Evidence-based incorporation of serum sodium concentration into MELD. Gastroenterology. 2006;130(6):1652-60.
69. Luca A, Angermayr B, Bertolini G, Koenig F, Vizzini G, Ploner M, et al. An integrated MELD model including serum sodium and age improves the prediction of early mortality in patients with cirrhosis. Liver Transpl. 2007;13(8):1174-80.
70. Sharma P, Schaubel DE, Sima CS, Merion RM, Lok ASF. Re-weighting the model for end-stage liver disease score components. Gastroenterology. 2008;135(5):1575-81.
71. Heuman DM, Mihas AA, Habib A, Gilles HS, Stravitz RT, Sanyal AJ, et al. MELD-XI: a rational approach to "sickest first" liver transplantation in cirrhotic patients requiring anticoagulant therapy. Liver Transpl. 2007;13(1):30-7.
72. Mahmud N, Fricker Z, Panchal S, Lewis JD, Goldberg DS, Kaplan DE. External Validation of the VOCAL-Penn Cirrhosis Surgical Risk Score in 2 Large, Independent Health Systems. Liver Transpl. 2021;27(7):961-70.
73. Mahmud N, Fricker Z, Hubbard RA, Ioannou GN, Lewis JD, Taddei TH, et al. Risk Prediction Models for Post-operative Mortality in Patients with Cirrhosis. Hepatology. 2021;73(1):204-18.
74. Newman KL, Johnson KM, Cornia PB, Wu P, Itani K, Ioannou GN. Perioperative Evaluation and Management of Patients With Cirrhosis: Risk Assessment, Surgical Outcomes, and Future Directions. Clin Gastroenterol Hepatol. 2020;18(11):2398-414.e3.
75. Bhangui P, Laurent A, Amathieu R, Azoulay D. Assessment of risk for non-hepatic surgery in cirrhotic patients. J Hepatol. 2012;57(4):874-84.
76. Pathare P, Elbayomi M, Weyand M, Griesbach C, Harig F. MELD-score for risk stratification in cardiac surgery. Heart Vessels. 2023;38(9):1156-63.
77. Abbas N, Fallowfield J, Patch D, Stanley AJ, Mookerjee R, Tsochatzis E, et al. Guidance document: risk assessment of patients with cirrhosis prior to elective non-hepatic surgery. Frontline Gastroenterol. 2023;14(5):359-70.

78. Rashid A, Gupta A, Adiamah A, West J, Grainge M, Humes DJ. Mortality following appendicectomy in patients with liver cirrhosis: a systematic review and meta-analysis. World J Surg. 2022;46(3):531-41.
79. Cohen SM, Te HS, Levitsky J. Operative risk of total hip and knee arthroplasty in cirrhotic patients. J Arthroplasty. 2005;20(4):460-6.
80. Onochie E, Kayani B, Dawson-Bowling S, Millington S, Achan P, Hanna S. Total hip arthroplasty in patients with chronic liver disease: a systematic review. SICOT J. 2019;5:40.
81. Simegn AE, Melesse DY, Bizuneh YB, Alemu WM. Perioperative management of patients with liver disease for non-hepatic surgery: a systematic review. Ann Med Surg (Lond). 2022;75:103397.
82. Moreau R, Jalan R, Gines P, Pavesi M, Angeli P, Cordoba J, et al. Acute-on-chronic liver failure is a distinct syndrome that develops in patients with acute decompensation of cirrhosis. Gastroenterology. 2013;144(7):1426-37,1437.e1-9.
83. Johnston DE. Special considerations in interpreting liver function tests. Am Fam Physician. 1999;59(8):2223-30.
84. Bleszynski MS, Bressan AK, Joos E, Hameed SM, Ball CG. Acute care and emergency general surgery in patients with chronic liver disease: how can we optimize perioperative care? A review of the literature. World J Emerg Surg. 2018;13:32.
85. Jalan R, Mookerjee R, Cheshire L, Williams R, Davies N. Albumin Infusion for Severe Hyponatremia in Patients with Refractory Ascites: A Randomized Clinical Trial. J Hepatol. 2007;46:S95.
86. Intagliata NM, Argo CK, Stine JG, Lisman T, Caldwell SH, Violi F. Concepts and Controversies in Haemostasis and Thrombosis Associated with Liver Disease: Proceedings of the 7th International Coagulation in Liver Disease Conference. Thromb Haemost. 2018;118(08):1491-506.
87. Davis JPE, Northup PG, Caldwell SH, Intagliata NM. Viscoelastic Testing in Liver Disease. Ann Hepatol. 2018;17(2):205-13.
88. Canillas L, Pelegrina A, Álvarez J, Colominas-González E, Salar A, Aguilera L, et al. Clinical Guideline on Perioperative Management of Patients with Advanced Chronic Liver Disease. Life (Basel). 2023;13(1):132.
89. Grilo-Bensusan I, Pascasio-Acevedo JM. Hepatopulmonary syndrome: What we know and what we would like to know. World J Gastroenterol. 2016;22(25):5728-41.
90. Hickman L, Tanner L, Christein J, Vickers S. Non-Hepatic Abdominal Surgery in Patients with Cirrhotic Liver Disease. J Gastrointest Surg. 2019;23(3):634-42.
91. Nadim MK, Durand F, Kellum JA, Levitsky J, O'Leary JG, Karvellas CJ, et al. Management of the critically ill patient with cirrhosis: a multidisciplinary perspective. J Hepatol. 2016;64(3):717-35.
92. Hoste EA, Maitland K, Brudney CS, Mehta R, Vincent JL, Yates D, et al. Four phases of intravenous fluid therapy: a conceptual model. Br J Anaesth. 2014;113(5):740-7.
93. Simonetto DA, Gines P, Kamath PS. Hepatorenal syndrome: pathophysiology, diagnosis, and management. BMJ. 2020;370:m2687.
94. Gilbert-Kawai N, Hogan B, Milan Z. Perioperative management of patients with liver disease. BJA Educ. 2022;22(3):111-7.

95. Zanetto A, Northup P, Roberts L, Senzolo M. Haemostasis in cirrhosis: Understanding destabilising factors during acute decompensation. J Hepatol. 2023;78(5):1037-47.
96. Chandok N, Watt KDS. Pain management in the cirrhotic patient: the clinical challenge. Mayo Clin Proc. 2010;85(5):451-8.
97. Verbeeck RK. Pharmacokinetics and dosage adjustment in patients with hepatic dysfunction. Eur J Clin Pharmacol. 2008;64(12):1147-61.
98. Mcclain RL, Ramakrishna H, Aniskevich S, Cartwright JA, Phar LGW, Pai SL, et al. Anesthetic pharmacology and perioperative considerations for the end stage liver disease patient. Curr Clin Pharmacol. 2015;10(1):35-46.
99. Gelman S. General anesthesia and hepatic circulation. Can J Physiol Pharmacol. 1987;65(8):1762-79.
100. Soon-Ho NAM. Liver function and inhaled anesthetics. J Korean Med Assoc. 2006;49(12):1126.
101. Moon AM, Jiang Y, Rogal SS, Tapper EB, Lieber SR, Barritt AS 4th. Opioid prescriptions are associated with hepatic encephalopathy in a national cohort of patients with compensated cirrhosis. Aliment Pharmacol Ther. 2020;51(6):652-60.
102. Dershwitz M, Hoke JF, Rosow CE, Michalowski P, Connors PM, Muir KT, et al. Pharmacokinetics and Pharmacodynamics of Remifentanil in Volunteer Subjects with Severe Liver Disease. Anesthesiology. 1996;84(4):812-20.
103. Craig RG, Hunter JM. Neuromuscular blocking drugs and their antagonists in patients with organ disease. Anaesthesia. 2009;64 Suppl 1:55-65.
104. van Miert MM, Eastwood NB, Boyd AH, Parker CJ, Hunter JM. The pharmacokinetics and pharmacodynamics of rocuronium in patients with hepatic cirrhosis. Br J Clin Pharmacol. 1997;44(2):139-44.
105. Kiamanesh D, Rumley J, Moitra VK. Monitoring and managing hepatic disease in anaesthesia. Br J Anaesth. 2013;111(Suppl 1):i50-61.

CHAPTER 14

Acute Kidney Disease and Anesthesia

Sophia TH Chew

ABSTRACT

Acute kidney injury (AKI) is a common and severe complication in surgical patients associated with increased morbidity and mortality. The financial impact and overall incremental annual index hospitalization costs related to AKI exceed $1 billion in the United States alone. Adding to the financial burden is the increased risk of short and long-term complications, including chronic kidney disease and end-stage renal disease. The pathogenesis of AKI is multifaceted and complex. Although novel biomarkers may help detect the early onset of AKI, treatment remains elusive. Prevention of AKI is essential to managing AKI with strategies including maintenance of renal perfusion and avoidance of nephrotoxins and blood transfusion-related insults.

Keywords: Acute kidney injury; Postoperative complications; Renal biomarkers; Surgery; Diagnosis; Treatment

KEY POINTS

- Postoperative AKI is a well-recognized cause of significant morbidity and mortality.
- Early identification of the at-risk patient with proper triage and timely escalation of care remains critical to management.
- Management of the AKI patient involves a bundled care strategy to avoid further damage and mitigate the downstream effects of AKI.
- Follow-up of the AKI patient is essential as it is associated with adverse long-term outcomes.

INTRODUCTION

Acute kidney injury (AKI) is a severe complication after surgery that can lead to a significant increase in mortality, risk of chronic kidney disease, and end-stage renal disease with the need for long-term dialysis with a corresponding increase in healthcare utilization and costs.[1-4] The incidence of AKI varies between 7 and 40%, with the highest incidence reported in cardiac surgeries.

In cardiac surgical patients who developed AKI requiring dialysis, the mortality can exceed 60-70%.[5-7]

■ DEFINITION OF ACUTE KIDNEY INJURY

Acute kidney injury is defined by an increase in serum creatinine and/or a decrease in urine output. In 2004, the Acute Dialysis Quality Initiative group classified the level of kidney dysfunction based on the elevation of serum creatinine (SCr) concentration, reduction in glomerular filtration rates (GFRs), urine output, and clinical outcomes.[2] This staging is also known as the Risk, Injury, Failure, Loss, and End-stage (RIFLE) criteria. It is divided into Risk of renal dysfunction, Injury to the kidney, Failure of kidney function, Loss of kidney function, and End-stage kidney disease.[8] The classification that is based on the worst criteria should be used.

The staging system for AKI proposed by Acute Kidney Injury Network (AKIN) incorporated the three functional stages characterized by the RIFLE criteria with modifications to include minor changes in SCr concentration. It excludes changes in GFR.[9] Changes in SCr concentration (increased by at least 1.5 times baseline) and urine output (<0.5 mL/kg/h for at least 6 hours) formed the basis of the two classifications **(Table 1)**. The AKIN and RIFLE criteria provide robust and accurate risk assessment for in-hospital mortality when patients are classified appropriately. The AKIN criteria are advantageous as it does not require a baseline creatinine concentration and measurement of urine output.[10]

The Kidney Disease Improving Global Outcomes (KDIGO) group proposed a standard definition and staging system.[11] It defines AKI as an increase in SCr concentration ≥0.3 mg/dL (26.5 μmol/L) within 48 hours or an increase in SCr concentration ≥1.5 × baseline that is known or presumed to have occurred within the previous 7 days or urine volume <0.5 mL/kg/h for 6 hours. The KDIGO criteria for AKI staging demonstrate greater sensitivity to detect AKI and can predict associated in-hospital mortality compared with the RIFLE or AKIN criteria.

Surgical registries and databases have yet to formally accept these consensus classifications with different societies using slightly different criteria.[12-15] The serum creatinine cut-off of ≥309 μmol/L (3.5 mg/dL) is used by the American College of Surgeons Committee on Trauma to define AKI. The Society of Thoracic Surgeons Quality Performance Measures defines postoperative renal failure as a serum creatinine of ≥354 μmol/L (4.0 mg/dL) or 3x the last preoperative creatinine value. An increase in serum creatinine >177 μmol (2 mg/dL) from baseline or need for the renal replacement therapy (RRT) is the criteria used by the American College of Surgeons National Surgical Quality Improvement Project (NSQIP) for AKI. A low incidence of AKI but high mortality rates is reported by studies based on the American

TABLE 1: Staging of AKI (different workgroups).

Workgroup	Acute dialysis quality initiative group	AKI network	Kidney disease global outcome
Criteria	Serum creatinine, urinary output, glomerular filtration rate, and clinical outcome	Serum creatinine and urinary output	Serum creatinine and urinary output
Staging	**Risk:** • Serum creatinine increased by 1.5x • Urinary output <0.5 mL/kg/h for 6 hours • eGFR decreased by >25% within 7days **Injury:** • Serum creatinine increased by 2.0x • Urinary output <0.5 mL/kg/h for 12 hours • eGFR decreased by >50% **Failure:** • Serum creatinine increased by 3.0x Or • Serum creatinine ≥4 mg/dL (354 μmol/L) with acute rise ≥0.5 mg/dL (44 μmol/L) • Urinary output <0.3 mL/kg/h for 24 hours or anuria for 12 hours • eGFR decreased by >75% **Loss:** • Complete loss of kidney function >4 weeks • End-stage kidney disease total loss of kidney function >3 months	**Stage 1:** • Serum creatinine increased ≥0.3 mg/dL (26.5 μmol/L) Or • Serum creatinine increased by 1.5–2.0x • Urinary output <0.5 mL/kg/h for 6 hours **Stage 2:** • Serum creatinine increased by >2.0–3.0x • Urinary output <0.5 mL/kg/h for >12 hours **Stage 3:** • Serum creatinine increased by >3.0 Or • Serum creatinine ≥4 mg/dL (354 μmol/L) with acute rise of >0.5 mg/dL (44 μmol/L) • Urinary output <0.5 mL/kg/h for >24 hours or anuria for 12 hours	**Stage 1:** • Serum creatinine increased ≥0.3 mg/dL (26.5 μmol/L) within 48 hours Or • Serum creatinine increased by 1.5–1x, which is known or presumed to have occurred within 7 days • Urinary output <0.5 mL/kg/h for 6–12 hours **Stage 2:** • Serum creatinine increased by >2.0–2.9x • Urinary output <0.5 mL/kg/h for ≥12 hours **Stage 3:** • Serum creatinine increased by >3.0 or serum creatinine >4 mg/dL (354 μmol/L) other initiation of renal replacement therapy • Urinary output <0.3 mL/kg/h for ≥24 hours or anuria for ≥12 hours • eGFR <35 mL/min/1.73 m² in patients <18 years

(AKI: acute kidney injury; eGFR: estimated glomerular filtration rate)

College of Surgeons NSQIP database, giving the impression that AKI is rare in surgical patients. There is a need to follow one global AKI scoring system to benchmark, audit, research, and improve quality.

■ NORMAL PHYSIOLOGY OF THE KIDNEYS

The kidneys receive 20% of the cardiac output, with most of the blood in the cortex directed to glomerular filtration. The complex peritubular microcirculation with the counter-current system is designed to deliver oxygen, reabsorb water and solutes to the systemic circulation, and crucially allow for water conservation. The renal blood flow is maintained by autoregulation within a mean arterial pressure (MAP) range of 60-100 mm Hg. The sympathetic nervous system, nitric oxide, prostaglandin E2 and angiotensin, adenosine, and endothelin are involved in autoregulation.[16]

■ PATHOPHYSIOLOGY OF ACUTE KIDNEY INJURY

The pathogenesis of AKI after surgery is complex, multifactorial, and incompletely understood. Several injury pathways contribute to the development of AKI to differing extents in different patients. These include etiologies such as renal hypoperfusion, tissue ischemic reperfusion injury, and inflammatory and nephrotoxic mechanisms.[17]

Renal Hypoperfusion

The initial insult in AKI is often renal hypoperfusion. It occurs due to reduced blood flow to the highly metabolic renal medulla, which is vulnerable to risk of hypoxia and hypoperfusion. The delicate balance of oxygen delivery to demands in the renal medulla is disrupted easily by reduced supply or increased demands, leading to cell injury and organ failure.

Numerous studies have demonstrated an association between intraoperative hypotension and developing postoperative AKI.[18-25] A retrospective analysis of >30 noncardiac surgeries found intraoperative hypotension (MAP <55 mm Hg) to be an independent risk factor for AKI.[21] The risk magnitude depends on the duration of hypotension, and even short episodes of low blood pressure for 1-5 minutes are significant. Another analysis of 57,000 patients corroborated that intraoperative hypotension (MAP below 65 mm Hg for a few minutes) increased the risk of AKI.[23]

Blood pressure is essential in renal perfusion and is a surrogate marker of the adequacy of oxygen delivery. Oxygen delivery to the renal medulla depends on a complex interplay among pressure, flow, and oxygen content. In cardiac surgery, Ranucci et al. studied the role of nadir oxygen delivery, nadir hematocrit, and pump flow during cardiopulmonary bypass (CPB) and the risks of AKI.[26,27] It was reported that a nadir oxygen delivery (DO_2) of <262 mL/min/m^2 during CPB is associated independently with AKI stage 2.

The nadir DO_2 level is also associated significantly with prolonged intensive care unit (ICU) and postoperative hospital length of stay. Although increasing pump flow rates may improve oxygen delivery, excessive renal blood flow paradoxically may lead to increased energy consumption, aggravating hypoxic stress, cell injury, and kidney impairment.

Microcirculatory Dysfunction

An intact microcirculation ensures the adequacy of perfusion of the renal tubules. In sepsis, microcirculatory dysfunction results in maladaptive flow and hypoperfusion in the kidney areas. Endothelial dysfunction further disrupts this maldistribution in the microcirculation by capillary leak, transmigration of leucocytes, and proinflammatory cytokines release.[28]

Inflammatory Response

The systemic inflammatory response during surgery triggers the immune system and vascular endothelium, proinflammatory cytokines, and free radicals to cause renal tubular injury.[28] Renal autoregulation is adversely affected by vasodilatation, capillary permeability increase, and the systemic inflammatory response. Cytokine-activated macrophages, neutrophils, and lymphocytes migrate into the renal parenchyma, enhancing renal injury.[29] Ischemia and reperfusion induce reactive oxygen species production, which causes an inflammatory response from the upregulation of proinflammatory transcription factors, such as nuclear factor kappa B.[30] The immune cells can infiltrate the parenchymal cells and contribute to long-term fibrosis.[31]

■ FORMATION OF MICROVASCULAR THROMBI

Endothelial cells inhibit blood coagulation under normal conditions by interacting with protein C and thrombomodulin. Natural anticoagulants, including protein C, are degraded, or their production is reduced in the inflammatory response. This causes a prothrombotic state with the formation of microthrombi, leading to capillary plugging. This phenomenon is typical of the response to sepsis and conditions associated with complement activation.[28] In cardiac surgery, blood interfaces with nonendothelial surfaces during cardiopulmonary bypass, activating the coagulation cascade and forming microthrombi.

Drugs Affecting Renal Function

Diuretic therapy, antibiotics (gentamicin and trimethoprim), antihypertensives [angiotensin-converting enzyme (ACE) inhibitors and angiotensin-receptor blockers], nonsteroidal anti-inflammatory drugs (NSAIDs), and contrast media can affect the renal function. There is a concern that renin-angiotensin-aldosterone system blockers impair kidney autoregulation, leading to decreased GFR. This is of concern in patients with heart failure, but this reduction in GFR is usually slight, and treatment with these drugs need not be withheld perioperatively.[32,33]

Aminoglycosides are bactericidal antibiotics. They can cause direct kidney injury by inhibiting oxidative phosphorylation and the synthesis of adenosine triphosphate.[34] Deterioration of renal function is associated with the duration of gentamicin treatment. Using gentamicin in the perioperative period has been linked to an increased risk of postoperative dialysis.[35]

Nonsteroidal anti-inflammatory drugs inhibit cyclooxygenase enzymes and can cause renal ischemia with a subsequent decrease in glomerular filtration. By blocking prostaglandin synthesis, extreme and protracted outer medullary hypoxia has been demonstrated with the injudicious use of NSAIDs.[36]

Patients requiring urgent or emergent surgery often need angiography, which exposes them to radiocontrast-induced nephropathy. Renal vasoconstriction or a direct cytotoxic effect of the agent has been postulated as the mechanism of contrast-induced nephropathy (CIN).[37]

Genetic Predisposition

Many genetic polymorphisms have been associated with AKI and its outcomes.[38] In cardiac surgery, the apolipoprotein E e4 allele, which is responsible for lipoprotein metabolism, tissue repair, and immunomodulation, was found to be protective of AKI and associated with a lower peak SCr concentration and a reduction in postoperative SCr concentration elevation in patients undergoing cardiac surgery.[39] Polymorphism of 174G>C in the interleukin 6 (*IL6*) gene is associated with higher postoperative plasma IL-6 concentrations and the development of AKI.

A genome-wide association study of AKI after CABG surgery found genome-wide significance at two new susceptibility loci: (1) GRM7|LMCD1-AS1 locus and (2) BBS9 52. These results suggest that these two new loci may be involved in the pathogenesis of perioperative AKI.[40]

■ RISK PREDICTION MODELS

Early identification of patients at high risk of AKI using risk prediction models enables clinicians to monitor these patients closely and to initiate effective preventive and therapeutic strategies to reduce the incidence of AKI. However, several validated risk prediction models for AKI were developed using older definitions of AKI and for selected populations, e.g., cardiac surgery. Most of these risk factors utilize static risk that includes male sex, the advanced age of >50, multiple comorbidities [for example, hypertension, preexisting ascites, chronic kidney disease, intraperitoneal surgery, heart failure, emergent surgery, use of an ACE inhibitor or angiotensin receptor blocker (ARB) polypharmacy and a higher American Society of Anesthesiologists physical status classification score]. In patients in the ICU after surgery, the risk factors for AKI are related to those of critical illness and are often associated with shock and sepsis.

Biomarkers

Diagnosis of AKI in patients with stable chronic kidney disease is based on changes in SCr concentration and a reasonable estimate of the GFR. However, it functions poorly during the acute stages of kidney injury. Serum creatinine concentrations and GFR do not have a linear relationship and a significant decline in GFR of >50% occurs before any increase in SCr concentration. There is also a lag phase between the initial kidney injury and the rise in the SCr concentration. Serum creatinine concentration is also influenced by sex, age, protein intake, and medications.[41]

Given the limitations of SCr concentration, the use of novel biomarkers to aid in diagnosing AKI has been explored **(Table 2)**. These detect the early onset of renal injury before functional damage, reflected by a rising SCr concentration. Several urine and blood biomarkers have been examined to indicate kidney injury, and the rise of these biomarkers precedes a rise in SCr concentration.[42,43] Most of the AKI biomarkers research has aimed to discover a "kidney troponin" that correlates with renal injury, a key research area identified by the American Society of Nephrology. However, unlike myocardial infarction, the etiology of AKI is multifaceted, and thus a single biomarker is unlikely to have all the ideal characteristics of a "kidney troponin".[44]

About 276 patients at high risk of AKI, identified by a positive cell cycle arrest biomarker 4 hours after cardiac surgery, were randomized to a standard of care or a bundled intervention based on the KDIGO guidelines.[45] The KDIGO bundle included optimizing volume status and hemodynamics, closely monitoring creatinine levels and urine output, glucose levels, minimizing contrast exposure, and avoiding nephrotoxins. At 72 hours, there was a significant reduction in absolute risk of AKI by 17% and a reduction in AKI stages 2 and 3 of 15%. Göcze et al. followed a targeted approach without functional hemodynamic optimization in a study on major noncardiac surgery patients at risk of AKI.[46] They demonstrated a 13% reduction in AKI stages 2 and 3 ($p = 0.04$), although the decrease in the overall incidence of AKI at seven days was not significant. Both studies demonstrated the utilization of novel cell cycle arrest AKI biomarkers to aid in the early detection of kidney injury, allowing for the prompt and effective execution of an AKI care bundle in at-risk patients to reduce the incidence of AKI following major surgery.

TABLE 2: Comparison of some common biomarkers of AKI.

AKI biomarker	Characteristics	Origin in the kidney
• Alanine aminopeptidase • Alkaline phosphatase gamma-glutamyl-transpeptidase	Enzymes located on the brush border villi of the proximal tubular cells	Released from tubular brush border after injury to proximal tubular cells
Calprotectin	Cytosolic calcium-binding complex of two proteins of the S100 group; derived from neutrophils and monocytes	Detected in urine following intrinsic AKI
Chitinase 3-like protein 1	39-kDa soluble intracellular protein of glycoside hydrolase family 18 expressed by macrophages, endothelial cells, chondrocytes, neutrophils, smooth muscle, and cancer cells	Undergoes glomerular filtration. In addition it is also secreted by macrophages within the kidneys in the event of renal stress or damage
Cystatin-C	13-kDa protein and cysteine protease inhibitor made by most nucleated human cells and released into plasma at constant rate	Freely filtered in glomeruli and completely absorbed and catabolized by proximal tubular cell. There is no tubular resorption or secretion
Alpha-glutathione-S-transferase (α-GST)	47–51 kDa cytoplasmic enzyme in proximal tubule	Released into urine following tubular injury
π-glutathione S-transferase	47–51 kDa cytoplasmic enzyme in distal tubules	Released into urine after tubular injury
Hepatocyte growth factor	Antifibrotic cytokine produced by mesenchymal cells. Involved in tubular cell regeneration after acute kidney injury	Released into urine after tubular injury
Hepcidin	2.78-kDa peptide hormone predominantly produced in hepatocytes, kidney, brain, and heart. It is a regulator of iron metabolism	Freely filtered followed by tubular uptake and catabolism

Contd...

AKI biomarker	Characteristics	Origin in the kidney
Combination of insulin-like growth factor-binding protein-7 (IGFBP) and tissue inhibitor of metalloproteinase-2 (TIMP-2)	• *IGFBP-7*: 29-kDa secreted protein, bind to and inhibit signaling through IGF-1 receptors which are involved in G1 cell cycle arrest • *TIMP-2*: 21-kDa protein, endogenous inhibitor of metalloproteinase activities involved in cell cycle arrest	• Released into urine following tubular cell stress. • Raised urine TIMP-2 and IGFBP-7 showed pooled AUROC of 0.857 (0.789–0.925)
Interleukin-18	• 18-kDa proinflammatory cytokine • Produced by multiple tissues including macrophages, monocytes, proximal tubular epithelial cells, and collecting ducts	• Released into urine by proximal tubular cells after tubular injury • Lack of definite agreement on cut off level of IL-18 for AKI
Kidney injury molecule-1	Transmembrane glycoprotein produced by proximal tubular cells following ischemic or nephrotoxic injury	• Released into urine after ischemic or nephrotoxic tubular damage • Urinary KIM-1 concentrations increase with age in healthy human individuals
Urinary liver-type fatty acid-binding protein	14-kDa intracellular carrier protein produced in proximal tubular cells and hepatocytes	Freely filtered in glomeruli. Reabsorbed and catabolized in proximal tubular cells. Increased urinary excretion after tubular cell damage
α_1-microglobulin	Low molecular weight protein produced in liver	Freely filtered in glomeruli. Reabsorbed and catabolized in proximal tubular cells. Increased urinary excretion after tubular cell dysfunction
β_2-microglobulin	12-kDa light chain of major histocompatibility Class I expressed on cell surface of every nucleated cell	Freely filtered in glomeruli. Reabsorbed and catabolized in proximal tubular cells. Increased urinary excretion after tubular cell dysfunction

Contd...

AKI biomarker	Characteristics	Origin in the kidney
MicroRNA	Endogenous single-stranded molecules of noncoding nucleotides	Upregulated following tubular injury and detectable in plasma and urine
Monocyte chemoattractant peptide-1	Peptide expressed in renal mesangial cells and podocytes	Released into urine
N-acetyl-β-D-glucosaminidase	>130-kDa lysosomal enzyme; produced in proximal and distal tubular cells and nonrenal cells	• Too large to undergo glomerular filtration • Released into urine after tubular damage
Neutrophil gelatinase-associated lipocalin	At least three different types: 1. Monomeric 25-kDa glycoprotein produced by neutrophils and epithelial tissues, including renal tubular cells 2. Homodimeric 45-kDa protein produced by neutrophils 3. Heterodimeric 135-kDa protein produced by renal tubular cells	• 25 and 45 kDa NGAL undergo glomerular filtration. Reabsorbed by healthy tubular cells • 25 and 135 kDa NGAL are released into urine following tubular damage
Netrin-1	50–75 kDa laminin-related molecule minimally expressed in proximal tubular epithelial cells of normal kidneys	• Expressed in injured proximal tubules and released into urine • Not specific to the kidneys
Proenkephalin	Endogenous polypeptide hormone in adrenal medulla, nervous system, immune system, and renal tissue	Cleared by glomerular filtration

(AKI: acute kidney injury; AUROC: area under the receiver operating characteristic; IL–18: interleukin-18; kDa: kilodalton; KIM-1: kidney-injury-molecule 1; NGAL: neutrophil gelatinase-associated lipocalin; RNA: ribonucleic acid)

PERIOPERATIVE PATIENT MANAGEMENT

Prevention of AKI remains the key as there are no current therapeutic interventions to treat AKI associated with surgery specifically.

Preoperative Preparation

The primary preoperative goals include correcting intravascular depletion, optimizing cardiac output, and avoiding nephrotoxic agents. Drugs such as NSAIDs, ACE inhibitors, and intravenous contrast preoperatively can increase the risk of AKI. To avoid perioperative hypotension, it is common to discontinue ACE inhibitors and ARBs before surgery. However, limited data supports this practice. An analysis of data from 949 patients undergoing major gastrointestinal or hepatobiliary surgery found no difference in the rates of AKI between patients who continued with ACE inhibitors withheld versus those who continued it perioperatively.[47]

Nonsteroidal anti-inflammatory drugs are commonly given for pain relief in the perioperative period but are best avoided in patients at high risk of AKI, such as those with sepsis or hypovolemia. Although NSAIDS are used in patients with normal renal function, their role in increasing the risk of AKI postoperatively is unclear.[48]

Administration of single-shot aminoglycosides, as in antibiotic prophylaxis for cardiac surgery, is not opposed by the European Renal Best Practice (ERBP) working group. If more than one dose is required, they recommend using aminoglycoside antibiotics for as short a duration as possible.[49]

Some patients may undergo scans requiring contrast before surgery. The contrast medium is nephrotoxic as it can cause crenation of red cells and release of free oxygen radicals. The toxicity is not just related to the type and dose of contrast medium but is also influenced by the patient's age, underlying renal function, and hydration status. Current guidelines recommend using intravenous isotonic fluid fluids for hydration to reduce the risk of CIN.[49]

Intraoperative Maintenance of Renal Perfusion and Renal Function

Maintenance of renal blood flow and adequate perfusion pressure is the mainstay of perioperative management for preventing AKI. A perioperative quality initiative study found an increased risk of AKI and death associated with an intraoperative mean arterial blood pressure below 60–70 mm Hg.[50] Both the magnitude and duration of intraoperative hypotension were significant risk factors. A retrospective cohort analysis reported that one-third of all intraoperative hypotension at a single institution occurred between the induction of anesthesia and surgical incision. Hypotension before and after surgical incision was associated with kidney and myocardial injuries.[51]

In a study involving 298 high-risk abdominal surgeries, patients were randomized to tight blood pressure control (systolic pressure was maintained within 10% baseline with norepinephrine) or minimal blood pressure control (ephedrine was administered if systolic pressure fell to <40% below baseline or <80 mm Hg) during surgery and for four hours postoperatively showed that patients assigned to tight blood pressure treatment developed significantly lower rates of organ-specific morbidity, including AKI.[52]

The optimal systemic pressure that prevents AKI is variable and differs between patients, but a reasonable target would be a systemic MAP of between 65 and 75 mm Hg. Furthermore, the goals for arterial pressure should be individualized according to the normal baseline blood pressure, particularly in patients with preexisting hypertension or kidney impairment. To date, it remains uncertain which vasopressor is most effective in preventing AKI. In low cardiac output states, renal perfusion pressures may improve using both inotropes and vasopressors. The ERBP recommends utilizing vasopressor therapy (norepinephrine or vasopressin) to improve renal perfusion in volume-resuscitated patients rather than extra fluid.[11]

Cardiac output monitoring and optimizing the increase in global oxygen delivery are part of goal-directed therapy and effectively reduce the risk of AKI. A meta-analysis of 65 randomized controlled trials in high-risk patients undergoing major abdominal and orthopedic surgery found that goal-directed hemodynamic therapy improved renal perfusion and oxygenation with judicious maintenance of fluids and inotropes.[53]

The fluid volume administered for adequate intravascular volume replacement should be individualized. In the RELIEF (Restrictive versus Liberal Fluid Therapy in Major Abdominal Surgery) randomized control trial (RCT), 3,000 patients undergoing noncardiac surgery were randomized to either restrictive aerofluid balance or moderately liberal fluid balance target. An increased risk of AKI was found in the restrictive zero fluid-balance group.[54] A fluid regimen with an overall positive fluid balance of 1–2 L at the end of surgery is recommended to mitigate the risk of AKI.[55]

The type of intravenous fluids used can also impact AKI. Normal saline (0.9%) is associated with an increased risk of AKI as compared with balanced crystalloids. Large volumes of 0.9% saline can lead to hyperchloremic acidosis and AKI and should not be used during major surgery.[56] Starch-based colloids have been shown to increase the risk of AKI in critically ill patients and sepsis. Although concern has been raised about the use of starch-based colloids, the data is limited. A recent trial reported no significant difference in the composite outcome of postoperative complications or death between patients who received colloids within 14 days after major abdominal surgery.[57]

Diuretic therapy is not recommended to prevent AKI (level 1B); however loop diuretic agents are useful to promote diuresis as part of the management of volume overload.[11]

Perioperative anemia with hemoglobin levels <8 g/dL is a risk factor for perioperative AKI. Treatment options to correct anemia include iron and erythropoietin given preoperatively. The effectiveness of oral iron is limited by gastrointestinal side effects. The duration of therapy may be prolonged which is not possible for time-sensitive surgery. Intravenous iron may be a better alternative to treat anemia and may be considered in combination with erythropoiesis-stimulating agents.

Red blood cell transfusion as therapy for anemia increases the risk of AKI. In cardiac surgery, it was demonstrated that restricting blood transfusion is not inferior to a liberal transfusion strategy in preventing AKI.[58] Current clinical guidelines recommendations by various societies maintain that a restrictive perioperative allogeneic red blood cell transfusion is preferred to a liberal transfusion strategy for perioperative blood conservation, as it reduces both transfusion rates and units of allogeneic red blood cells without increased risk of mortality or morbidity (Class I, level A). Antifibrinolytic agents (lysine analogs such as epsilon-aminocaproic acid and tranexamic acid) are recommended to reduce total blood loss and decrease the number of patients who require a blood transfusion during cardiac surgery (Class I, level of evidence A).[59]

Glycemic Control

Hyperglycemia is detrimental in critically ill and is associated with increased mortality and morbidity, including AKI and the need for dialysis. The 2001 Van den Berghe study demonstrated that intensive glycemic control (80–110 mg/dL and 4.4–6.1 mmol/L) was associated with a significant decrease in the need for RRT, other morbidity, and mortality in critically ill surgical patients versus conventional glycemic control (180–200 mg/dL and 10–11.1 mmol/L).[60] In 2009, the Normoglycemia in Intensive Care Evaluation-Survival Using Glucose Algorithm Regulation study compared intensive (blood glucose: 80–110 mg/dL and 4.4–6.1 mmol/L) with conventional (blood glucose ≤180 mg/dL and 10 mmol/L) glycemic control. It found no difference between the two groups in the need for RRT or incidence of other ICU morbidities. There was a significant increase in the incidence of severe hypoglycemia in the intensive glucose control group with an associated increase in 90-day mortality.[61] The KDIGO workgroup recommends that the average blood glucose should not exceed 150 mg/dL (8.3 mmol/L) but that insulin therapy should not be used to lower blood glucose to <110 mg/dL (6.1 mmol/L). These thresholds are interpolated from a comparison of trials that compared intensive and conventional glycemic control regimens, and close glycemic monitoring is necessary.

KDIGO Bundle

The KDIGO clinical practice guideline for AKI recommends supportive measures, such as volume optimization, maintaining adequate blood pressure, and avoiding nephrotoxins. Two RCTs demonstrated that, once biomarkers are identified after surgery, implementing the bundle in high-risk patients significantly reduced the incidence of AKI; however, the studies were not adequately powered to examine differences in longer-term patient outcomes.[45,46]

RENAL REPLACEMENT THERAPY

In established AKI, RRT is initiated for the treatment of volume overload, uremia, severe metabolic acidosis, and hyperkalemia. There is a considerable debate on the optimal timing of starting RRT in patients with AKI. The proponents of early initiation of RRT proposed that early therapy reduces the incidence of AKI and improve outcomes in patients with cardiac disease. However, RRT is associated with increased risk of complication, healthcare costs, and clinical workload.

The STARRT-AKI study showed that early commencement of RRT based on AKI criteria without conventional indications does not improve survival. Furthermore, early RRT may unnecessarily expose patients to dialysis which can lead to an increased risk of dialysis dependency at 90 days as compared to a conservative strategy for initiating RRT [odds ratio for mortality with early RRT 1.20; 95% confidence interval (CI), 0.91–1.59].[62]

Modality of Renal Replacement Therapy

Various modalities of RRT have been used in AKI, including continuous renal replacement therapy (CRRT), intermittent hemodialysis, and extended dialysis. Intermittent hemodialysis may be of shorter duration with less anticoagulation requirements but potentially more hemodynamically unstable. CRRT offers better hemodynamic stability, with the KDIGO guidelines suggesting using CRRT in hemodynamically unstable patients (Class 2B; not graded). Extended dialysis may also be suitable for treatment in this setting.[11]

OUTCOMES OF ACUTE KIDNEY INJURY AND ACUTE KIDNEY DISEASE

Acute kidney injury is associated with a higher risk of morbidity, short- and long-term mortality, increased resource utilization, and costs.[3-7,12] Patients with AKI admitted in an ICU for at least 24 hours following major surgery, had worse survival over 10 years.[63]

Patients with AKI are susceptible to postoperative complications, such as infection, cardiovascular events, and prolonged mechanical ventilation. An analysis of noncardiac patients, who underwent noncardiac and nonvascular surgery, found that 6.7% met the RIFLE criteria for AKI. AKI patients were at significantly higher risk of cardiovascular events, including acute coronary syndrome, acute heart failure, and arrhythmias.[64]

Patients with AKI are at increased risk of acute kidney disease and progressive deterioration of kidney function, including chronic kidney disease and end-stage renal disease. In patients undergoing major surgery those who developed AKI, the incidence of kidney failure at 1 year was 0.94% versus as compared to 0.05% of those who did not.[65] Using a competing risk model, adjusted progression to kidney failure during 10 years of follow-up was 0.4, 2.3, 7.3, and 15.7% for the patients with no kidney disease, AKI with no CKD, CKD with no AKI, and AKI with CKD, respectively ($p < 0.001$).

■ POSTOPERATIVE MONITORING AND MANAGEMENT

Acute kidney injury is best considered a clinical syndrome with short- and long-term complications that may persist long after the initial insult. Monitoring pathways must be developed in collaboration with nephrologists. A detailed kidney health assessment is highly recommended, including an integrated assessment for structural kidney damage, prognostication of AKI, and risk assessment for the progression of AKI to CKD. Based on the focused assessment, appropriate care pathways, including the frequency of screening, must be established for early detection of deterioration and early treatment. This, in turn, will impact the longer-term outcomes of AKI.

■ CONCLUSION

Acute kidney injury is a multifaceted complex syndrome associated with significant morbidity and mortality. Prevention remains crucial to management which is best achieved through a multidisciplinary approach with intensivists, nephrologists, surgeons, and anesthesiologists. A targeted approach should include serial assessments of AKI risk, prognostication, and long-term follow-up of patients at risk of long-term sequelae.

■ REFERENCES

1. Zarbock A, Koyner JL, Hoste EAJ, Kellum JA. Update on perioperative acute kidney injury. Anesth Analg. 2018;127(5):1236-45.
2. Meersch M, Schmidt C, Zarbock A. Perioperative acute kidney injury: an under-recognized problem. Anesth Analg. 2017;125(4):1223-32.
3. Schurle A, Koyner JL. CSA-AKI: incidence, epidemiology, clinical outcomes, and economic impact. J Clin Med 2021;10(24):5746.
4. Alshaikh HN, Katz NM, Gani F, Nagarajan N, Canner JK, Kacker S, et al. Financial impact of acute kidney injury after cardiac operations in the United States. Ann Thorac Surg. 2018;105(2):469-75.
5. Machado MN, Nakazone MA, Maia LN. Prognostic value of acute kidney injury after cardiac surgery according to kidney disease: Improving global outcomes definition and staging (KDIGO) criteria. PLoS One. 2014;9(5):e98028.

6. Rydén L, Ahnve S, Bell M, Hammar N, Ivert T, Holzmann MJ. Acute kidney injury following coronary artery bypass grafting: Early mortality and postoperative complications. Scand Cardiovasc J. 2012;46(2):114-20.
7. Srivastava V, D'Silva C, Tang A, Sogliani F, Ngaage DL. The impact of major perioperative renal insult on long-term renal function and survival after cardiac surgery. Interact Cardiovasc Thorac Surg. 2012;15(1):14-7.
8. Bellomo R, Ronvo C, Kellum JA, Mehta RL, Palevsky P. Acute Dialysis Quality Initiative workgroup. Acute renal failure—Definition, outcome measures, animal models, fluid therapy and information technology needs: The Second International Consensus Conference of the Acute Dialysis Quality Initiative (ADQI) Group. Crit Care. 2004;8(4):R204-12.
9. Mehta RL, Kellum JA, Shah SV, Molitoris BA, Ronco C, Warnock DG, et al. Acute kidney injury network: Report of an initiative to improve outcomes in acute kidney injury. Crit Care. 2007;11(2):R31.
10. Robert AM, Kramer RS, Dacey LJ, Charlesworth DC, Leavitt BJ, Helm RE, et al. Cardiac surgery-associated acute kidney injury: a comparison of two consensus Criteria. Ann Thorac Surg. 2010;90(6):1939-43.
11. Kellum JA, Lameire N, Aspelin P, Barsoum RS, Burdmann EA, Goldstein SL, et al. Kidney disease: Improving global outcomes (KDIGO) acute kidney injury work group. KDIGO clinical practice guideline for acute kidney injury. Kidney Int Suppl. 2012;2(1):1-138.
12. Bihorac A, Brennan M, Ozrazgat Baslanti T, Bozorgmehri S, Efron PA, Moore FA, et al. National Surgical Quality Improvement Program underestimates the risk associated with mild and moderate postoperative acute kidney injury. Crit Care Med. 2013;41(11):2570-83.
13. Vascular Quality Initiative. (2023). Quality improvement. [online] Available from: https://www.vqi.org/quality-improvement [Last accessed September, 2023].
14. Dixon JL, Papaconstantinou HT, Hodges B, Korsmo RS, Jupiter D, Shake J, et al. Redundancy and variability in quality and outcome reporting for cardiac and thoracic surgery. Proc (Bayl Univ Med Cent). 2015;28(1):14-7.
15. Cronenwett JL, Kraiss LW, Cambria RP. The society for vascular surgery vascular quality initiative. J Vasc Surg. 2012;55(5):1529-37.
16. Ergin B, Kapucu A, Demirci-Pansei C, Ince C. The renal microcirculation in sepsis. Nephrol Dial Transplant. 2015;30(2):169-77.
17. Okusa MD. The inflammatory cascade in acute ischemic renal failure. Nephron. 2002;90(2):133-8.
18. Tang Y, Zhu C, Liu J, Wang A, Duan K, Li B, et al. Association of intraoperative hypotension with acute kidney injury after noncardiac surgery in patients younger than 60 years old. Kidney Blood Press Res. 2019;44(2):211-21.
19. Mathis MR, Naik BI, Freundlich RE, Shanks AM, Heung M, Kim M, et al. Preoperative risk and the association between hypotension and postoperative acute kidney injury. Anesthesiology. 2020;132(3):461-75.
20. Kanji HD, Schulze CJ, Hervas-Malo M, Wang P, Ross DB, Zibdawi M, et al. Difference between pre-operative and cardiopulmonary bypass mean arterial pressure is independently associated with early cardiac surgery-associated acute kidney injury. J Cardiothorac Surg. 2010;5:71.
21. Walsh M, Devereaux PJ, Garg AX, Kurz A, Turan A, Rodseth RN, et al. Relationship between intraoperative mean arterial pressure and clinical outcomes

after noncardiac surgery: toward an empirical definition of hypotension. Anesthesiology. 2013;119(3):507-15.
22. Sun LY, Wijeysundera DN, Tait GA, Beattie WS. Association of intraoperative hypotension with acute kidney injury after elective noncardiac surgery. Anesthesiology. 2015;123(3):515-23.
23. Salmasi V, Maheshwari K, Yang D, Mascha EJ, Singh A, Sessler DI, et al. Relationship between intraoperative hypotension, defined by either reduction from baseline or absolute thresholds, and acute kidney and myocardial injury after noncardiac surgery: a retrospective cohort analysis. Anesthesiology. 2017;126(1):47-65.
24. Jang WY, Jung JK, Lee DK, Han SB. Intraoperative hypotension is a risk factor for postoperative acute kidney injury after femoral neck fracture surgery: a retrospective study. BMC Musculoskelet Disord. 2019;20(1):131.
25. Vedel AG, Holmgaard F, Rasmussen LS, Langkilde A, Paulson OB, Lange T, et al. High-target versus low-target blood pressure management during cardiopulmonary bypass to prevent cerebral injury in cardiac surgery patients: a randomized controlled trial. Circulation. 2018;137(17):1770-80.
26. Ranucci M, Romitti F, Isgrò G, Cotza M, Brozzi S, Boncilli A, et al. Oxygen delivery during cardiopulmonary bypass and acute renal failure after coronary operations. Ann Thorac Surg. 2005;80(6):2213-20.
27. de Somer F, Mulholland JW, Bryan MR, Aloisio T, Van Nooten GJ, Ranucci M. O_2 delivery and CO_2 production during cardiopulmonary bypass as determinants of acute kidney injury: Time for a goal-directed perfusion management? Crit Care. 2011;15(4):R192.
28. Zafrani L, Payen D, Azoulay E, Ince C. The microcirculation of the septic kidney. Semin Nephrol. 2015;35(1):75-84.
29. Gando S. Microvascular thrombosis and multiple organ dysfunction syndrome. Crit Care Med. 2010;38(2 Suppl):S35-42.
30. Zhang WR, Garg AX, Coca SG, Devereaux PJ, Eikelboom J, Kavsak P, et al. Plasma IL-6 and IL-10 concentrations predict AKI and long-term mortality in adults after cardiac surgery. J Am Soc Nephrol. 2015;26(12):3123-32.
31. Liu KD, Glidden DV, Eisner MD, Parsons PE, Ware LB, Wheeler A, et al. Predictive and pathogenetic value of plasma biomarkers for acute kidney injury in patients with acute lung injury. Crit Care Med. 2007;35(12):2755-61.
32. Mason NA. Angiotensin-converting enzyme inhibitors and renal function. DICP. 1990;24(5):496-505.
33. Clark H, Krum H, Hopper I. Worsening renal function during renin-angiotensin-aldosterone system inhibitor initiation and long-term outcomes in patients with left ventricular systolic dysfunction. Eur J Heart Fail. 2014;16(1):41-8.
34. Bentley ML, Corwin HL, Dasta J. Drug-induced acute kidney injury in the critically ill adult: recognition and prevention strategies. Crit Care Med. 2010;38(6 Suppl):S169-74.
35. Nielsen DV, Hjortdal V, Larsson H, Johnsen SP, Jakobsen CJ. Perioperative aminoglycoside treatment is associated with a higher incidence of postoperative dialysis in adult cardiac surgery patients. J Thorac Cardiovasc Surg. 2011;142(3):656-61.
36. Hörl WH. Nonsteroidal anti-inflammatory drugs and the kidney. Pharmaceuticals (Basel). 2010;3(7):2291-321.

37. Persson PB, Hansell P, Liss P. Pathophysiology of contrast medium-induced nephropathy. Kidney Int. 2005;68(1):14-22.
38. Vilander LM, Kaunisto MA, Pettilä V. Genetic predisposition to acute kidney injury—a systematic review. BMC Nephrol. 2015;16:197.
39. Chew ST, Newman MF, White WD, Conlon PJ, Saunders AM, Strittmatter WJ, et al. Preliminary report on the association of apolipoprotein E polymorphisms, with postoperative peak serum creatinine concentrations in cardiac surgical patients. Anesthesiology. 2000;93(2):325-31.
40. Stafford-Smith M, Li YJ, Mathew JP, Li YW, Ji Y, Phillips-Bute BG, et al. Genome-wide association study of acute kidney injury after coronary bypass graft surgery identifies susceptibility loci. Kidney Int. 2015;88(4):823-32.
41. Ostermann M. Diagnosis of acute kidney injury: Kidney Disease Improving Global Outcomes criteria and beyond. Curr Opin Crit Care. 2014;20(6):581-7.
42. Cruz DN, Mehta RL. Acute kidney injury in 2013: Breaking barriers for biomarkers in AKI–progress at last. Nat Rev Nephrol. 2014;10(2):74-6.
43. Klein SJ, Brandtner AK, Lehner GF, Ulmer H, Bagshaw SM, Wiedermann CJ, et al. Biomarkers for prediction of renal replacement therapy in acute kidney injury: a systematic review and meta-analysis. Intensive Care Med. 2018;44(3):323-36.
44. Parikh CR, Han G. Variation in performance of kidney injury biomarkers due to cause of acute kidney injury. Am J Kidney Dis. 2013;62(6):1023-6.
45. Meersch M, Schmidt C, Hoffmeier A, Van Aken H, Wempe C, Gerss J, et al. Prevention of cardiac surgery-associated AKI by implementing the KDIGO guidelines in high risk patients identified by biomarkers: the PrevAKI randomized controlled trial. Intensive Care Med. 2017;43(11):1551-61.
46. Gőcze I, Jauch D, Götz M, Kennedy P, Jung B, Zeman F, Gnewuch C, et al. Biomarker-guided intervention to prevent acute kidney injury after major surgery: the prospective randomized BigpAK study. Ann Surg. 2018;267(6):1013-20.
47. STARSurg Collaborative. Association between peri-operative angiotensin-converting enzyme inhibitors and angiotensin-2 receptor blockers and acute kidney injury in major elective non-cardiac surgery: a multicentre, prospective cohort study. Anaesthesia. 2018;73(10):1214-22.
48. Bell S, Rennie T, Marwick CA, Davey P. Effects of peri-operative nonsteroidal anti-inflammatory drugs on post-operative kidney function for adults with normal kidney function. Cochrane Database Syst Rev. 2018;11(11):CD011274.
49. Fliser D, Laville M, Covic A, Fouque D, Vanholder R, et al. A European Renal Best Practice (ERBP) position statement on the Kidney Disease Improving Global Outcomes (KDIGO) Clinical Practice Guidelines on Acute Kidney Injury: Part 1: Definitions, conservative management and contrast-induced nephropathy. Nephrol Dial Transplant. 2012;27(12):4263-72.
50. Sessler DJ, Bloomstone JA, Aronson S, Berry C, Gan TJ, Kellum JA, et al. Perioperative quality initiative consensus statement on intraoperative blood pressure, risk and outcomes for elective surgery. Br J Anaesth. 2019;122(5):563-74.
51. Maheshwari K, Turan A, Mao G, Yang D, Niazi AK, Agarwal D, et al. The association of hypotension during non-cardiac surgery, before and after skin incision, with postoperative acute kidney injury: a retrospective cohort analysis. Anaesthesia. 2018;73(10):1223-8.
52. Futier E, Lefrant J-Y, Guinot P-G, Godet T, Lorne E, Cuvillon P, et al. Effect of individualized vs standard blood pressure management strategies on

postoperative organ dysfunction among high-risk patients undergoing major surgery: a randomized clinical trial. JAMA. 2017;318(14):1346-57.
53. Giglio M, Dalfino L, Puntillo F, Brienza N. Hemodynamic goal-directed therapy and postoperative kidney injury: an updated meta-analysis with trial sequential analysis. Crit Care. 2019;23(1):232.
54. Myles PS, Bellomo R, Corcoran T, Forbes A, Peyton P, Story D, et al. Restrictive versus liberal fluid therapy for major abdominal surgery. N Engl J Med. 2018;378(24):2263-74.
55. Miller TE, Myles PS. Perioperative fluid therapy for major surgery. Anesthesiology. 2019;130(5):825-32.
56. Shaw AD, Bagshaw SM, Goldstein SL, Scherer LA, Duan M, Schermer CR, et al. Major complications, mortality, and resource utilization after open abdominal surgery: 0.9% saline compared to Plasma-Lyte. Ann Surg. 2012;255(5):821-9.
57. Kabon B, Sessler DI, Kurz A; Crystalloid-Colloid Study Team. Effect of intraoperative goal-directed balanced crystalloid versus colloid administration on major postoperative morbidity: a randomized trial. Anesthesiology. 2019;130(5):728-44.
58. Garg AX, Badner N, Bagshaw SM, Cuerden MS, Fergusson DA, Gregory AJ, et al. Safety of a restrictive versus liberal approach to red blood cell transfusion on the outcome of AKI in patients undergoing cardiac surgery: a randomized clinical trial. J Am Soc Nephrol. 2019;30(7):1294-304.
59. Tibi P, McClure RS, Huang J, Baker RA, Fitzgerald D, Mazer CD, et al. STS/SCA/AmSECT/SABM Update to the Clinical Practice Guidelines on Patient Blood Management. Ann Thorac Surg. 2021;112(3):981-1004.
60. van den Berghe G, Wouters P, Weekers F, Verwaest C, Bruyninckx F, Schetz M, et al. Intensive insulin therapy in critically ill patients. N Engl J Med. 2001;345(19):1359-67.
61. NICE-SUGAR Study Investigators, Finfer S, Chittock DR, Su SY, Blair D, Foster D, et al. Intensive versus conventional glucose control in critically ill patients. N Engl J Med. 2009;360(13):1283-97.
62. STARRT-AKI Investigators; Canadian Critical Care Trials Group; Australian and New Zealand Intensive Care Society Clinical Trials Group; United Kingdom Critical Care Research Group; Canadian Nephrology Trials Network; Irish Critical Care Trials Group; et al. Timing of initiation of renal-replacement therapy in acute kidney injury. N Engl J Med. 2020;383(3):240-51.
63. Bihorac A, Yavas S, Subbiah S, Hobson CE, Schold JD, Gabrielli A, et al. Long-term risk of mortality and acute kidney injury during hospitalization after major surgery. Ann Surg. 2009;249(5):851-8.
64. Biteker M, Dayan A, Tekkeşin Aİ, Can MM, Taycı İ, İlhan E, et al. Incidence, risk factors, and outcomes of perioperative acute kidney injury in noncardiac and nonvascular surgery. Am J Surg. 2014;207(1):53-9.
65. Gameiro J, Neves JB, Rodrigues N, Bekerman C, Melo MJ, Pereira M, et al. Acute kidney injury, long-term renal function and mortality in patients undergoing major abdominal surgery: a cohort analysis. Clin Kidney J. 2016;9(2):192-200.

CHAPTER 15

Perioperative Management and Anesthetic Implications of Drug Addiction and Substance Abuse

Puneet Khanna

ABSTRACT

The prevalence of substance abuse and addiction to recreational drugs has increased the probability that anesthesiologists encounter patients who are acutely intoxicated and addicted to various recreational drugs or might be on deaddiction programs.

Nearly all aspects of the perioperative management are impacted by chronic substance abuse, beginning with difficulty securing an intravenous line, attaching monitors, induction of general anesthesia, and intraoperative and postoperative analgesia. The broad spectrum of problems associated with opioid abuse range from the rapid development of tolerance, physical addiction, psychological dependence, narcotic abstinence syndrome, and issues relating to the route of administration, intravenous, and subcutaneous. Acute perioperative pain management can be particularly challenging for opioid abusers about the significantly elevated postoperative opioid requirement for pain control. E-cigarette or vaping use-associated lung injury is an acute or subacute lung injury, a known complication found in young males using e-cigarettes. Nicotine overdose is another prominent adverse effect, as the nicotine content mentioned in e-cigarettes is highly unreliable. E-cigarette use is associated with increased inflammation and irritability of airway mucosa and a high risk of intraoperative bronchospasm.

Keywords: Physical dependence; Psychological dependence; Opioid use disorders; Vaping; *Cannabis*; Nicotine

■ KEY POINTS

- The incidence of various substance abuse is on an alarming rise, significantly upscaling the probability of anesthesiologists encountering a substance abuser in the intensive care unit, routine, and emergency operation theaters, and the emergency department.
- Opioid addicts have difficult peripheral venous access, reduced intravascular volume, and are prone to hemodynamic instability.

- Among the many risk factors associated with persistent postoperative use as well as misuse, those which are most relevant to us are a history of current opioid use, current or previous substance use disorder, previous history of opioid use, younger age, smoking, more medical comorbidities history of chronic pain, and coexisting psychiatric disease.
- Considering the poor pain control and high postoperative morbidity in patients who are chronic opioid users, it has been suggested to taper opioids preoperatively, over 10–12 weeks, particularly doses equivalent to or higher than 90 mg morphine orally.
- E-cigarette or vaping use-associated lung injury is an acute or subacute lung injury, a known complication found in young males using e-cigarettes. Nicotine overdose, increased inflammation, and irritability of airway mucosa associated with a high risk of intraoperative bronchospasm and cardiovascular adverse effects are among the other adverse effects of vaping.
- *Cannabis* synergistically acts with volatile agents, causing profound myocardial depression. It also exaggerates the respiratory depressant effects of opioids.
- Nicotine significantly inhibits pulmonary gas exchange, causes ciliary hypomotility, and exaggerates sputum production. This, in turn, increases airway reactivity and causes a higher incidence of bronchospasm and perioperative adverse respiratory events.

INTRODUCTION

The prevalence of substance abuse and addiction to recreational drugs has increased the probability that anesthesiologists encounter patients who are acutely intoxicated and addicted to various recreational drugs or might be on deaddiction programs. Chronic abuse of these substances has equally prominent anesthetic implications. The purpose of this chapter is to elaborate on all the problems that an anesthesiologist might encounter in the perioperative and postoperative period regarding chronic illicit drug use in the patient.

Nearly all aspects of perioperative management are impacted by chronic substance abuse beginning with difficulty securing an intravenous line, attaching monitors, induction of general anesthesia, and intraoperative and postoperative analgesia. Addiction is when a person develops physical and psychological dependence on a substance. It includes dependence, tolerance as well as withdrawal symptoms. Physical dependence produces symptoms, such as vomiting and tremors. Psychological dependence has a far outreached impact, the intensity of which varies from the user's physical condition and the type, amount, and duration of drug abuse.[1]

■ SCREENING FOR SUBSTANCE ABUSE

In any patient suffering from chronic substance abuse, the importance of a detailed history cannot be understated. The history taking should be performed with empathy, and a patient at any point in time should not feel that he is being judged. Testing should be considered, and also suggests routine screening should be done.

Amongst various substances being abused by patients nowadays, we discuss the most frequently encountered, such as alcohol, marijuana, opioids, stimulants such as cocaine and amphetamines, and caffeine. The commonly abused drugs in India include alcohol, *Cannabis*, and opioids.[2]

■ OPIOID USE DISORDERS

The incidence of opioid use disorders worldwide is on an alarming rise. This has been implicated in the utilization of opioids in noncancer pain, resulting in a surge in the consumption of opioids and an increased prevalence of opioid overdose deaths. From 1999 to 2016, >200,000 people died in the United States due to opioid overdose.[3] Nonprescription pain medicine disorders such as heroin use disorders and fentanyl-like drug use continue to be on the rise. Opioid use disorders have been widely described in outpatients, but their manifestation, concerns, and complication in inpatients, especially perioperatively, have been scarcely described in the literature.

The broad spectrum of problems associated with opioid abuse range from the rapid development of tolerance, physical addiction, psychological dependence, narcotic abstinence syndrome, and issues relating to the route of administration, intravenous, and subcutaneous. Opioid use disorders have also been associated with other comorbidities such as psychiatric diagnoses, human immunodeficiency virus, and hepatitis C.[4] Patients in withdrawal present with sympathetic overstimulation resulting in restlessness, insomnia, mydriasis, tachycardia, tachypnea, and hypertension, the peak occurring approximately 48–72 hours after the last opioid dose. Opioid addicts have difficult peripheral venous access, reduced intravascular volume, and are prone to hemodynamic instability. Whereas acute opioid abuse reduces the minimum alveolar concentration (MAC) of volatile anesthetics amongst chronic opioid users, a cross-tolerance to all central nervous system (CNS) depressants, including volatile anesthetics and benzodiazepines, has been observed.[5] For the same reason, acute perioperative pain management can be particularly challenging in these patients of the significantly elevated postoperative opioid requirement for pain control. Considering the poor pain control and high postoperative morbidity in patients who are chronic opioid users, it has been suggested to taper opioids preoperatively, over 10–12 weeks, particularly doses equivalent to or higher than 90 mg morphine orally.[6]

Currently, medications that are Food and Drug Administration have approved to treat opioid use disorder (OUD) are buprenorphine, methadone, and naltrexone. Therefore, it is important to consider drug interactions with these drugs in patients with OUDs. In patients who are on buprenorphine, it has been suggested to reduce the dose to 8-12 mg sublingually, perioperatively, keeping into account that buprenorphine being a potent agonist of μ-receptor; can reduce opioid receptor binding by 85-90% and make postoperative analgesia challenging.[7]

Lastly, as anesthesiologists, we should be able to identify patients who are at risk of persistent postoperative use or misuse. Among the many risk factors associated with persistent postoperative use, those which are most relevant to us are a history of current opioid use, current or previous substance use disorder, previous history of opioid use, younger age, smoking, more medical comorbidities history of chronic pain, and coexisting psychiatric disease (particularly anxiety and depression).

ALCOHOL

Alcohol abuse is the leading cause of thiamine deficiency worldwide. Deficiency of this vitamin leads to Wernicke's encephalopathy, a syndrome characterized by the classic triad of encephalopathy, ophthalmoplegia, and ataxia. Any acute stressor such as critical illness and major trauma can precede the development of encephalopathy in chronic alcoholics. Intravenous thiamine should be administered to all the patients with a history of alcohol abuse. *Folate deficiency* is another known vitamin deficiency associated with these patients, leading to a high prevalence of megaloblastic anemia, a high incidence of postoperative wound infections, and poor healing. *Metabolic acidosis* in the form of alcoholic ketoacidosis and lactic ketoacidosis is the most commonly encountered metabolic disturbance. *Hypophosphatemia* and *hypomagnesemia* are the most commonly associated electrolyte abnormalities in these patients. Hepatic dysfunction is commonly seen in chronic alcoholics, ranging from alcoholic fatty liver, alcoholic hepatitis, or alcohol-related cirrhosis.

Chronic alcohol ingestion leads to cardiovascular morbidity in the form of alcoholic cardiomyopathy characterized by cardiomegaly and reduced ejection fraction, as well as a significantly high association with hypertension and cerebrovascular disease.[8] Acute alcohol intoxication is associated with high gastric volume and acidity, suppression of laryngeal reflexes, and a significantly increased risk of aspiration of gastric contents. Patients in acute alcohol withdrawal may present with symptoms including generalized tremor, tachycardia, cardiac arrhythmias, hypertension, nausea, vomiting, confusion, agitation, and hallucinations.

Chronic alcohol abuse is associated with resistance to all the central nervous system depressants, increasing the induction dose of intravenous anesthesia agents and MAC of volatile agents. However, in acute alcohol intoxication, decreased dosing of volatile and intravenous induction agents is required. About opioids, decreased metabolism has been observed in chronic alcoholics, significantly increasing the risk of accumulation with repeated doses. Neuromuscular agents with organ-independent elimination such as atracurium should be preferred. Paracetamol dose adjustment also may be needed in case of known hepatic dysfunction. In the postoperative period, nonopioid drugs should be preferred for postoperative analgesia. A high degree of suspicion for alcohol withdrawal is required to detect and treat in the postoperative period promptly.[9]

CANNABIS

Cannabis leads to sympathetic overstimulation leading to tachycardia, hypertension, and tremors. Cross tolerance has been observed with alcohol, barbiturates, benzodiazepines, and phenothiazines, wherein higher induction doses of intravenous anesthesia agents have been required. It synergistically acts with volatile agents, causing profound myocardial depression. It also exaggerates the respiratory depressant effects of opioids, therefore warranting their extremely judicious use in *Cannabis* abusers. There is a higher incidence of chronic bronchitis and emphysema in chronic *Cannabis* users. In the postoperative period, one must be vigilant about the high probability of withdrawal symptoms. Recent evidence also demonstrates higher pain scores and significantly higher analgesic consumption in *Cannabis* users.[10]

NICOTINE

It is the most widely used ingredient in cigarettes producing dependence and a broad spectrum of respiratory adverse effects. It significantly inhibits pulmonary gas exchange, causes ciliary hypomotility, and exaggerates sputum production. This increases airway reactivity, and a higher incidence of bronchospasm and perioperative adverse respiratory events may be present. Ideally, smoking abstinence should be advised for at least 4–6 weeks to gain mucociliary function and thus reduce the incidence of perioperative respiratory events. In nicotine abusers, regional anesthesia is the preferred mode of anesthesia as it avoids airway manipulation and hemodynamic fluctuations.

VAPING SUBSTANCES

The use of vaping substances or e-cigarettes is on a steep rise in developed countries like the UK after reports from the Royal College of Physicians stated that e-cigarettes are associated with not > 5% risk as compared to combustible cigarettes.[11] A group that is increasingly vaping is the youth who have used combustible cigarettes. It is implicated that they have a high chance of converting to smokers later.

Vaping is not free from harmful effects. E-cigarette or vaping use is associated with lung injury. Acute and subacute lung injuries are known complications in young males using e-cigarettes. Nicotine overdose is another prominent adverse effect, as the nicotine content mentioned in e-cigarettes is highly unreliable. Burns injuries due to explosion trauma due to thermal runaway malfunction of the lithium-ion batteries are also on the rise. E-cigarette use is associated with increased inflammation and irritability of airway mucosa and a high risk of intraoperative bronchospasm.[12] Cardiovascular effects of e-cigarette use are increased heart rate and blood pressure, which is more consistent with nicotine use.[13]

Nicotine- and tetrahydrocannabinol (THC)-containing e-liquids in e-cigarettes lead to pharmacological effects of the same substances taken through other routes. Volatile compounds like toluene are produced, leading to CNS depression, which may lead to reduced anesthetic requirement.

CONCLUSION

Taking into account the rapid lifestyle changes in the form of urbanization, migration, and lack of traditional family support system, the incidence of various substance abuse is on an alarming rise, significantly upscaling the probability of anesthesiologist encountering a substance abuser in the intensive care unit, routine, and emergency operation theaters as well as an emergency department. As perioperative physicians, we should efficiently manage postoperative pain to decrease the incidence of persistent postoperative opioid use and thus make an impact at the level of society and the nation.

REFERENCES

1. Malenks RC, Nestler EJ, Hyman SE. Reinforcement and addictive disorders. In: Sydor A, Brown RY (Eds). Molecular Neuropharmacology: A Foundation for Clinical Neurosciences. New York: McGraw-Hill Medical; 2009. pp. 364-8.
2. Ray R. (2004). The Extent, Pattern and Trends of Drug Abuse in India, National Survey, Ministry of Social Justice and Empowerment, Government of India and United Nation's Office on Drugs and Crime, Regional Office for South Asia. 2004. [online] Available from: https://www.unodc.org/pdf/india/presentations/india_national_survey_2004.pdf [Last accessed September, 2023].
3. Hedegaard H, Miniño AM, Warner M. (2018). Drug Overdose Deaths in the United States, 1999-2017. [online] Available from: https://www.cdc.gov/nchs/data/databriefs/db329-h.pdf [Last accessed September, 2023].
4. Blanco C, Volkow ND. Management of opioid use disorder in the USA: Present status and future directions. Lancet. 2019;393(10182):1760-72.
5. Rudra A, Bhattacharya A, Chatterjee S, Sengupta S, Das T. Anaesthetic implications of substance abuse in adolescent. Indian J Anaesth. 2008;52(2):132-9.

6. Bohnert ASB, Guy GP Jr, Losby JL. Opioid prescribing in the United States before and after the Centers for Disease Control and Prevention's 2016 opioid guideline. Ann Intern Med. 2018;169(6):367-75.
7. Warner NS, Warner MA, Cunningham JL, Gazelka HM, Hooten WM, Kolla BP, et al. A practical approach for the management of the mixed opioid agonist-antagonist buprenorphine during acute pain and surgery. Mayo Clin Proc. 2020;95(6):1253-67.
8. Laonigro I, Correale M, Di Biase M, Altomare E. Alcohol abuse and heart failure. Eur J Heart Fail. 2009;11(5):453-62.
9. Tønnesen H. Alcohol abuse and postoperative morbidity. Dan Med Bull. 2003;50(2):139-60.
10. Liu CW, Bhatia A, Buzon-Tan A, Walker S, Ilangomaran D, Kara J, et al. Weeding out the problem: the impact of preoperative cannabinoid use on pain in the perioperative period. Anesth Analg. 2019;129(3):874-81.
11. Royal College of Physicians. (2016). Nicotine without smoke: tobacco harm reduction. [online] Available from: https://www.rcplondon.ac.uk/projects/outputs/nicotine-without-smoke-tobacco-harm-reduction [Last accessed September, 2023].
12. Gotts JE, Jordt SE, McConnell R, Tarran R. What are the respiratory effects of e-cigarettes? BMJ. 2019;366:l5275.
13. Qasim H, Karim ZA, Rivera JO, Khasawneh FT, Alshbool FZ. Impact of Electronic Cigarettes on the Cardiovascular System. J Am Heart Assoc. 2017;6(9):e006353.

CHAPTER 16

Anticoagulation and Regional Anesthesia

Eric King, Harsimran Kaur, Shalini Dhir

ABSTRACT

Many patients benefit from regional anesthesia techniques. Some of them are anticoagulated with potent antithrombotic drugs, increasing the risks of hemorrhagic complications. Vertebral canal hematoma (VCH) in anticoagulated patients undergoing neuraxial intervention will lead to permanent disability if not recognized immediately. Deep plexus blocks carry similar risks. Superficial plexus blocks done at compressible sites do not carry similar risks. A guidelines-based approach for patients at bleeding risk is essential when considering regional anesthesia. This review summarizes guidelines from the 2018 American Society of Regional Anesthesia and Pain Medicine (ASRA) and 2022 European Society of Anaesthesiology and Intensive Care/European Society of Regional Anaesthesia (ESAIC/ESRA). Like any recommendations, they are subject to change as we gain more knowledge.

Keywords: Anticoagulation; Regional anesthesia; Neuraxial anesthesia; Vertebral canal hematoma

■ KEY POINTS

- Although rare, there is a significant risk of vertebral canal hematoma (VCH) in anticoagulated patients.
- Hemorrhage in deep peripheral nerve blocks can have serious consequences.
- Superficial blocks done at compressible sites have a low risk of bleeding complications, and time intervals do not apply for such blocks.
- Refer to guidelines for time intervals before/after neuraxial blockade or catheter insertion/removal in perioperative patients.

■ INTRODUCTION

It is not uncommon for many patients presenting for surgery to be on some form of anticoagulation or antiplatelet agents. These agents pose a significant conflict for clinicians when considering neuraxial and peripheral nerve block techniques, as the risk of significant bleeding must be weighed against the procedure's benefit. Overall, hemorrhagic complications, such as neuraxial or deep plexus hematomas, are rare based on limited clinical data. However rare, these complications can result in significant patient morbidity and mortality and add secondary investigations and invasive interventions. With the ongoing addition of new anticoagulants with unique pharmacokinetic profiles, various regional techniques, and patient risk factors, and knowing when the risks outweigh the benefits has become even more challenging.

The American Society of Regional Anesthesia and Pain Medicine (ASRA)[1] as well as the European Society of Anaesthesiology and Intensive Care and European Society of Regional Anaesthesia (ESAIC/ESRA)[2] have published guidelines that aid in making these difficult clinical decisions. Many other anesthesiology societies have also published similar recommendations or consensus guidelines on regional anesthesia for patients on anticoagulation. These guidelines do not replace clinical judgment regarding specific patient scenarios. Clinicians must understand the specific agents' pharmacokinetics, appreciate the regional procedure's risks and benefits for each patient, and know how to manage the complications. This chapter will focus on the considerations one must have before performing any regional procedure on a patient taking anticoagulation, complications, pharmacologic review of common anticoagulants, and management of high- and low-risk regional techniques.

CONSIDERATIONS BEFORE REGIONAL ANESTHESIA FOR PATIENTS ON ANTICOAGULATION

In addition to the usual routine anesthetic evaluation, patient risk factors that may influence bleeding disposition and/or drug pharmacokinetics should be investigated. A thorough history and physical examination should look for signs and symptoms suggesting a bleeding disorder (recurrent nosebleeds, petechiae, mucosal bleeding, purpura, ecchymoses).[1] History of renal or hepatic dysfunction may significantly influence anticoagulation pharmacokinetics and are a significant consideration for perioperative planning. Reviewing relevant radiographic imaging may also help identify and understand anatomic difficulties.

As with any medication, understanding the indication for anticoagulation is essential. Common indications include atrial fibrillation, prophylaxis, and treatment for venous thromboembolism (VTE), pulmonary embolism (PE), prosthetic or mechanical heart valves, treatment of acute coronary syndrome (ACS), among others. The specific anticoagulant or antiplatelet agent, its route of administration, dose, and frequency should be identified as well as other medications or supplements that may have additional anticoagulation properties. Periprocedural management of anticoagulation must always

TABLE 1: Risk factors for vertebral canal hematoma (VCH).

Patient-related	Elderly, female, coagulopathy, thrombocytopenia, spinal anatomic abnormalities, and renal/hepatic insufficiencies
Procedure-related	Catheter insertion/removal, traumatic procedure (multiple attempts), presence of blood in the needle or catheter during insertion/removal, indwelling epidural catheter > single-shot epidural block > single-shot spinal block (in descending order of severity)
Drug-related	Anticoagulation/antiplatelet/fibrinolytic presence, immediate anticoagulant administration (pre- and postneuraxial block) dual anticoagulant/antiplatelet therapies

Source: Adapted from Poredoš P.[3]

balance the risk of bleeding with developing thrombosis. With certain conditions, such as recent coronary stents or mechanical heart valves, it may not be safe to withhold anticoagulation or antiplatelet agents for extended periods. In cases of significant thrombosis risk, a multidisciplinary approach (medicine, surgery, and anesthesia) is recommended for consideration of bridging therapy with low-molecular-weight heparin (LMWH) or unfractionated heparin (UFH). Depending on the anticoagulant, dose, and procedure, laboratory investigations may also be relevant. These tests include international normalized ratio (INR), activated partial thromboplastin time (aPTT), activated clotting time (ACT), platelet count, anti-Xa level, and specific blood levels for certain drugs.[2]

Given the above considerations, one must question the risk factors for bleeding complications in an anticoagulated patient **(Table 1)**, the time of holding anticoagulation before the procedure, catheter removal, and subsequent restarting of the anticoagulation. The available guidelines may guide the answer to these questions but require each clinician to exercise judgment with each clinical scenario.

■ COMPLICATIONS

The risk of complications can differ drastically depending on patient factors and the specific regional technique used. Technical factors that influence complication rate include type and size of the needle, multiple attempts and needle passes, bloody tap, use of indwelling catheters, and operator experience.[3,4] VCH is the most significant hemorrhagic complication due to bleeding in a noncompressible, concealed space that may lead to spinal cord compression, ischemia, and neurologic damage. Because there is no mandatory reporting system or centralized registry, the true incidence of neurologic complications following neuraxial procedures is not well defined. Retrospective studies vary widely in incidence depending on the study and patient demographics. In one study, incidences ranged from 1:18,000 after epidural anesthesia and 1:158,000 after spinal anesthesia, 1:3,600 in elderly women undergoing knee arthroplasty, and 1:200,000 in obstetric patients.[5] Other studies also report similar incidences of VCH.[6,7] Therefore, guidelines continue to use conservative thresholds for anticoagulation cessation due to the significant consequences of VCH. Identified patient risk factors associated with VCH after neuraxial anesthesia are mentioned in **Table 1**.[3,8]

The primary complications related to peripheral nerve blocks in anticoagulated patients include hemorrhage and hematoma, causing compression of nearby structures. A systematic review in 2018 showed that the overall estimated incidence of bleeding complications associated with peripheral regional anesthesia in patients treated with anticoagulant and/or antiplatelet agents was 0.67% in observational studies and 0.82% when case reports were included.[9] Vast majority of the complications were local hematomas without neurologic compromise. However, there were 15 severe bleeding complications, with 1 death secondary to a retroperitoneal hematoma following a lumbar plexus block. Overall, the safety of peripheral nerve blocks is not well defined and is limited by poor-quality evidence and lack of reporting. Safety will vary depending on site compressibility, vascularity, block depth, body habitus, adjacent critical structures, and whether bleeding or hematomas are easy to assess and treat.[4] The ASRA guidelines recommend considering any perineuraxial, deep plexus, or deep peripheral nerve block to be treated similarly to neuraxial techniques.[1] Clinical judgment for other plexus or peripheral techniques should be exercised based on the abovementioned factors. European guidelines, however, have not placed any restrictions on compressible site peripheral nerve blocks.[2] **Table 2** combines this risk stratification for individual blocks from the ESAIC guidelines and additional recommendations, further facilitating appropriate clinical decision-making.[2,4]

■ COMMON ANTICOAGULANTS

As mentioned before, it is imperative to understand the pharmacologic properties of anticoagulants commonly used. Below is a list of commonly used anticoagulants and antiplatelet agents, along with a few clinical considerations. This list is not exhaustive, and reference to the ASRA/ESRA guidelines for specific periprocedural management or uncommonly used anticoagulants is advised.[1,2]

Heparin (UFH, LMWH)

Heparins contain an active polysaccharide sequence that exerts their anticoagulation effect via binding to antithrombin III, potentiating its ability to inactivate thrombin, factors Xa, XIa, XIIa, and IXa.[1,10]

TABLE 2: Types of blocks.

	Deep blocks	Superficial blocks
Antithrombotic drug withdrawal	Mandatory	Not mandatory
Site	Deep, non-compressible	Superficial, compressible
Bleeding risks	Clinically significant	Clinically nonsignificant
Location of blocks		
Head, neck	• Stellate ganglion • Deep cervical plexus • Paravertebral	• Occipital • Peribulbar • Sub-tenon • Superficial cervical plexus
Upper limb	• Infraclavicular	• Interscalene • Supraclavicular • Axillary • Suprascapular • Ulnar, radial, medial
Thorax	• Epidural • Paravertebral	• Parasternal intercostal plane • Serratus anterior • Erector spinae plane (ESP) • Intercostal • Interpectoral plane and pectoserratus plane
Abdomen, pelvic		• Ilioinguinal • Iliohypogastric • Transversus abdominis plane (TAP) • Rectus sheath • Genital branch of genitofemoral nerve • Pudendal nerve
Lower limb, back	• Lumbar plexus • Psoas compartment • Lumbar sympathectomy • Lumbar paravertebral • Quadratus lumborum • Fascia transversalis • Sacral plexus • Pericapsular nerve group (PENG) • Sciatic (proximal) • Spinal, epidural	• Femoral • Adductor canal • Sciatic (popliteal) • Fascia iliaca lateral cutaneous nerve of the thigh • Femoral branch of genitofemoral nerve • *Ankle:* Sural, saphenous, tibial, peroneal

Unfractionated heparin is available in intravenous and subcutaneous routes. Common indications for UFH include ACS, treatment or prevention of VTE, bridge therapy for atrial fibrillation, or cardioversion.[10] Intraoperatively, low doses are often used in vascular surgery during cross-clamping of arterial vessels (5,000–10,000 units) or high doses in cardiopulmonary bypass (300–400 IU/kg). Subcutaneous UFH is commonly used for VTE prophylaxis in the perioperative period with doses of 5,000 units BID or TID. The half-life is dose-dependent, approximately 60 minutes after 100 IU/kg doses and up to 150 minutes with 400 IU/kg doses.[11] UFH can be monitored using the aPTT, anti-factor Xa, or ACT if given higher doses. The reversal agent for UFH is protamine which binds to heparin, forming a stable ion pair.

Low-molecular-weight heparin is primarily used for prophylaxis and treating arterial and VTE, bridge therapy, and ACS. LMWH reduces inhibitory activity against thrombin relative to factor Xa.[12] As its response is predictable, laboratory monitoring is usually unnecessary, though anti-Xa monitoring can be used with high doses.[10] The half-life is significantly longer than UFH at 3–6 hours after subcutaneous injection, which is dose-independent.[12] LMWHs are predominantly cleared renally, so the half-life may be prolonged in patients with renal insufficiency.

Anti-factor Xa Agents (Fondaparinux, Rivaroxaban, Apixaban, Edoxaban)

Fondaparinux is a synthetic analog of the naturally occurring pentasaccharide found in heparins. Fondaparinux will selectively and irreversibly bind to antithrombin to enhance its reactivity with factor Xa, with no effect on thrombin.[12] Though not commonly used, it is an alternative in heparin-induced thrombocytopenia for VTE prevention.[10] Its half-life after subcutaneous injection is prolonged at 17–21 hours, allowing for once-daily doses without coagulation monitoring. Fondaparinux is almost completely renally cleared and is contraindicated in patients with renal insufficiency. No specific antidote for fondaparinux is available, but recombinant activated factor VII can be considered.

Direct Oral Anticoagulants

Direct oral anticoagulants (DOACs) are further divided into direct oral factor-Xa inhibitors and direct thrombin inhibitors (DTIs).

Direct oral factor-Xa inhibitors, such as rivaroxaban, apixaban, and edoxaban, are highly selective direct competitive factor Xa inhibitors and have become popular. They are relatively new anticoagulants approved for preventing stroke in nonvalvular atrial fibrillation, preventing VTE after hip replacement surgery, and preventing and treating recurrent VTE and PE.[13] These agents are at least as effective as vitamin K antagonists (VKAs), with a safer risk profile for bleeding, rapid onset, short half-life, and require no routine laboratory monitoring. All DOACs are contraindicated in patients with severe hepatic disease, with Warfarin being the recommended alternative.[13] The prothrombin time (PT) and aPTT are unreliable laboratory tests for monitoring their effect. Instead, chromogenic anti-factor Xa assays developed using specific calibrators for the agent in question is the test of choice but may not be commonly available. The effects of the direct factor-Xa inhibitors can be inhibited with the reversal agent andexanet alfa [rivaroxaban and apixaban have Food and Drug Administration (FDA) approval].[14]

The half-life of rivaroxaban is 7-11 hours in healthy adults, and is prescribed once or twice daily dosing.[15] Approximately 35% of the rivaroxaban is renally eliminated, so dose reductions are required in patients with renal impairment.[13] The half-life of apixaban is 9-14 hours in healthy adults and increases to 17.5 hours in patients with moderate-to-severe renal impairment, and is prescribed as twice daily dosing.[1,15] Apixaban is approximately 73% reliant on the hepatic/biliary system for drug elimination.[13] The remaining 27% is renally eliminated and is the DOAC of choice in patients with end-stage renal disease.[13] The half-life of edoxaban is 9-11 hours in healthy adults and prescribed as once-daily dosing.[15] Edoxaban is 50% renally eliminated, so it also requires dose reductions in patients with renal dysfunction.[13]

Direct thrombin inhibitors such as dabigatran are direct competitive free and clot-bound thrombin inhibitors. It has a terminal half-life of 12-17 hours in healthy patients but increases to 28 hours in severe renal insufficiency and is prescribed as once or twice daily dosing.[16] Dabigatran is 80% renally cleared, and significant dose adjustments must be made for patients with renal disease.[13] The effects of dabigatran can be reversed during emergency surgery or life-threatening bleeding with idarucizumab (praxbind),[17] a monoclonal antibody fragment that binds and neutralizes its effect.

Vitamin K Antagonists

Warfarin is the most common VKA. It produces its anticoagulant effect by competitively inhibiting the conversion of vitamin K to its active form, thus inhibiting the production of vitamin K-dependent clotting factors (II, VII, IX, and X).[10] Warfarin is indicated for the prevention and treatment of VTE, prevention of thrombosis in prosthetic heart valves, atrial fibrillation, and prevention of stroke, recurrent myocardial infarction (MI), or death in patients with acute MI.[10] Warfarin is administered as once-daily dosing, with a highly variable dose response and range, and is monitored using INR nomograms. Prothrombin has a half-life of 60-72 hours, so it often takes several days for warfarin to reach therapeutic levels.[18] Conversely, it takes several days for the anticoagulant effect to wear off after discontinuation. The perioperative management of patients on warfarin remains controversial, and bridging therapy with LMWH or UFH may be required if the risk of thrombosis is significant.[18] If emergency reversal is required for severe bleeding, intravenous vitamin K and prothrombin complex concentrate (PCC) or fresh frozen plasma can be given to reverse its effect.

Antiplatelet Agents (NSAIDs, Thienopyridine Derivatives, Platelet P2Y$_{12}$ Receptor Antagonists)

Nonsteroidal anti-inflammatory drugs (NSAIDs) exert their antiplatelet action by inhibiting platelet cyclooxygenase 1 (COX-1), which prevents the synthesis of thromboxane A2 and decreases platelet aggregation.[19] Low-dose aspirin (60–325 mg) is primarily prescribed for primary or secondary prevention of thromboembolic cardiovascular and cerebrovascular disease. The definition of low dose is also controversial (<325 mg ASRA, <200 mg ESRA). Aspirin irreversibly inhibits the COX-1 enzyme, so its anti-platelet effect will persist for the platelet's lifespan. Other NSAIDs such as ibuprofen, diclofenac, and indomethacin reversibly inhibit COX-1, so the antiplatelet effect is negligible after 24 hours.[20]

Thienopyridine derivatives, such as ticlopidine, clopidogrel, and prasugrel, irreversibly inhibit the P2Y$_{12}$ receptors on platelet membranes, preventing adenosine diphosphate (ADP) from binding and thus reducing platelet aggregation.[19] They are prodrugs that must undergo hepatic metabolism through the cytochrome P450 (CYP) enzymatic pathway before exerting their effect. These agents are indicated for primary prevention of thromboembolism in atrial fibrillation, medical management of ACS and coronary stents, and secondary prevention of MI, cerebrovascular disease, and peripheral vascular disease.[21] They are often administered in combination with aspirin.

Ticagrelor is a nonthienopyridine agent that also inhibits the P2Y$_{12}$ receptor, but its action is reversible and does not require hepatic metabolism to exert its effect.[19] Its antiplatelet effect can be observed within 30 minutes, with the maximum effect at 2 hours.[1] Ticagrelor is used for secondary prevention in ACS, in combination with aspirin.

Management of regional anesthesia in patients receiving some of the common anticoagulants is in **Table 3**. For restarting them after the intervention, published guidelines for postoperative VTE prophylaxis may be referred to. For infrequently used drugs, appropriate guidelines need to be consulted.

MANAGEMENT OF ANTITHROMBOTIC THERAPY IN OBSTETRIC PATIENTS

Though the anesthetic management of the anticoagulated parturient is outside the scope of this review, specific attention to the obstetric population is worth discussing, as neuraxial blocks are crucial in peripartum care. Because VTE is a significant source of morbidity and mortality in the obstetric population, thromboprophylaxis is not uncommon, especially in high-risk parturients. Due to limited clinical data, ASRA guidelines recommend applying the same guidelines for neuraxial and peripheral blocks to the obstetric population.[1] They do, however, mention that in certain patients, the

TABLE 3: Management of common anticoagulants in high-risk bleeding blocks.

Drug and dose	Stop before procedure Low/high dose	Target laboratory value at intervention	Restart medication after procedure Low/high dose
VKA: Warfarin	5 days	INR <1.4 (ASRA); < normal as per local lab (ESAIC/ESRA)	No delay: Monitor INR daily
DXI Rivaroxaban Apixaban	24 hours/72 hours 36 hours/72 hours	No testing No testing Consider DXI levels <30 ng/mL if renal dysfunction	6 hours 6 hours • Consider longer if bloody tap • Remove catheter prior to restarting
DTI: Dabigatran	48 hours/72 hours	No testing/normal TT time	6 hours/24 hours • Remove catheter prior to restarting (follow postoperative VTE prophylaxis guidelines)
LMWH	12 hours/24 hours (24 hours/48 hours if CrCl < 30 mL/min)	No testing/anti-Xa <0.1 IU/mL	12 hours/24–72 hours • Remove catheter prior to restarting high dose (follow postoperative VTE prophylaxis guidelines)
UFH	IV: 4 hours/6 hours SC: 6 hours/12 hours (48 hours if CrCl < 30 mL/min)	No testing/aPTT, anti-Xa or ACT per local laboratory	Immediately/1 hour IV, 6–12 hours SC • Remove catheter prior to restarting high dose
Aspirin Note: Low dose [<200 mg (ESAIC/ESRA), <325 mg (ASRA)]	0 days/3–7 days	No testing/specific platelet function tests	Per dose interval/6 hours
Thienopyridine derivatives: Clopidogrel	5–7 days	Platelet count and/or aggregation test	Immediately/6 hours • Can keep catheter 1–2 days

(ACT: activated clotting time; ASRA: American Society of Regional Anesthesia and Pain Medicine; aPTT: activated partial thromboplastin time; CrCl: creatinine clearance; DTI: direct thrombin inhibitor; DXI: direct Xa inhibitors; ESAIC: European Society of Anaesthesiology and Intensive Care; ESRA: European Society of Regional Anaesthesia; INR: international normalized ratio; IV: intravenous; LMWH: low-molecular-weight heparin; SC: subcutaneous; TT: thrombin time; UFH: unfractionated heparin; VKA: vitamin K antagonist; VTE: venous thromboembolism) risks of general anesthesia may be more significant than those of neuraxial anesthesia and that exceptions or modifications may be appropriate. Fortunately, the incidence of VCH after neuraxial blockade in the obstetric patient appears to be lower than in the general population.[5,22] Additionally, a systematic review of published studies and the US Closed Claims Project Database between 1990 and 2013 found no spinal epidural hematomas associated with neuraxial anesthesia in obstetric patients treated on UFH or LMWH for thromboprophylaxis.[23] In a small proportion of these patients, the neuraxial procedure was done with the continuation of thromboprophylaxis or with a shorter time interval than the minimum ASRA recommended time for anticoagulation cessation. Until more high-quality evidence is available, the authors recommend a multidisciplinary approach between the obstetric and anesthesia teams regarding the anticoagulation dosing and timing and weigh the relative risks of performing a neuraxial procedure. Although the incidence of spinal hematoma after neuraxial intervention is difficult to arbitrate, it is reported to be less than the nonobstetric population; nonetheless,[5,7] as the pharmacological data regarding anticoagulation in pregnancy is sparse, and there are no large published series in this group, both ASRA and ESAIC/ESRA suggest using recommendations used for nonpregnant population.

■ CONCLUSION

Time intervals before and after neuraxial/deep plexus intervention should be followed depending on the type and dose of anticoagulation, patient factors, including but not limited to renal function, and whether the traumatic procedure influences the time interval required. If regional anesthesia's benefits outweigh general anesthesia's risks, drug-specific reversal agents may be required. Peripheral nerve blocks at a compressible site are considered safe and do not require time intervals. The threshold for suspecting a hemorrhagic complication and nerve tissue compression should be low in anticoagulated patients.

Due to multifactorial complexity, decisions about RA in patients receiving antithrombotic/prophylactic therapy must be made on an individual basis depending on:
- Risk of complications versus benefits of regional anesthesia
- Following dosing guidelines
- Alternative anesthetic/analgesic techniques for patients with unacceptable risks
- Coagulation status optimization at the time of block and catheter placement
- Indwelling catheters removal times should be respected under therapeutic anticoagulation.

- Until the guidelines for the obstetric population are published, those meant for the nonobstetric population should be followed.

REFERENCES

1. Horlocker TT, Vandermeulen E, Kopp SL, Gogarten W, Leffert LR, Benzon HT. Regional Anesthesia in the Patient Receiving Antithrombotic or Thrombolytic Therapy: American Society of Regional Anesthesia and Pain Medicine Evidence-Based Guidelines (Fourth Edition). Reg Anesth Pain Med. 2018;43(3):263-309.
2. Kietaibl S, Ferrandis R, Godier A, Llau J, Lobo C, MacFarlane AJ, et al. Regional anaesthesia in patients on antithrombotic drugs: Joint ESAIC/ESRA guidelines. Eur J Anaesthesiol. 2022;39(2):100-32.
3. Poredoš P. Peripheral Nerve Blocks in Patients on Antithrombotic Drugs: a Rescue or an Unnecessary Risk? Acta Clin Croat. 2022;61(Suppl 2):67-77.
4. Tsui BCH, Kirkham K, Kwofie MK, Tran Q, Wong P, Chin KJ, et al. Practice advisory on the bleeding risks for peripheral nerve and interfascial plane blockade: evidence review and expert consensus. Can J Anaesth. 2019;66(11):1356-84.
5. Moen V, Dahlgren N, Irestedt L. Severe neurological complications after central neuraxial blockades in Sweden 1990-1999. Anesthesiology. 2004;101(4):950-9.
6. Ehrenfeld JM, Agarwal AK, Henneman JP, Sandberg WS. Estimating the incidence of suspected epidural hematoma and the hidden imaging cost of epidural catheterization: a retrospective review of 43,200 cases. Reg Anesth Pain Med. 2013;38(5):409-14.
7. Bateman BT, Mhyre JM, Ehrenfeld J, Kheterpal S, Abbey KR, Argalious M, et al. The risk and outcomes of epidural hematomas after perioperative and obstetric epidural catheterization: a report from the Multicenter Perioperative Outcomes Group Research Consortium. Anesth Analg. 2013;116(6):1380-5.
8. Working Party; Association of Anaesthetists of Great Britain & Ireland; Obstetric Anaesthetists' Association; Regional Anaesthesia UK. Regional anaesthesia and patients with abnormalities of coagulation: the Association of Anaesthetists of Great Britain & Ireland The Obstetric Anaesthetists' Association Regional Anaesthesia UK. Anaesthesia. 2013;68(9):966-72.
9. Joubert F, Gillois P, Bouaziz H, Marret E, Iohom G, Albaladejo P. Bleeding complications following peripheral regional anaesthesia in patients treated with anticoagulants or antiplatelet agents: A systematic review. Anaesth Crit Care Pain Med. 2019;38(5):507-16.
10. Alquwaizani M, Buckley L, Adams C, Fanikos J. Anticoagulants: A Review of the Pharmacology, Dosing, and Complications. Curr Emerg Hosp Med Rep. 2013;1(2):83-97.
11. Hirsh J, Raschke R, Warkentin TE, Dalen JE, Deykin D, Poller L. Heparin: mechanism of action, pharmacokinetics, dosing considerations, monitoring, efficacy, and safety. Chest. 1995;108(4 Suppl):258S-75S.
12. Garcia DA, Baglin TP, Weitz JI, Samama MM. Parenteral anticoagulants: Antithrombotic Therapy and Prevention of Thrombosis, 9th ed: American College of Chest Physicians Evidence-Based Clinical Practice Guidelines. Chest. 2012;141(2 Suppl):e24S-e43S.
13. Chen A, Stecker E, A Warden B. Direct Oral Anticoagulant Use: A Practical Guide to Common Clinical Challenges. J Am Heart Assoc. 2020;9(13):e017559.

14. Siegal DM, Curnutte JT, Connolly SJ, Lu G, Conley PB, Wiens BL, et al. Andexanet Alfa for the Reversal of Factor Xa Inhibitor Activity. N Engl J Med. 2015;373(25):2413-24.
15. Weitz JI, Eikelboom JW, Samama MM. New antithrombotic drugs: Antithrombotic Therapy and Prevention of Thrombosis, 9th ed: American College of Chest Physicians Evidence-Based Clinical Practice Guidelines. Chest. 2012;141(2 Suppl):e120S-e51S.
16. Stangier J, Rathgen K, Stähle H, Mazur D. Influence of renal impairment on the pharmacokinetics and pharmacodynamics of oral dabigatran etexilate: an open-label, parallel-group, single-centre study. Clin Pharmacokinet. 2010;49(4):259-68.
17. Pollack Jr CV, Reilly PA, Eikelboom J, Glund S, Verhamme P, Bernstein RA, et al. Idarucizumab for dabigatran reversal. N Engl J Med. 2015;373(6):511-20.
18. Hirsh J, Fuster V, Ansell J, Halperin JL; American Heart Association; American College of Cardiology. American Heart Association/American College of Cardiology foundation guide to warfarin therapy. Circulation. 2003;107(12):1692-711.
19. Passacquale G, Sharma P, Perera D, Ferro A. Antiplatelet therapy in cardiovascular disease: Current status and future directions. Br J Clin Pharmacol. 2022;88(6):2686-99.
20. Cronberg S, Wallmark E, Söderberg I. Effect on platelet aggregation of oral administration of 10 non-steroidal analgesics to humans. Scand J Haematol. 1984;33(2):155-9.
21. Mahmood H, Siddique I, McKechnie A. Antiplatelet drugs: a review of pharmacology and the perioperative management of patients in oral and maxillofacial surgery. Ann R Coll Surg Engl. 2020;102(1):9-13.
22. D'Angelo R, Smiley RM, Riley ET, Segal S. Serious complications related to obstetric anesthesia: the serious complication repository project of the Society for Obstetric Anesthesia and Perinatology. Anesthesiology. 2014;120(6):1505-12.
23. Leffert LR, Dubois HM, Butwick AJ, Carvalho B, Houle TT, Landau R. Neuraxial Anesthesia in Obstetric Patients Receiving Thromboprophylaxis with Unfractionated or Low-Molecular-Weight Heparin: A Systematic Review of Spinal Epidural Hematoma. Anesth Analg. 2017;125(1):223-31.

CHAPTER 17

Clinical Outcome Scoring in Intensive Care

Pallavi Ahluwalia

ABSTRACT

Scoring systems describe the severity of a disease process and help predict patient outcomes clinically. Outcome scoring systems often use patient data, clinical health information, preexisting chronic diseases, and physiological and laboratory data to determine outcomes such as length of intensive care unit (ICU) and hospital stay and predict mortality. They have undergone many modifications for better adaptability, improved prediction power, ease of calculation, and universal application. Various models have been updated, and only some are in their third generation. Presently, there is no gold standard score. They must be chosen based on need, whether they are being used for outcome/mortality prediction, severity assessment, or workload assessment to monitor them based on efficacy and cost. Broadly, they can be categorized into the standard/multiorgan or single organ/disease-specific scoring systems. With rising healthcare costs and a scarcity of ICU beds, clinicians must use these predictive scores to appropriately triage patient admissions to ICU and avoid unnecessary expenditure and optimal bed utilization. Predictive scores do not help much in managing individual patients but greatly help researchers during clinical trials, institutions, and other healthcare administration officials to monitor ICU performance.

Keywords: Predictive/prognostic scores; APACHE score; SAPS score; SOFA score; MPM Score; MODS; LODS

KEY POINTS

- Using a scoring system in ICUs helps predict prognosis and indicates which therapies the research should focus on to improve outcomes in critically ill patients.
- APACHE (Acute physiologic and Chronic Health Evaluation) score is one of the most commonly used scoring systems worldwide and is declared the "gold standard" for evaluation in ICUs.
- The construction of a scoring system is determined by the population sample used for the calibration and subsequent validation of the model.

- Repetitive scores such as SOFA and MODS are primarily used to assess organ dysfunction.
- An ideal scoring model should include easily measurable variables and high levels of discrimination, be well calibrated and validated for use in all patients in ICUs, and be able to predict mortality and length of stay (LOS).
- Predictive scores are utilized by researchers in clinical trials, by institutions, and by healthcare officials to examine ICU performance.
- Scoring systems should be seen as complementary rather than competitive and mutually exclusive. If required, they can be combined for enhanced accuracy and prognostication.

INTRODUCTION

Scoring systems for critically ill patients can be broadly categorized into two main groups: organ or disease-specific scores, such as the Glasgow Coma Scale (GCS), and generic scores that can be applied to all intensive care unit (ICU) patients. Generic scores can be further divided into three broad categories. The first category includes scores that assess the severity of the disease upon admission and are used to predict outcomes. Examples of such scores are APACHE score, Simplified Acute Physiology Score (SAPS), and Mortality Probability Model (MPM). These scoring systems consider physiological variables, chronic health conditions, and other factors to assess the severity of the illness. The second category comprises scores that evaluate the presence and severity of organ dysfunction. These scores are designed to assess the functioning of various organs and help monitor the progression of organ failure. Examples of such scores include the Multiple Organ Dysfunction Score (MODS), Sequential Organ Failure Assessment (SOFA), and Logistic Organ Dysfunction Score (LODS). The third category encompasses scores that assess nursing care and evaluate nursing workload. These scoring systems, such as the Therapeutic Intervention Scoring System (TISS), the Nine Equivalents of Nursing Manpower Use Score (NEMS), and the Nursing Activity Score (NAS), focus on measuring the nursing interventions and workload required for patient care.

Specialized scoring systems are essential when dealing with specific patient populations such as pediatrics, burn victims, trauma patients, and those undergoing cardiac surgery. These populations have distinct physiological characteristics or treatment courses that differ from the general adult ICU patients. Organ or disease-specific predictive scoring systems cater to these unique needs. For instance, the Model for End-stage Liver Disease (MELD) score is designed to assess a patient with end-stage liver disease. Similarly, the GCS score is used for assessment following head trauma.

Scoring systems can also be categorized based on their timing of application. First-day scoring systems, including the APACHE, SAPS, and MPM, evaluate disease severity and predict outcomes upon admission. On the other hand, repetitive scoring systems are used to monitor patients over time. They include the SOFA, MODS, and LODS. These scoring systems assess the severity and presence of organ dysfunction, enabling healthcare providers to track the progression of organ failure and make informed treatment decisions.

Specialized scoring systems are necessary for specific patient populations with unique physiological characteristics or treatment courses. Organ or disease-specific scoring systems and the distinction between first-day and repetitive scoring systems provide valuable tools for predicting outcomes, monitoring organ dysfunction, and guiding medical interventions in the ICU setting.

■ VALIDATION AND TESTING MODEL PERFORMANCE

Calibration refers to how accurately a model or scoring system aligns with actual outcomes within its relevant range. To assess calibration, the Hosmer–Lemeshow goodness-of-fit test is commonly employed. This test involves dividing the data into risk subgroups, typically deciles, and comparing the number of observed outcomes with the predicted outcomes for each risk level. When the observed and expected outcomes closely match across the entire range of the model, the sum of chi-squares will be low, indicating good calibration.

Discrimination, on the other hand, measures the model's ability to predict outcomes correctly. The area under the receiver-operating characteristic (AUROC) curve, often called the C-statistic, summarizes sensitivity and specificity across all possible decision thresholds. A higher area under the curve indicates better discrimination, with a theoretical maximum value of 1.0. Generally, an AUROC above 0.7 is considered acceptable, while values above 0.8 are considered excellent, and those above 0.9 are considered outstanding. It is important to note that receiver-operating characteristic (ROC) analysis is only valid when a model has demonstrated good calibration and is used to compare different scoring systems.

■ OUTCOME PREDICTION SCORES USED IN HEALTHCARE

Acute Physiology and Chronic Health Evaluation I–IV Systems

There are three key factors that impact the outcomes in critically ill patients: (1) Preexisting chronic diseases, (2) the patient's physiological resilience, and (3) the severity of their current illness. The APACHE scoring system considers physiological variables, chronic health conditions, admission type (emergency/elective), and postoperative/nonoperative status. The most abnormal measurements recorded during the initial 24 hours of ICU stay are used to calculate the score.[1]

In 1981, the APACHE score was developed to categorize patients based on illness severity. It consisted of a physiology score that assessed the degree of acute illness and a preadmission evaluation that assessed the patient's chronic health status.[1] In 1985, the score was revised and simplified to create APACHE II, a widely used scoring system worldwide. APACHE II[2] incorporates only 12 physiological variables compared to the original score of 34. Age and chronic health conditions are included and weighted according to their effect, resulting in a single score. The maximum value of the score is 71. The most extreme values observed for each physiological variable within 24 hours of ICU admission are considered. The primary diagnosis that led to admission in ICU is also factored in as a weight and predicted mortality is calculated using the patient's APACHE II score and the provisional diagnosis during admission. Although preexisting health status and acute physiological dysfunction may be similar, the most critical variable in predicting mortality is the reason leading to ICU admission.

In 1991 the APACHE III[3] system was developed, further improving prognostication, discrimination, and calibration. It expanded the score range from 0 to 299 and included 16 variables. Later in 2006, the APACHE IV system came into existence, based on a large dataset and incorporated more variables, providing increased accuracy. However, APACHE IV is primarily used within the United States and is considered more complex and less frequently utilized due to its significant number of physiologic variables. Overall, the APACHE score is a valuable tool for clinicians and researchers to assess illness severity, predict mortality risk, guide clinical decision-making, and evaluate the performance of ICU units.

Advantages of using APACHE Score in ICU

It can help in predicting mortality risk. It can guide clinical decision-making by providing an objective measure of disease severity. It can help clinicians to identify patients requiring more aggressive management, such as mechanical ventilation or vasoactive medications, or those who may benefit from palliative care. It can be used for assessment of the performance of ICU units over time. By comparing the actual mortality rates with the expected mortality rates based on the APACHE score, clinicians can identify areas for improvement and evaluate the efficacy of therapies. As a result, it facilitates better communication between doctors and ensures all patients receive the same quality care. The APACHE score has been used extensively in clinical research to assess the efficacy of interventions and compare outcomes between different patient populations.

Disadvantages

It is a complex scoring system that requires significant data to be collected and analyzed, which may be challenging. Clinicians unfamiliar with it may need help to calculate and understand it. The existence or absence of organ failure and the degree of mental status impairment are clinical characteristics open to interpretation. Due to this subjectivity, there may be discrepancies in ratings between doctors or hospitals. It is calculated 24 hours after ICU admission, which might limit its utility in guiding early interventions or decision-making. APACHE was developed using data from a broad range of patient populations. It may not accurately predict mortality risk in specific patient populations, such as those with certain comorbidities or those receiving specific treatments. This score is based on a single point in time and may not accurately reflect changes in patient status over time. The score should not be used as the sole criterion for making clinical decisions, and clinicians should also consider the patient's clinical condition while interpreting the score.

Simplified Acute Physiology Score

Intensive care unit patients can have their 24-hour mortality risk predicted using SAPS. Originally developed in France in 1984,[4] using 13 weighted physiological indicators and the patient's age (as a variable), SAPS I was designed to predict mortality in ICU patients. European and North American patients and chronic health issues were incorporated into the later SAPS II (1993) developed by Le Gall and colleagues using logistic regression analysis, which also had improved calibration and discrimination. There are 17 factors included, including the patient's age, the type of admission, the underlying ailment they were diagnosed with, and 12 physiological characteristics (measured during the initial 24 hours of ICU admission). Values for SAPS II are between 0 and 163. A logistic regression analysis is performed to calculate expected mortality. Patients with burns or an underlying heart problem as well as those under the age of 18 are excluded from its use.[5,6] Based on worldwide patient data, SAPS III was released in 2005 with 20 variables (preadmission, inhospital, and acute physiological derangements).

Advantages

Simplified Acute Physiology Score gives an excellent predictive value for assessing mortality risk in ICU patients. It can help identify patients at greater risk of adverse outcomes early. This objective tool uses measurable physiological variables to calculate a patient's risk. This can help to standardize care and reduce the potential for bias or variability in clinical decision-making. It is easy to use and can be calculated quickly. This is important in the ICU setting, where time is often of the essence. It can be used extensively in research studies to evaluate the effectiveness of treatments and interventions in critically ill patients. This can help to improve our understanding of critical care and guide the development of new treatment strategies. It can be used to compare outcomes across different ICUs or patient populations, which can help identify areas for improvement and optimize resource allocation.

Disadvantages

Simplified Acute Physiology Score only considers physiological variables and does not consider other factors influencing a patient's prognosis, such as comorbidities or social determinants of health. There can be variability in how different clinicians score the SAPS variables, which can impact the overall score's accuracy and reliability. It is only suitable for the first day in the ICU, so it may not provide an accurate picture of a patient's prognosis over a longer time frame. It does not consider how patients respond to treatment or interventions, which could impact their overall prognosis. While the SAPS score has been validated in many settings, it may need to be more reliable in specific patient populations or ICU settings.

Mortality Prediction Model

The MPM (1985)[7] determines the likelihood of hospital mortality based on variables (present or absent) at the time of admission and within the initial 24 hours. To predict outcomes at 24, 48, and 72 hours, the MPM II (Revised Mortality Prediction Model II) was developed in 1993 and employed the same data set as SAPS II. All variables are scored as present or missing except for the actual age in years and assigned a 1 or 0 in MPM II. The likelihood of dying while hospitalized can then be determined with the use of MLR. Additionally, MPM II has two scores: MPM0 (admission model) and MPM24 (24-hour model) for patients who will have longer ICU stays (>24 hours). The admission model has variables (16), and includes three physiological parameters recorded within the first hour postadmission. The MPM0 predicts the likelihood of death until hospital discharge based on the patient's status before ICU admission. Advantages include the identification of high-risk patients. This can help clinicians prioritize their care and allocate resources more effectively and efficiently, improving overall patient outcomes and reducing costs. MPM uses objective criteria to predict outcomes, which can help reduce bias and variability in decision-making. It can be used as a research tool. MPM can provide prognostic information to their families, helping them make more informed decisions about their care and treatment options. It can track and evaluate the effectiveness of interventions and quality improvement initiatives to improve patient outcomes.

Discussion: **Table 1** compares outcome prediction scores, i.e., APACHE, SAPS, and MPM. Various studies have compared scoring systems. Observed

TABLE 1: Comparison of APACHE I, II, III, and IV; SAPS I, II, and III; and MPM I, II, III.

	APACHE	SAPS	APACHE II	MPM	APACHE III	SAPS II	MPM II	SAPS III	APACHE IV	MPM III
Years	1981	1984	1985	1985	1991	1993	1993	2005	2006	2007
Countries	1	1	1	1	1	12	12	35	1	1
ICUs	2	8	13	1	40	137	140	303	104	135
Number of patients	705	679	5,815	2,783	17,440	12,997	19,124	16,784	110,558	124,855
Variables as per their weights	POE	POE	POE	MLR	MLR	MLR	MLR	MLR	MLR	MLR
Variables	–	–	–	–	–	–	–	–	–	–
Age	N	Y	Y	Y	Y	Y	Y	Y	Y	Y
Origin	N	N	N	N	Y	N	N	Y	Y	N
Surgical history	N	N	Y	Y	Y	Y	Y	Y	Y	Y
Chronic health conditions	Y	N	Y	Y	Y	Y	Y	Y	Y	Y
Physiology status	Y	Y	Y	Y	Y	Y	Y	Y	Y	Y
Acute diagnosis	N	Y	N	Y	N	Y	Y	Y	Y	Y
Number of variables	34	14	17	11	26	17	15	20	142	16
Score	Y	Y	Y	Y	Y	Y	N	Y	Y	N
Mortality prediction	N	N	Y	Y	Y	Y	Y	Y	Y	Y

(APACHE: Acute Physiology and Chronic Health Evaluation; MLR: multiple logistic regression; MPM: Mortality Probability Model; POE: panel of experts; SAPS: Simplified Acute Physiology Score; Y: yes; N: no) mortality differed significantly from what was predicted by all models, but Livingston et al.[8] stated that all models exhibited good discrimination. The discrimination power of APACHE IV was slightly better than the other scores (AUROC curve of 0.892 for APACHE IV, 0.873 calculated for SAPS II, and 0.809 for MPM0 III, p value 0.001). This was noted by Kuzniewicz et al.[9] According to Sakr et al.[10] SAPS III, APACHE II, and SAPS II all have comparable discriminative ability (an AUROC of 0.80 was computed for APACHE II, 0.83 was determined for SAPS II, and 0.84 was calculated for SAPS III). The Intensive Care National Audit and Research Centre (ICNARC) model was established by Harrison et al.[11] but it has yet to be compared to any other models. The APACHE scoring system is the only one shown to be adequately discriminatory and better calibrated for predicting mortality and ICU stay, according to an analysis of 11,300 patients from 35 California hospitals, done retrospectively.[12] They also showed that MPM outperformed other methods when forecasting how long a patient would need ventilator support and how long they would be in the ICU. Minimizing ICU and hospital stays and cutting expenses is a top priority for the healthcare system. There were 12 significant predictors of major complications according to APACHE II and SAPS II scores taken at the time of ICU admission. Regarding discriminating power, MPM II at 7 days was superior to SOFA (at 7 days) and MPM II at 48 days. Calibration was best for MPM II at 7 days, followed by SOFA and then APACHE II.[13]

Limitations: First, these scores work best when the study group is matched with the development population. Second, accuracy depends upon the quality of input data. Third, there is an inherent bias as many are based on limited ICU patients and are focused explicitly on measuring ICU performance. Fourth, a majority of researchers, use patient data noted at hospital discharge rather than ICU discharge, and the values may differ and influence the accuracy of scores.

ORGAN DYSFUNCTION SCORES

Sequential Organ Failure Score

In 1994, the European Society of Intensive Care Medicine[14] created the SOFA. The SOFA score was amended in 1996. Initially, only for sepsis-related organ dysfunction, it was later validated for nonsepsis organ dysfunction. Its original use was for describing the sequence of organ dysfunction/failure in septic patients admitted to ICU and understanding the progression of failure of organs and various interactions among organ failures. It accurately predicts mortality in ICU patients without sepsis-related organ failure. Scores range from 0 (poor) to 4 (excellent) across six organ systems: lungs, heart, kidneys, liver, brain, and coagulation profile. The SOFA score differs significantly from other scores in that it employs a treatment-related variable (the dose of vasopressor drugs) instead of the cardiovascular component's composite variable. Sequential evaluation of organ failure in the first few days of ICU admission provides valuable prognostic information. The average number of SOFA points earned throughout a patient's ICU hospitalization is the mean SOFA score. Nonsurvivors have a considerably higher ten-day ICU-SOFA score. A student's delta SOFA score is their maximum minus their entrance SOFA score. The qSOFA (quick SOFA) score is based on the following three factors with each worth 1 point: (1) GCS score of 14 indicates an altered mental state; (2) hypotension is a systolic blood pressure (SBP) of ≤100 mm Hg; (3) breathing rate <22 breaths/min. Patients who meet two or more of the above criteria are at high risk for developing sepsis.

The Modified SOFA (MSOFA) score was proposed and published by Grissom et al.[15] This is a stream-lined explanation. Measurements of PaO_2/FiO_2 (partial pressure of arterial oxygen/fraction of inspired oxygen) and serum bilirubin levels are replaced by the SpO_2 (pulse oximeter saturation)/FiO_2 ratio and jaundice assessment in the MSOFA. Despite its apparent ease, further verification is needed. While daily scoring of individual and composite scores is possible throughout an ICU stay, no such technique exists for predicting death. It is commonly employed as a secondary endpoint in clinical studies due to its simplicity and the fact that it considers supportive interventions in assessing patient morbidity.

Interpretation

Irrespective of the initial SOFA score, an increase in the score in ≤48 hours of ICU stay implies a mortality rate of ≥50%, and an unchanged score implies a mortality rate of between 27 and 35% (if the initial score was <8) and 60% mortality prediction (if the initial score was ≥8), whereas a decreasing score correlates with a lesser mortality rate of <6% (if initial score was <8) and 27% (if the initial score was ≥8).[16]

Multiple Organ Dysfunction Score

The MODS was created in 1995 after researchers analyzed data from 30 studies that defined organ dysfunction using criteria.[17,18] There were originally seven components: the respiratory, cardiovascular system (CVS), renal, hematological, hepatic, central nervous system (CNS), and gastrointestinal systems. Due to the absence of a perfect gastrointestinal descriptor, the later gastrointestinal system was cut from the final model. Based on the day's initial measurements, the six organs can receive a score between 0 (standard) and 4 (highest dysfunction). 24 is the maximum score. Although MODS were not developed for this purpose, it does correlate strongly with ICU mortality as it rises. The delta MODS is a more accurate predictor of outcome than any single score.[17]

Logistic Organ Dysfunction Score

In 1996, researchers used a database of 13,152 admissions to 137 ICUs across 12 countries to generate the LODS.[19] Using a set of 12 predetermined factors, multiple logistic regression (MLR) was used to evaluate the functionality of six organ systems (the nervous system, cardiovascular system, kidneys, lungs, blood, and liver). Each system is given a score between 0 (no dysfunction) and 5 (highest dysfunction), based on the worst value for each variable during the initial 24 hours after admission. In contrast to the SOFA and MODS scores, LODS uses a weighted method, with the respiratory and coagulation systems, each receiving a maximum of 3 points and the liver receiving 1 point. Therefore, the value of LODS can be anything between 0 and 22. A logistic regression equation (LRE) can be used to translate scores into mortality risk estimates. A higher score or severity of organ dysfunction was associate with higher mortality and LODS score of 22 was associated with 99.7% mortality.[19,20]

Discussion: Various studies have compared organ dysfunction scores. In a single-center investigation, Pettilä et al.[21] found that APACHE III, SOFA, LODS, and MODS had comparable discriminative abilities for inhospital mortality prediction. In a study of 949 patients in the general ICU, Peres Bota et al.[22] observed no significant differences between the mortality prediction accuracy of MODS and SOFA. Timsit et al.[20] found that the SOFA and LODS were highly reliable and valid in a multicenter investigation. A Canadian study of 1,436 ICU patients[23] found that SOFA and MODS were only somewhat effective at separating the living from the dead. SOFA demonstrated superior discriminative performance over MODS in predicting hospital mortality and adverse neurologic prognosis in patients with brain damage.[24] **Table 2** shows their comparison. As a global score that summarizes organ dysfunction across many body systems and an LRE that transforms the score into a probability model, the LODS bridges the gap between a score for predicting mortality and an organ failure score.[25]

SEVERITY ASSESSMENT BASED ON IMPACT ON NURSES' WORKLOAD

Therapeutic Intervention Scoring System

Therapeutic Intervention Scoring System was created to assess disease severity and quantify the workload for ICU staff. The original score had 57 items, later reduced to a daily collection of 76 items (interventions and therapies) in 1983. TISS-76 was criticized as being excessively time-consuming and challenging. Thus, a more straight-forward version was developed in 1996, employing advanced statistical methods.[26] TISS-28 consists of only 28 things organized into seven categories: support for

TABLE 2: Comparison of organ dysfunction scores.[14]

Characteristics	LODS	MODS	SOFA
Publication year	1996	1995	1996
Variables and their weights selection	MLR	Literature review and logistic	POE
Variables used for organ dysfunction assessment:			
Neurologic	GCS	GCS	GCS
Cardiovascular	HR, SBP	Pressure-adjusted HR	MAP Vasopressor use
Renal	Serum urea or urea nitrogen, creatinine, urine output	Serum creatinine	Serum creatinine, urine output
Respiratory	PaO_2/FiO_2 ratio, mechanical ventilation	PaO_2/FiO_2 ratio	PaO_2/FiO_2 ratio, mechanical ventilation
Hematologic	WBC count	Platelet count	Platelet count
Hepatic	Serum bilirubin, prothrombin time	Serum bilirubin	Serum bilirubin

(FiO_2: fraction of inspired oxygen; GCS: Glasgow Coma Scale; HR: heart rate; LODS: Logistic Organ Dysfunction Score; MAP: mean arterial pressure; MLR: multiple logistic regression; MODS: Multiple Organ Dysfunction Score; PaO_2: partial pressure of arterial oxygen; POE: panel of experts; SBP: systolic blood pressure; SOFA: Sequential Organ Dysfunction Score; WBC: white blood cell)

breathing, circulation, kidney function, nerve function, metabolism, and other vital organs. Total 78 points after weighting each category. TISS can be used as a tool for resource allocation (accounting). It is a reliable indicator to monitor nursing and medical activity but unreliable for assessing illness severity.

Nine Equivalents of Nursing Manpower Use Score

The TISS-28 was the basis for creating the more user-friendly and widely deployed NEMS.[27] There are nine types of nursing care provided in the ICU, including essential monitoring, intravenous medication advice, mechanical ventilation, supplemental ventilation, single/multiple vasoactive drugs, dialysis procedures, and specialty treatments. They are all given different point values, and the sum is 56. NEMS is validated in a sizable population of ICU patients, is user-friendly, and produces negligible interobserver variability.[28] Once again, this method can objectively categorize ICUs according to the volume of care supplied rather than the complexity of care delivered to analyze the efficiency with which nurses handle their workloads within those units.[29]

Nursing Activity Score

The Nursing Activities Score (NAS) is derived from the TISS-28 and accounts for various nursing tasks unrelated to patients' illnesses. A cross-sectional observational research lasting 1 week was used to calculate how long each activity takes on average, and the results were compared (across 15 countries, in a cohort of 99 ICUs) to those of the TISS-28 items.

Discussion: Intensive care unit nurse staffing is primarily evaluated using these scores. However, greater scores predict poorer results.[30,31] They help estimate total expenditures for groups of ICU patients, but scores are less reliable when applied to one patient.

■ SINGLE ORGAN OR DISEASE-SPECIFIC SCORING SYSTEMS

The MELD score[32] characterizes advanced liver disease severity. The severity of liver disease and the need for a liver transplant are quantified numerically (from 6 to 40 for the MELD score). It calculates serum creatinine, bilirubin levels, and international normalized ratio (INR). It is used to predict death and problems in the first 3 months after receiving a liver transplant from a deceased donor. A GCS score[33] estimates the likelihood of survival following a head injury. The GCS scale ranges from 3 to 15, with 3 being the worst and 15 the best. Best E refers to best eye response, best V indicates best verbal response, and best M refers to the best motor response. Mild brain injury is indicated by a score of ≥13, moderate injury by a score of 9–12, and severe brain injury by a score of ≤8. An unresponsive score that considers brainstem reflexes and breathing is an alternative to GCS and a more reliable predictor of mortality.[34] European systems for cardiac operative risk evaluation (EUROSCORE) is used to predict mortality after cardiac surgery.[35] The intracerebral hemorrhage (ICH) score is used to evaluate the severity of intracerebral bleeding. The Ranson's and BISAP ("B" for blood urea nitrogen, "I" for impaired mental status, "S" for systemic inflammatory response syndrome, "A" for age, and "P" for pleural effusion) scores measure the severity of acute pancreatitis.

■ DO WE HAVE AN IDEAL SCORING SYSTEM?

Desired Characteristics of an Ideal Scoring System

The scoring system must be based on easily measurable characteristics and be calibrated and tested across ICUs. They should be widely applicable (in different countries, with different health systems, and with diverse patient cohorts), have a high level of discrimination, and be able to be used with any ICU patient group to predict the LOS in hospital and/or mortality. They should be able to foretell the patient's functional status or quality of life after being released from the ICU. Taking into account comorbidities and organizational factors are also desirable qualities. The score should provide a standardized terminology and evaluation framework for critical care practices and procedures. Finally, comparing groups in clinical trials should be made possible. Numerous prognostic scoring methods may indicate that the best one has yet to be developed.[36] This is why different people have different favorite methods of scoring. Patients treated in US ICUs informed the development of APACHE and MPM, while about 35 countries are represented in SAPS.[37,38]

WHY DO WE NEED A SCORING SYSTEM IN ICU?

Application of Scoring Systems

Patients are stratified for clinical trials using scoring systems, ICU performance is compared to other ICUs, mortality and prognosis are predicted, LOS are measured for both individuals and groups, and resources are allocated based on the severity at presentation using scoring systems. A score can be created using scoring methodologies to indicate the seriousness of the condition requiring ICU admission. A standardized mortality ratio (SMR) compares actual deaths to the population's projected death rate. Scoring methods allow for its estimation. In clinical trials, they allow for the stratification and comparison of populations. They can also be used to compare the hazards of different groups against a common baseline. Expected and actual performance can be compared with the help of a scoring system. They help forecast the duration of stay and the resources needed to manage the patient's illness severity at admission. They can be used to examine the efficiency and effectiveness of ICUs over time.

PROBLEMS OF USING SEVERITY OF ILLNESS SCORES TO COMPARE OUTCOMES BETWEEN ICUs

Different methods of data collection, different standards, and different time frames could be used. Audits and reviews of scoring by knowledgeable individuals should be conducted regularly. It is possible that diagnostic groups underestimate or overestimate the degree of heterogeneity in patient populations. Multiple organs may be involved, making diagnosis and categorization difficult. Concerns about missing data, erroneous data, bias, or fraud may arise due to funding competition. Variation in the data is possible due to its frequent comparison throughout time. It is not just the ICU staff that has a role in determining the severity of an outcome; other on-site resources, such as imaging, laboratories, and the availability of surgical specialists, also play a role. One significant restriction is the potential for erroneous score interpretation. The chance of dying while hospitalized, as determined by a given score, should be understood in the context of a group of patients rather than an individual. It is essential to update scoring systems to prevent the gradual loss of discrimination and calibration, which reduces their predictive power over time. Currently, no scoring method predicts outcome or morbidity after ICU discharge. Outcome predictors are designed for groups rather than individuals. Estimates of mortality probability range from 0 to 1.0, although each patient will live or die. Mortality predictions differ depending on when the data was obtained geographically and momentarily. ICU or hospital discharge results do not always correlate with 30-, 60-, or 365- day outcomes. The use of scoring systems to guide therapeutic decisions has yet to be thoroughly investigated, and risk adjustment systems should never be used as the primary criterion for directing or withholding therapy in an individual patient.

CONCLUSION

Clinical outcome prediction models can neither assess the severity of organ dysfunctions, nor can the patients' progression over time be monitored. Even though organ dysfunction scores may correlate with outcomes, predicting outcomes is best left to systems like the APACHE and SAPS scores. Care in ICU costs three times as much as care in the wards. Therefore keeping tabs on ICU efficiency is a wise use of hospital resources. While SMR can be used for large patient groups, it cannot predict individual patient outcomes or evaluate therapy responses. When assessing the quality of intensive care, the APACHE score is accepted universally as the "gold standard".[39] The ability of APACHE and SOFA to accurately predict mortality in the ICU and hospital settings has been directly compared.[40] Again, different authors report contrasting data; some authors emphasize the APACHE score at admission more than others. When comparing the SOFA score to the APACHE II score at the time of hospital admission, the former was found to have slightly better discrimination and calibration in 2007.[41]

REFERENCES

1. Zimmerman JE, Kramer A, McNair DS, Malila FM. Acute Physiology and Chronic Health Evaluation (APACHE) IV: hospital mortality assessment for today's critically ill patients. Crit Care Med. 2006;34(5):1297-310.
2. Knaus WA, Zimmerman JE, Wagner DP, Draper EA, Lawrence DE. APACHE-acute physiology and chronic health evaluation: a physiologically based classification system. Crit Care Med. 1981;9:591-7.
3. Knaus WA, Draper EA, Wagner DP, Zimmerman JE. APACHE II: A severity of disease classification system. Crit Care Med. 1985;13:818-29.
4. Salluh JI, Soares M. ICU severity of illness scores: APACHE, SAPS and MPM. Curr Opin Crit Care. 2014;20(5):557-65.
5. Metnitz PGH, Moreno RP, Almeida E, Jordan B, Bauer P, Campos RA, et al; SAPS 3 Investigators. SAPS 3—From evaluation of the patient to evaluation of the intensive care unit. Part 1: objectives, methods and cohort description. Intensive Care Med. 2005;31(10):1336-44.

6. Moreno RP, Metnitz P, Almeida E, Jordan B, Bauer P, Campos RA, et al; SAPS 3 Investigators. SAPS 3—From evaluation of the patient to evaluation of the intensive care unit. Part 2: development of a prognostic model for hospital mortality at ICU admission. Intensive Care Med. 2005;31(10):1345-55.
7. Lemeshow S, Teres D, Klar J, Avrunin JS, Gehlbach SH, Rapoport J. Mortality Probability Models (MPM II) based on an international cohort of intensive care unit patients. JAMA. 1993;270(20):2478-86.
8. Livingston BM, MacKirdy FN, Howie JC, Jones R, Norrie JD. Assessment of the performance of five intensive care scoring models within a large Scottish database. Crit Care Med. 2000;28(6):1820-7.
9. Kuzniewicz MW, Vasilevskis EE, Lane R, Dean ML, Trivedi NG, Rennie DJ, et al. Variation in ICU risk-adjusted mortality: impact of methods of assessment and potential confounders. Chest. 2008;133:1319-27.
10. Sakr Y, Krauss C, Amaral AC, Réa-Neto A, Specht M, Reinhart K, et al. Comparison of the performance of SAPS II, SAPS 3, APACHE II, and their customized prognostic models in a surgical intensive care unit. Br J Anaesth. 2008;101:798-803.
11. Harrison DA, Parry GJ, Carpenter JR, Short A, Rowan K. A new risk prediction model for critical care: the Intensive Care National Audit & Research Centre (ICNARC) model. Crit Care Med. 2007;35:1091-8.
12. Vasilevskis EE, Kuzniewicz MW, Cason BA, Lane RK, Dean ML, Clay T, et al. Mortality probability model III and simplified acute physiology score II: assessing their value in predicting length of stay and comparison to APACHE IV. Chest. 2009;136(1):89-101.
13. Sekulic AD, Trpkovic SV, Pavlovic AP, Marinkovic OM, Ilic AN. Scoring systems in assessing survival of critically ill ICU Patients. Med Sci Monit. 2015;21:2621-9.
14. Vincent JL, Moreno R, Takala J, Willatts S, De Mendonça A, Bruining H, et al. The SOFA (Sepsis-related Organ Failure Assessment) score to describe organ dysfunction/failure. On behalf of the Working Group on Sepsis-related Problems of the European Society of Intensive Care Medicine. Intensive Care Med. 1996;22:707-10.
15. Grissom CK, Brown SM, Kuttler KG, Boltax JP, Jones J, Jephson AR, et al. A modified sequential organ failure assessment score for critical care triage. Disaster Med Public Health Prep. 2010;4(4):277-84.
16. Ferreira FL, Bota DP, Bross A, Melot C, Vincent JL. Serial evaluation of the SOFA score to predict outcome in critically ill patients. JAMA. 2001;286(14):1754-8.
17. Marshall JC, Cook DJ, Christou NV, Bernard GR, Sprung CL, Sibbald WJ. Multiple organ dysfunction score: a reliable descriptor of a complex clinical outcome. Crit Care Med. 1995;23:1638-52.
18. Marshall JC. Multiple organ dysfunction syndrome. In: Sibbald WJ, Vincent JL (Eds). Clinical Trials for the Treatment of Sepsis. Heidelberg: Springer-Verlag; 1995. pp. 122-38.
19. Le Gall JR, Klar J, Lemeshow S, Saulnier F, Alberti C, Artigas A, et al; ICU Scoring Group. The logistic organ dysfunction system: a new way to assess organ dysfunction in the intensive care unit. JAMA. 1996;276:802-10.
20. Timsit JF, Fosse JP, Troché G, De Lassence A, Alberti C, Garrouste-Orgeas M, et al. Calibration and discrimination by daily logistic organ dysfunction scoring comparatively with daily sequential organ failure assessment scoring

for predicting hospital mortality in critically ill patients. Crit Care Med. 2002;30:2003-13.
21. Pettilä V, Pettila M, Sarna S, Voutilainen P, Takkunen O. Comparison of multiple organ dysfunction scores in the prediction of hospital mortality in the critically ill. Crit Care Med. 2002;30:1705-11.
22. Peres Bota D, Melot C, Lopes FF, Nguyen Ba V, Vincent JL. The Multiple Organ Dysfunction Score (MODS) versus the Sequential Organ Failure Assessment (SOFA) score in outcome prediction. Intensive Care Med. 2002;28:1619-24.
23. Zygun DA, Laupland KB, Fick GH, Sandham JD, Doig CJ. Limited ability of SOFA and MOD scores to discriminate outcome: a prospective evaluation in 1,436 patients. Can J Anaesth. 2005;52:302-8.
24. Zygun D, Berthiaume L, Laupland K, Kortbeek J, Doig C. SOFA is superior to MOD score for the determination of non-neurologic organ dysfunction in patients with severe traumatic brain injury: a cohort study. Crit Care. 2006;10(4):R115.
25. Vincent JL, Moreno RP. Clinical review: scoring systems in the critically ill. Crit Care. 2010;14(2):142-311.
26. Miranda DR, de Rijk A, Schaufeli W. Simplified Therapeutic Intervention Scoring System: the TISS-28 items—results from a multicenter study. Crit Care Med. 1996;24:64-73.
27. Reis MD, Moreno R, Iapichino G. Nine equivalents of nursing manpower use score (NEMS). Intensive Care Med. 1997;23:760-5.
28. Rothen HU, Küng V, Ryser DH, Zürcher R, Regli B. Validation of "nine equivalents of nursing manpower use score" on an independent data sample. Intensive Care Med. 1999;25:606-11.
29. Moreno R, Reis MD. Nursing staff in intensive care in Europe: the mismatch between planning and practice. Chest. 1998;113:752-8.
30. Padilha KG, Sousa RM, Kimura M, Miyadahira AM, da Cruz DA, Vattimo Mde F, et al. Nursing workload in intensive care units: a study using the Therapeutic Intervention Scoring System-28 (TISS-28). Intensive Crit Care Nurs. 2007;23:162-9.
31. Padilha KG, de Sousa RM, Queijo AF, Mendes AM, Reis Miranda D. Nursing Activities Score in the intensive care unit: analysis of the related factors. Intensive Crit Care Nurs. 2008;24:197-204.
32. Kamath PS, Wiesner RH, Malinchoc M, Kremers W, Therneau TM, Kosberg CL, et al. A model to predict survival in patients with end-stage liver disease. Hepatology. 2001;33(2):464-70.
33. Zuercher M, Ummenhofer W, Baltussen A, Walder B. The use of Glasgow Coma Scale in injury assessment: a critical review. Brain Inj. 2009;23(5):371-84.
34. Wijdicks EF, Bamlet WR, Maramattom BV, Manno EM, McClelland RL. Validation of a new coma scale: The FOUR score. Ann Neurol. 2005;58(4):585-93.
35. Nashef SA, Roques F, Hammill BG, Peterson ED, Michel P, Grover FL, et al; EurpSCORE Project Group. Validation of European System for Cardiac Operative Risk Evaluation (EuroSCORE) in North American cardiac surgery. Eur J Cardiothorac Surg. 2002;22(1):101-5.
36. Boniatti MM, Friedman G, Castilho RK, Vieira SR, Fialkow L. Characteristics of chronically critically ill patients: comparing two definitions. Clinics (Sao Paulo). 2011;66(4):701-4.

37. Vincent JL, Opal SM, Marshall JC. Ten reasons why we should NOT use severity scores as entry criteria for clinical trials or in our treatment decisions. Crit Care Med. 2010;38:283-7.
38. Higgins TL, Teres D, Copes WS, Nathanson BH, Stark M, Kramer AA. Assessing contemporary intensive care unit outcome: an updated Mortality Probability Admission Model (MPM0-III). Crit Care Med. 2007;35(3):827-35.
39. Bouch C, Thompson J. Severity scoring systems in the critically ill. Continuing Education in Anaesthesia. Critical Care and Pain. 2008;8(5):181-5.
40. Ho KM, Lee KY, Williams T, Finn J, Knuiman M, Webb SA. Comparison of acute physiology and chronic health evaluation (APACHE) II score with organ failure scores to predict hospital mortality. Anaesthesia. 2007;62:466-73.
41. Minne L, Hanna AA, de Jonge E. Evaluation of SOFA-based models for predicting mortality in the ICU: A systematic review. Crit Care. 2008;12(6):R161.

CHAPTER 18

Extracorporeal Membrane Oxygenation Support in Intensive Care

Vivek Gupta, GS Wander

ABSTRACT

The use of extracorporeal membrane oxygenation (ECMO) is rapidly increasing worldwide. This increase has been possible because of technological advancement and rapidly growing interest among acute and critical care physicians in exploring newer indications for using this novel technology for life-threatening but reversible cardiac, respiratory, or cardiorespiratory dysfunction. The availability of a cannula for percutaneous placement safely, a centrifugal pump, a miniature membrane lung, and significant advancement in critical care management allow ECMO initiation and management in the intensive care unit (ICU). However, robust monitoring and interpretation of patient and ECMO parameters ensure safe ECMO management. The complications during ECMO may be attributed to the pre-ECMO critical condition, or they may have a new onset. The common complications include bleeding, vascular injuries, sepsis, acute kidney injury (AKI), and neurological insult. Successful ECMO management requires a multidisciplinary team of medical specialties, perfusionists, physiotherapists, occupational therapists, nutritionists, psychologists, and critical care nurses.

Keywords: ECMO, extracorporeal membrane oxygenation; ICU

KEY POINTS

- Extracorporeal membrane oxygenation (ECMO) in the intensive care unit (ICU) is a valuable modality for severe but reversible respiratory, cardiac, or cardiorespiratory failure, even after maximizing the available support in the ICU armamentarium.
- The ECMO is most commonly used as a bridge to recovery; however, its use as a bridge to procedure/surgery, bridge to another bridge, or bridge to transplant is rising.
- The basic configuration of ECMO is venoarterial (VA) for cardiac/cardiorespiratory support and venovenous (VV) for respiratory support; however, hybrid ECMO may be required in complex situations.

- A careful selection of patients must be made, excluding contraindications, before initiating ECMO since it is a resource-intensive and costly procedure associated with several complications.
- Understanding the ECMO physiology and vigilant monitoring of machine and human integration for optimizing hemodynamics, gas exchange, and metabolic parameters is vital to success during the ECMO run.

INTRODUCTION

The ICU is a highly specialized and dynamic area supporting critically ill patients with advanced monitoring and management to improve morbidity and mortality. Intensive care management is an approach to optimizing a patient's physiology, addressing the life-threatening situation ranging from prevention to providing required organ support with various degrees of severity and managing underlying pathological processes. Managing these critically ill patients is challenging and requires invasive and noninvasive intervention for diagnostic and therapeutic purposes.[1] Over the last two decades, extracorporeal life support (ECLS) has emerged as a promising therapy for severe but reversible respiratory, cardiac, or cardiorespiratory dysfunction unresponsive to conventional supports.[2] The advancement of ECMO technology, miniaturization of the oxygenator and circuit, and better cannula quality have allowed ECMO initiation and prolonged ECMO to run safely in the ICU.

WHAT IS EXTRACORPOREAL MEMBRANE OXYGENATION?

Extracorporeal membrane oxygenation is a term used to describe temporary support for severe myocardial and/or respiratory dysfunction using mechanical devices, including a pump (driving unit) and oxygenator (gas exchange device) with a circuit for blood flow. ECMO helps in augmenting oxygenation, ventilation, and cardiac output (CO). The configuration of ECMO, which supports the heart and lungs, is called VA ECMO or cardiac ECMO, and which supports only the lungs is called VV ECMO or respiratory ECMO **(Table 1)**.

PROGRESS OF ECMO

The ECMO was first used successfully in 1972 for respiratory support in an adult patient.[3] This encouraged the further use of ECMO in a child after a cardiac surgical procedure to support the heart without any complication at discharge and follow-up.[4] Bartlett and Gazzaniga, in 1975, used ECMO successfully for neonatal respiratory failure following meconium aspiration, and this encouraged the use of ECMO among newborns having persistent respiratory failure due to meconium aspiration syndrome, persistent fetal circulation, etc., with survival nearly 50% in this group of patients.[5] However,

TABLE 1: Salient difference—VA and VV ECMO.

VV ECMO	VA ECMO
Only respiratory support	Both cardiac and respiratory support
Only venous cannulation	Both arterial and venous cannulation
Relatively lower PaO_2 achieved	Higher PaO_2 achieved
The circuit connection is in series with the lungs	The circuit connection is parallel to the heart and lung
Higher blood flow is required to achieve oxygenation	Lower blood flow may be achieved
Unchanged pulmonary blood flow	Pulmonary circulation is bypassed, so it reduces pulmonary artery pressure
May lead to RV failure	It can be helpful in RV failure

(ECMO: extracorporeal membrane oxygenation; PaO_2: partial pressure of arterial oxygen; RV: right ventricle; VA: venoarterial; VV: venovenous)

a subsequent multicenter randomized controlled trial demonstrated poor outcome with multiple complications in adult patients with severe respiratory dysfunction supported with VA ECMO[6] and mechanical ventilation and mechanical ventilation alone. Therefore, using ECMO is restricted to highly specialized centers, especially for neonatal and pediatric patients. The recent era has seen a drastic increase in the use of ECMO, especially in adult patients.[7] This surge was observed during the H1N1 pandemic, and the famous multicenter randomized controlled CESAR trial demonstrated the usefulness of ECMO in severe but reversible respiratory failure.[8] The outcome with H1N1 severe acute respiratory distress syndrome (ARDS) supported with VV ECMO was encouraging, especially in specialized ECMO centers.[9] These promising results and better and safer hardware availability lead to increased ECMO usage for various ICU and emergency medicine indications. During the recent coronavirus disease 2019 (COVID-19) pandemic, the awareness and use of ECMO further increased with mixed results due to various confounding factors, including timings of initiation, age, comorbidities, development of acute kidney injury (AKI), etc.[10]

PHYSIOLOGY

Normal Gas Exchange Physiology

The metabolism in the body is directly associated with the amount of oxygen consumption per minute (VO_2), which is nearly 250 mL/min (5–8 mL/kg/min) at rest for an adult. However, the available oxygen in the blood is almost five times more than required. Mitochondrial utilization of oxygen facilitates substrate oxidation and produces energy and carbon dioxide. The carbon dioxide is transported through blood back to the lungs for exhalation.

The oxygen in the healthy lungs passes from the alveoli to the blood through passive diffusion efficiently.[11] The total arterial oxygen content (CaO_2) can be calculated as:

$$O_2 \text{ content} = (Hb \times SaO_2 \times 1.39) + (pO_2 \times 0.0031)$$

where Hb is hemoglobin, pO_2 is partial pressure of oxygen, and SaO_2 is arterial oxygen saturation.

Arterial oxygen content is approximately 20 mL/dL, and systemic oxygen delivery (DO_2) varies with changes in CO.

$$DO_2 = CaO_2 \times CO$$

Once oxygen is transferred to the tissues, the venous oxygen content (CvO_2) is calculated as:

$$CvO_2 = CaO_2 - VO_2/CO$$

This blood is transported to the lungs for oxygen enrichment.

Carbon dioxide production during aerobic metabolism is around 250 mL/min in a healthy person and passes through venous blood. Dissolved CO_2 contributes only 5% of total venous CO_2 content from carbonic acid in red blood cells and stays in equilibrium.

$$CO_2 + H_2O \leftrightarrow H_2CO_3 \leftrightarrow H^+ + HCO_3^-$$

Around 70% of venous CO_2 remains in the blood as bicarbonate, which is finally transported to the lung and expired to the atmosphere through the alveolar-capillary membrane.

Membrane Oxygenator: An Artificial Lung

During an ECMO run, the gas exchange is complex to understand as it depends on the gas exchange by the artificial lung, the gas exchange contributed by the native lung, and the patient's CO. The membrane oxygenator used for ECMO is made with polymethylpentene (PMP), a hydrophobic polymer. These microporous hollow fibers are tightly arranged to prevent plasma leakage even after prolonged use. These fibers act as an interface and allow sweep gas flow to pass through the inner lumen while blood passes on the outer surface of these fibers. The exchange of oxygen and carbon dioxide occurs due to a gradient on either side of the membrane, passing from the higher to the lower side. The higher surface area (150 m²) and thin alveolar membrane (1–3 μm) of native lung allow better gas exchange as compared to membrane lung surface area of around 1.2–1.9 m² and thickness of 10–30 μm.[12]

The DO_2 by the membrane lung is assessed by the rated flow depending upon the membrane surface area, the amount of mixing, the blood flow rate, and the oxygen-carrying capacity of the blood passing through the membrane lung. The diffusing capacity of CO_2 is much higher than oxygen, so the amount removed depends on the difference between the partial pressure of carbon dioxide (pCO_2) in the blood and the CO_2 in the sweep gas flow (ventilating gas in ECMO). The sweep gas flow is usually kept at a ratio of 1:1, which means equal to the ECMO blood flow. The quantity of CO_2 removed will be similar to the amount of oxygen added. However, if the sweep gas flow ratio increases, more CO_2 gets washed out, but oxygenation remains unchanged.

Venovenous ECMO: Gaseous Exchange and Hemodynamics

During VV ECMO, blood is drained from the venous system and returned to the venous system after gas exchange. Finally, the oxygenated blood is mixed with deoxygenated blood returned from the body. Consequently, the blood returning to the right heart is an admixture of the deoxygenated blood from systemic organs and the well-oxygenated extracorporeal blood, raising oxygen in the right heart. This mixed blood passes into the right ventricle, the lungs, and finally to systemic organs. In severe respiratory failure, the native lungs contribute none to gas exchange, so the arterial O_2 and CO_2 concentrations result from mixing the oxygenated ECMO blood with the deoxygenated systemic blood, resulting in the arterial saturation ranging from 60 to 90%. The desaturated arterial blood results in standard systemic DO_2 if the CO and hemoglobin concentration are sufficient. The oxygen supply from the membrane lung is dependent on the blood flow, the hemoglobin concentration, and the difference between the outlet minus inlet O_2 content, as follows:

$$VO_2 \text{ (mL)} = \text{Blood flow} \times (C_{out}O_2 - C_{in}O_2)$$

Blood flow depends on the resistance to flow in the drainage cannula, the suction produced by the pump, and the geometry of the cannulated vessel. CO_2 elimination is much easier during VV ECMO than achieving oxygenation. Hence, even lower blood flow can remove the CO_2 produced by the patient. VV ECMO is a hemodynamically neutral support since blood is not reinfused into the arterial system. Venous return and pulsatility are unaltered since drainage and reinfusion are balanced.

Venoarterial ECMO: Gaseous Exchange and Hemodynamics

Venoarterial ECMO is used predominantly in cardiopulmonary failure. In this configuration, blood is removed from the body by the venous drainage cannula, and oxygenated blood from the blood pump is perfused into the aorta, which mixes with blood from the left ventricle. If the lungs function well, the mixed blood is well-oxygenated and has normal pCO_2. If the lungs are not working well, the systemic blood gases will reflect the mixture of the cardiac and extracorporeal flows, resulting in lower oxygenation proximal to the mixing site.[13]

INDICATIONS AND PATIENT SELECTION

Every patient should be evaluated individually as a candidate for ECMO support. We must thoroughly evaluate for vascular disease to ensure smooth vascular access. Advanced age is associated with poor outcomes. However, elderly patients may be considered as per the indication, pre-ECMO conditions, and comorbidities.[14,15]

Circulatory Failure and ECMO

Venoarterial ECMO support may be helpful in acute circulatory failure classically characterized by hypotension (systolic blood pressure <90 mm Hg), tissue hypoperfusion despite optimal volume status, increased pulmonary wedge pressure >18 mm Hg, central venous pressure >12 mm Hg, cardiac index <1.8–2.0 L/min/m^2, and poor central venous oxygen saturation despite high doses of vasoactive drug administration and intra-aortic balloon counterpulsation support. High doses of vasoactive drugs are associated with increased mortality,[16] which can be reduced after ECMO. The primary aim of ECMO support in severe myocardial dysfunction is to stabilize circulation and perfusion as a bridge to cardiac function recovery, procedure/surgery, transplant, or another bridge. The usual indications to support these patients with VA ECMO include acute cardiogenic shock, acute myocarditis, postcardiotomy myocardial failure, postcardiac transplant or bridge to cardiac transplant, periprocedural support in cardiac catheterization, bridge to cardiac transplant/left ventricular assist device (LVAD), and extracorporeal cardiopulmonary resuscitation (E-CPR)[17] **(Table 2)**. These patients require VA cannulation (VA ECMO) usually peripheral approach however central approach is used in postcardiotomy patients.[18] This blood is drained from the right atrium and returned to the arterial system, which reduces preload but improves aortic blood flow and tissue perfusion. The current evidence has not shown any survival benefit with using intra-aortic balloon counter pulsation[19] for managing acute myocardial infarction (MI) with severe cardiogenic shock. VA ECMO support may be a promising mechanical circulatory support option in these acute MI patients with severe cardiogenic shock.

Respiratory Failure and ECMO

Venovenous ECMO support may be helpful in acute respiratory failure in various clinical settings, such as ARDS with different etiology, such as viral or bacterial pneumonia and aspiration pneumonitis. The other common indications are acute severe asthma pulmonary hemorrhage/diffuse alveolar hemorrhage, traumatic lung injury/contusion, smoke or toxic fume inhalation-induced acute lung injury,[20,21] candidate for lung transplant,[22] post-lung transplant graft dysfunction,[23] bronchopleural fistula, and assisted

TABLE 2: VA ECMO indications and possible destination.

VA ECMO indication	Clinical condition	Possible destination
Cardiogenic shock/myocarditis	• Acute coronary syndrome • Refractory arrhythmia • Acute fulminant myocarditis • Acute RV failure • Acute pulmonary embolism • Postpartum cardiomyopathy • Drug overdose leading to severe myocardial depression	Bridge to recovery
Postcardiotomy shock	Acute LV failure	Bridge to recovery
Periprocedural support/ECMO supported procedures	• High-risk percutaneous coronary intervention • Acute RV failure after insertion of LVAD	Bridge to recovery
Postcardiac transplant	• Primary graft failure • Hyperacute rejection following heart transplant	Bridge to recovery
LVAD	• Class IV/stage D heart failure • Chronic cardiomyopathies	Bridge to bridge
Extracorporeal cardiopulmonary resuscitation	Refractory cardiac arrest	Bridge to decision
Persistent ventricular arrhythmia storm	Antiarrhythmic resistant	Bridge to recovery/decision
Pulmonary hypertension with severe RV dysfunction	Hemodynamic instability	Bridge to recovery or bridge
Massive pulmonary embolism	Severe myocardial dysfunction/cardiac arrest	Bridge to recovery/procedure
Severe hypothermia	Persistent cardiac arrest	Bridge to recovery

(ECMO: extracorporeal membrane oxygen; LV: left ventricular; LVAD: left ventricular assist device; RV: right ventricular; VA: venoarterial)

airway or lung procedures.[24] The primary rationale for initiating VV ECMO is improving systemic oxygenation with adequate CO_2 removal while avoiding complications associated with mechanical ventilation. Various configurations of ECMO may be used in improving the gas exchange, primarily VV ECMO. However, in cases of cardiovascular collapse, VA ECMO or V-VA (access venous and return to both venous and arterial) ECMO will provide both respiratory support and hemodynamic stabilization. The beneficial role of ECMO has been demonstrated in patients with inhalation injuries and traumatic lung injuries **(Table 3)**.

TABLE 3: VV ECMO indications and possible destination.

VV ECMO indication	Clinical condition	Possible destination
Severe ARDS	Bacterial/viral/aspiration	Bridge to recovery
Traumatic lung injury/pulmonary contusion	Poor gas exchange	Bridge to recovery
Acute hypoxic/hypercapnic respiratory failure	• *Hypoxemia:* PaO_2/FiO_2 <80 mm Hg (adequate medical management) • Hypercapnia (pH <7.25 even after good ventilation) • Murray score >3	Bridge to recovery
Pulmonary embolism	Hemodynamically stable patient with severe hypoxemia	Bridge to recovery/procedure
Lung transplant	Waiting for transplant and not maintaining gas exchange	Bridge to transplant
Post-lung transplant graft dysfunction		Bridge to recovery
Inhalational fumes-induced acute lung injury	Poor gas exchange and acute lung injury	Bridge to recovery

(ARDS: acute respiratory distress syndrome; ECMO: extracorporeal membrane oxygen; FiO_2: fraction of inspired oxygen; PaO_2: partial pressure of arterial oxygen; VV: venovenous)

TABLE 4: Contraindications of VA and VV ECMO.

VA ECMO	VV ECMO

• *Absolute:*
  – Inability to achieve access due to peripheral vascular disease
  – Aortic dissection (unrepaired)
  – Severe aortic regurgitation
• *Relative:*
  – Contraindication to anticoagulation
  – Advanced age (>70 years)
  – Uncontrolled bleeding
	• *Absolute:* During CPR
	
	• *Relative:*
	  – Mechanical ventilation above 7 days
	  – Advanced age (>70 years)

(CPR: cardiopulmonary resuscitation; ECMO: extracorporeal membrane oxygen; VA: venoarterial; VV: venovenous)

■ CONTRAINDICATIONS

The absolute contraindications include "do not resuscitate" (DNR) orders, massive intracranial hemorrhage, multiorgan failure, or no chance of organ recovery without an option for transplant/assist devices. The contraindications specific to VA and VV ECMO are as follows **(Table 4)**.

However, in a persistent cardiac arrest situation, a decision regarding ECMO CPR should be made quickly and carefully after evaluating low flow (<60 minutes), no flow time (<5 minutes), poor cardiopulmonary resuscitation (CPR) quality (end-tidal carbon dioxide <10), unwitnessed cardiac arrest, or nonshockable initial rhythm.[25]

■ CIRCUIT CONFIGURATION AND DESIGN

The type and degree of support depend upon the patient's condition to initiate cardiopulmonary support (VA ECMO) or respiratory support (VV ECMO). However, the basic configuration of a typical circuit remains the same, irrespective of the type of support. The drainage of blood through a major vein, which passes through a pump (usually centrifugal) followed by a membrane oxygenator connected through an oxygen blender, which provides gas flow for gas exchange, and blood is returned to a major artery (VA ECMO) or vein (VV ECMO) after gas exchange **(Fig. 1)**. The currently used PMP oxygenators are well suited for long-term use and reduce inflammatory response and transfusion requirements **(Figs. 2A to D)**. The plastic tubing of the circuit is made up of polyvinyl chloride (PVC). The number of connectors and stopcocks should be as low as possible to reduce the risk of turbulent flow and blood stasis to minimize the complication. The temperature is maintained using a heater–cooler unit to prevent hypothermia due to inadvertent heat loss through the extracorporeal circuit. There may be several ports to take samples and check pressure to ensure circuit efficacy, efficiency, and patient safety.

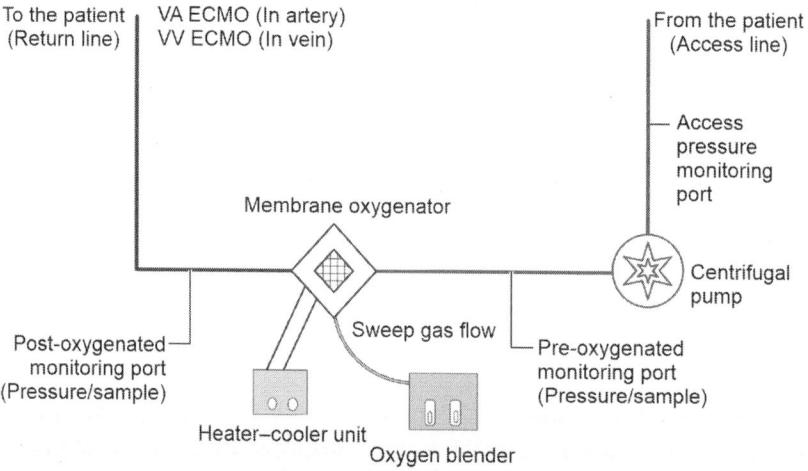

Fig. 1: Basic extracorporeal membrane oxygenation (ECMO) configuration. (VA: venoarterial; VV: venovenous)

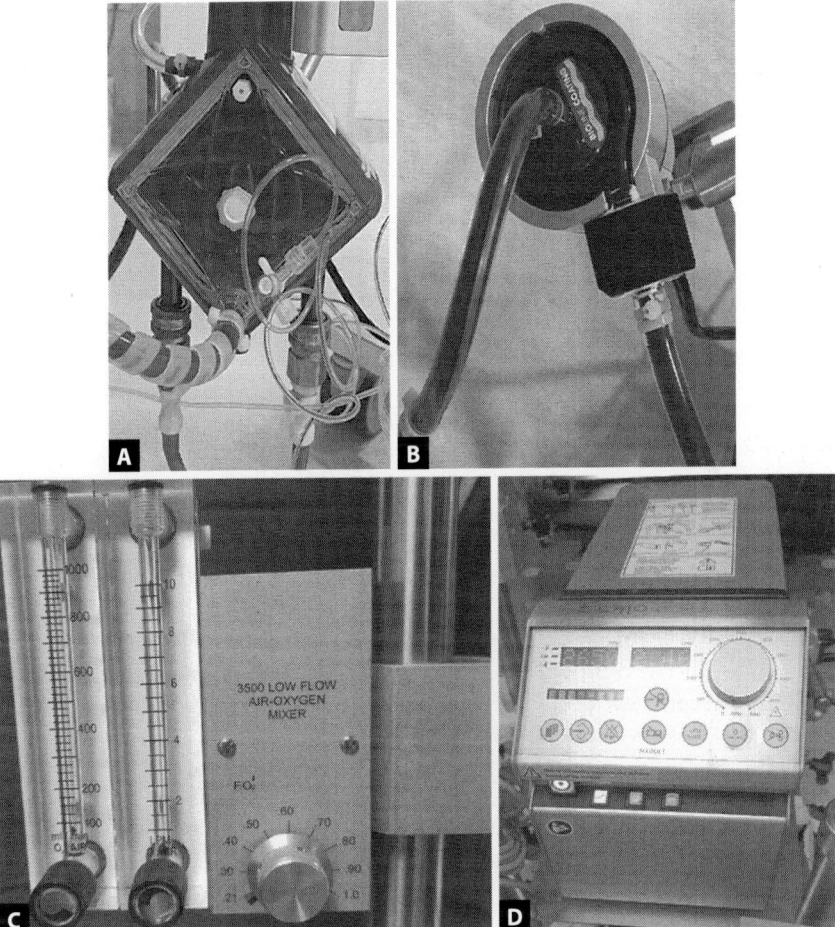

Figs. 2A to D: ECMO components. (A) Membrane oxygenator; (B) centrifugal pump with cone; (C) oxygen blender; (D) console.

■ MANAGEMENT STRATEGY DURING ECMO

The management approach includes ensuring the safety, efficacy, and efficiency of the ECMO system and managing fluids, anticoagulation, medications (e.g., antibiotics, sedatives, and muscle relaxants), mechanical ventilation strategy, and left ventricular venting during ECMO.

Hemodynamic Monitoring

Advanced hemodynamic monitoring during ECMO helps assess cardiovascular functions, adequate tissue perfusion, and ECMO effectiveness.[26] Hemodynamic monitoring during VV ECMO is similar to any ICU patient, whereas, during VA ECMO, the hemodynamic assessment requires echocardiographic, CO measurement, and venous oxygen saturation

TABLE 5: Role of echocardiography during ECMO.

Timings	Evaluation	Interpretation
Pre-ECMO	Cardiac function	• Choosing VA or VV ECMO • Excluding contraindications such as severe aortic regurgitation
After ECMO initiation	• Volume status • Cannula position	• Fluid administration • Correct part or placement of the venous cannula • Distance between access and return cannula to prevent recirculation
During ECMO support	• Cardiac function • Cannula position • Pericardial effusion	• Myocardial recovery • Onset or worsening of myocardial function/LV thrombus • RV dysfunction • Adequacy of flow • Obstructive shock
Recovery and weaning	Cardiac function recovery	• Ejection fraction • Aortic velocity time integral (above 10 cm) • Lateral mitral annular peak systolic velocity (above 6 cm)

(ECMO: extracorporeal membrane oxygenation; LV: left ventricular; RV: right ventricular; VA: venoarterial; VV: venovenous)

(SvO_2). Adequate tissue perfusion is evaluated by metabolic correction, improving lactate levels and urine output. Patients on VV ECMO may develop right ventricular dysfunction due to increased pulmonary blood flow and vascular resistance. The effectiveness of VV ECMO is assessed by monitoring the gas exchange.[27]

Echocardiography noninvasively provides a quick and real-time cardiac function assessment, especially during VA ECMO; however, its role during VV ECMO cannot be underestimated **(Table 5)**.

The major complication associated specifically with VA ECMO include differential hypoxemia (DH), dual circulation, North-South syndrome, or Harlequin syndrome.[28] In this condition, the upper and lower body's saturation differs due to two parallel circulations (native cardiac and ECMO circulation).[29] This phenomenon is commonly encountered during femoral-femoral VA ECMO, where ECMO blood flows retrograde in the aorta through the iliac artery. The antegrade blood flow ejected from the left ventricle meets this retrograde ECMO flow. The mixing of both flows occurs in the aorta, and the level depends upon the native cardiac function and degree of ECMO support. The upper body oxygenation depends on native lung function, while the membrane lung determines the lower region oxygenation. In case of deranged lung function, oxygenation of the upper body will be severely impaired, including coronary and cerebral oxygenation, leading to fulminant differential hypoxemia (FDH).[30] This DH leading to cerebral hypoperfusion is associated with poor neurological outcomes.[31]

Venoarterial ECMO augments the native CO, maintains the perfusion pressure, and improves tissue oxygenation even during a cardiac standstill. However, the pooled blood may lead to distension and myocardial stunning in a poorly or nonejecting left ventricle. The rising pressure in the left heart increases pressure in pulmonary capillaries, which may lead to pulmonary edema or hemorrhage. The stasis of blood in the left ventricle may also lead to thrombus formation. The persistent left ventricular distension may need left ventricular venting by pharmacological, nonsurgical, or surgical interventional methods. This includes dobutamine infusion, intra-aortic balloon pump, percutaneous left atrial venting, or surgical apical venting for cases unresponsive to less invasive management.

Monitoring Perfusion and Metabolism

Monitoring and interpreting arterial blood gases (ABG) during VV ECMO is the same as for any ICU patient. Continuous oxygen saturation monitoring reduces frequent ABG sampling. During the initial phase of VV ECMO, the shunt fraction is almost 100% in the native lung, and the partial pressure of oxygen is nearly similar to SvO_2. During VV ECMO, lower oxygen saturation (around 85%) may be acceptable if DO_2 is adequate, which is kept at least three times more than oxygen consumption to avoid tissue hypoxia.

The most common peripheral VA ECMO configuration is the femoral artery and femoral vein. Monitoring the right arm oxygen saturation or placing a right radial arterial cannula for ABG analysis is used to guide the adequacy of upper body oxygenation. An adequate balance must be ensured between DO_2 and oxygen consumption. A low venous saturation may reflect low CO and rising lactate levels, and signs of other organ hypoperfusion may warrant increasing ECMO flow for optimizing DO_2. The sublingual microcirculatory monitoring by measuring perfused vessel density (PVD), small-vessel densities (SVD), and percent perfused vessels (PPV) in patients with VA ECMO may be a future tool for assessing outcomes as well as weaning from VA ECMO.[32]

Monitoring and Management of Anticoagulation

Without standardized management protocols for anticoagulation during ECMO, there is significant variation in monitoring and management practices. Unfractionated heparin (UFH) is the most commonly used and most studied anticoagulant during ECMO. UFH prevents thrombus formation by binds with antithrombin (AT) and impairs thrombin activity by several thousandfold.[33] The loading dose of UFH at the time of cannulation is usually 50-100 units/kg bolus followed by 20-40 units/kg/h targeting an activated clotting time (ACT) of 180-200.[34] However, the dose may also be titrated on activated partial thromboplastin time (aPTT) or anti-Xa values[35,36] **(Table 6)**.

TABLE 6: Anticoagulation during ECMO.

Anticoagulants	Advantages	Disadvantages	Monitoring and targets	Doses
Heparin				
UFH	• Cheap • Vast experience • Antagonist available	• Unpredictable effect • Risk of heparin resistance • HIT	• ACT: 180–200 • aPTT: 50–70 • Anti-Xa: 0.3–0.7	• Bolus 50–100 U/kg • Infusion: 15–25 U/kg/h
LMWH	• No dependency on at • More predictable effect than UFH	• Longer half-life • Antagonist not available • Difficult to titrate	Anti-Xa: 0.5–1.0	No specific dose recommendations
Fondaparinux[37]	• Used in HIT • No dependency on AT	• Longer half-life • Antagonist not available	Anti-Xa: 0.4–0.7	Loading dose 5 mg S/C followed by 2.5 mg S/C 2–3 times a day
Direct thrombin inhibitors				
Bivaluridin[38]	• Shorter half-life • Used during HIT/resistance	• Not to be used in renal dysfunction • Risk of thrombus formation at the places of stasis/low flow	aPTT: 60–70	• Bolus 0.4–0.5 mg/kg • Infusion 0.05–0.5 mg/kg/h
Argatroban[39]	• Adequate half-life • Safely used in renal dysfunction • There is no risk of thrombosis at stasis/low flow area	Risk of bleeding, especially in hepatic dysfunction	aPTT: 45–60	• No bolus dose • Infusion 0.02–0.2 µg/kg/min

(ACT: activated clotting time; aPTT: activated partial thromboplastin time; AT: antithrombin; ECMO: extracorporeal membrane oxygenation; HIT: heparin-induced thrombocytopenia; LMWH: low-molecular-weight heparin; S/C: subcutaneous; UFH: unfractionated heparin)

Mechanical Ventilation during ECMO

Respiratory support during VV ECMO is required because the ECMO blood flow is insufficient, and a significant amount of blood passes through the diseased native lung. During VV ECMO, the primary aim is to give rest to the lung while preventing collapse. There is no consensus regarding optimal ventilation; however, restricting plateau airway pressures below 25 cmH$_2$O, keeping a low ventilatory rate around 4-10 breaths/min, maintaining PEEP around 10-15 cmH$_2$O, and minimizing FiO$_2$ with a target of 0.3 has helped reduce further lung injury. A low tidal volume ventilation (<6 mL/kg predicted body weight) prevents further lung injury. In a meta-analysis, driving pressures have been demonstrated as an essential factor associated with mortality during ECMO.[40]

Drug Dosing during ECMO

Critically ill patients pose a significant challenge in drug dosing due to the dynamic and unpredictable variation in pharmacokinetics (PK), increased volume of distribution, and decreased clearance.[41] These PK changes are more evident during ECMO, primarily due to inflammatory activation, increased volume of distribution, blood exposure to foreign material, and drug sequestration in the circuit.[42] These changes significantly alter the antibiotic concentration and half-life. The ideal way to choose the correct antibiotic dosing is therapeutic drug monitoring. However, it may not be available routinely. Meropenem PK has been studied during ECMO, and an initial higher dose is recommended due to the increased volume of distribution. While β-lactam antibiotics PK has shown variability and requires individualized antibiotic dosing.[43]

The other commonly used drugs are sedatives and analgesics during ECMO. Guidelines or optimal sedation regimens are still lacking due to dynamic changes in PK due to patient-specific variables. Moreover, there are no defined pharmacodynamic (PD) end points. The titration depends on clinical assessment such as subjective agitation and ventilator dysynchrony.[44]

ISSUES, CHALLENGES, AND COMPLICATIONS DURING ECMO

Extracorporeal membrane oxygenation is associated with several complications leading to increased morbidity and mortality. These complications are contributed by pre-ECMO critical condition, cannulation technique, circuit-related technical and mechanical issues, anticoagulation, sepsis, etc. VA ECMO is associated with higher complications with maximum complications related to ECMO CPR.

ECMO-associated Bleeding

The most common complication during ECMO is bleeding, with 10–30% incidence.[45] The incidence of bleeding in VA ECMO is double compared to VV ECMO. The bleeding may occur mainly due to systemic heparinization, hemodilution, platelet dysfunction, and systemic inflammatory response.[46] The bleeding usually occurs at the cannulation site, any other surgical site, gastrointestinal tract, retroperitoneal area, thoracic or abdominal cavity. The control of bleeding may need reducing or stopping anticoagulants, administering platelets and coagulation factors,[47] and controlling the bleeding point if possible. The pulmonary hemorrhage may require frequent bronchoscopy to clear the airway. Intracranial hemorrhage is associated with significant mortality in ARDS patients supported with VV ECMO.[48] It is crucial to maintain an appropriate balance between bleeding and thrombosis during ECMO using aPTT to improve outcomes.[49]

Challenges and Potential Complications of Cannulation

Successful cannulation is the first step for initiating ECMO, while complications during cannulation may lead to significant morbidity, including failure of ECMO initiation. The main aim during cannulation is to achieve in a simplified manner with minimum trauma and maintain adequate flow.[50] Vascular complications during ECMO reduce survival to discharge rate significantly.[51] Femoral artery and vein is the most common cannulation site during peripheral VA ECMO. Besides bleeding, other potential problems include differential perfusion of the upper and lower half of the body,[52] increasing afterload leading to left ventricular distension, and pulmonary edema. Another specific complication related to VA ECMO is lower limb ischemia due to inadequate distal blood flow due to femoral artery cannulation. A perfusion cannula is placed in the femoral artery distal to the cannula or retrograde cannula in the tibial artery to maintain the perfusion and reduce the risk of ischemia.[53] Central VA ECMO is restricted for cardiac surgical procedures and is associated with sternotomy-related complications. Other problems related to cannulation include arterial dissection, pseudoaneurysm, retroperitoneal bleeding, and risk of infection.[54]

Renal and Hepatic Involvement

The incidence of AKI during ECMO is quite common and is associated with significant morbidity, mortality, and increased therapy costs.[55] The AKI may be a new onset during ECMO or associated with pre-ECMO conditions such as severe sepsis, hypotension, low CO, high ventilator setting, nephrotoxic drug exposure, or high vasoactive drugs. ECMO-induced acute inflammatory response leading to leaky capillaries and intravascular volume depletion may also contribute to AKI. AKI may lead to oliguria and acute tubular necrosis and may progress to acute kidney disease, cortical necrosis, and irreversible loss of renal function.[56] The other critical etiological factors during ECMO are bleeding, sepsis, volume overload,[57] or nonpulsatile blood flow (during VA ECMO). Almost 50% of patients who develop AKI may need renal replacement therapy (RRT). The common indications for RRT initiation include Cumulative fluid overload (FO), prevention of FO, metabolic disturbances, uremia, and/or electrolyte imbalances. The FO during ECMO is associated with delayed recovery of lung function, prolonged weaning, and prolonged ECMO duration.[58] The other benefits of RRT initiation include adequate nutritional support, drugs, and blood product administration without a fear of FO. Moreover, overzealous diuretic use may be avoided to prevent its complications, given the lack of evidence for survival benefits.[59]

Hepatic dysfunction may occur due to pre-ECMO hemodynamic instability, which may recover later. However, raised bilirubin levels with thrombocytopenia may occur due to hemolysis, leading to elevated plasma-free hemoglobin (PFH) concentration.[60] Hyperbilirubinemia may lead to inflammation, oxidative stress, and apoptosis. Hemolysis during ECMO may lead to AKI.

Neurological Complications and Challenges

The neurological insult may occur due to pre-ECMO conditions such as hemodynamic instability (altered cerebral autoregulation), hypo-/hyperglycemia, fever, metabolic or electrolyte derangements, and cerebral emboli.[61] Moreover, cerebral infarction has been reported during ECMO gaseous microemboli or cannula-related microthrombus.[62] It is prudent to remember that sudden reduction in carbon dioxide at initiating VV ECMO in hypercapnic patients can lead to neurological insult. Another important cause of neurological insult during VA ECMO is upper body hypoxia and inadequate flow due to loss of pulsatile flow.[63] The common neurological complications include convulsion, intracranial hemorrhage, stroke, ischemic encephalopathy, etc.[64] Major and minor neurological complications may occur in almost 13% of patients on ECMO. Intracranial hemorrhage is associated with high mortality. Early identification of neurological events may be delayed due to the depth of sedation and challenges related to transportation for imaging during ECMO.

Infection and Sepsis

Sepsis is one of the most common complications encountered during ECMO, with an incidence as high as 40%.[65] The various factors predisposing to sepsis include increasing age, longer ECMO run,[66] higher disease severity score before ECMO, compromised immunity, comorbidities, especially autoimmune diseases, and multiple indwelling medical devices.[67] Sepsis is associated with higher mortality and morbidity by increasing the risk of coagulation abnormalities, gastrointestinal bleeding, metabolic derangements, seizure, and increased risk of circuit microthrombi warranting extracorporeal circuit replacement.[68] The usual sources of sepsis during ECMO include ventilator-associated pneumonia (VAP) and bloodstream infection due to indwelling vascular catheters. The incidence of catheter-associated urinary tract infections (CAUTI), pressure ulcer-associated infections, or *Clostridium difficile*-associated diarrhea is relatively lower.[65] The usually reported isolates related to sepsis include coagulase-negative *Staphylococcus* (CoNS), *Candida* species, *Pseudomonas aeruginosa*,[69] etc. However, data from Indian ICUs demonstrate a higher prevalence of gram-negative infections.[70]

■ CONCLUSION

Role of Anesthesiologists and Future Perspective
The use of ECMO is rapidly growing in the ICU and emergency room. One of the promising indications is the institution of VA ECMO as ECPR for refractory cardiac arrest to conventional CPR. This may facilitate rescue percutaneous cardiac intervention on VA ECMO. This requires a multidisciplinary team approach, such as emergency physicians, cardiologists, and intensivists, and a CPR team maintaining high-quality CPR prior to ECMO initiation.[71]

Extracorporeal membrane oxygenation is a sophisticated technology requiring extreme vigilance, training, and equipment maintenance to prevent mishaps due to error or equipment malfunction. Anesthesiologists, especially those trained in cardiac anesthesia, have a unique position in ECMO management due to their knowledge related to cardiopulmonary bypass, procedural skills, and skills of advanced hemodynamic monitoring.[72]

As a procedure, ECMO is a low-volume and high-risk clinical activity. There should be a simulation training program for professionals involved in ECMO management, both for beginners and to refresh their ECMO skills.[73] More focus must be given to improving team communication during ECMO crises for better outcomes. Moreover, an organization set up with the concept of an ECMO program director and a hospital administrator may help focus on quality and safety to maximize the benefits of ECMO.

■ REFERENCES

1. Jackson M, Cairns T. Care of the critically ill patient. Surgery (Oxf). 2021; 39(1):29-36.
2. Mosier JM, Kelsey M, Raz Y, Gunnerson KJ, Meyer R, Hypes CD, et al. Extracorporeal membrane oxygenation (ECMO) for critically ill adults in the emergency department: history, current applications, and future directions. Crit Care. 2015;19:431.
3. Hill JD, O'Brien TG, Murray JJ, Dontigny L, Bramson ML, Osborn JJ, et al. Prolonged extracorporeal oxygenation for acute post-traumatic respiratory

failure (shock-lung syndrome). Use of the Bramson membrane lung. N Engl J Med. 1972;286:629-34.
4. Bartlett RH, Gazzaniga AB, Jefferies MR, Huxtable RF, Haiduc NJ, Fong SW. Extracorporeal membrane oxygenation (ECMO) cardiopulmonary support in infancy. Trans Am Soc Artif Intern Organs. 1976;22:80-93.
5. Bartlett RH, Gazzaniga AB, Huxtable RH, Worcester C, Rucker R, Wetmore N, et al. Extracorporeal membrane oxygenation (ECMO) in newborn respiratory failure: technical consideration. Trans Am Soc Artif Intern Organs. 1979;25:473-5.
6. Zapol WM, Snider MT, Hill JD, Fallat RJ, Bartlett RH, Edmunds LH, et al. Extracorporeal membrane oxygenation in severe acute respiratory failure. A randomized prospective study. JAMA. 1979;242:2193-6.
7. Extracorporeal Life Support Organization. (2023). ECLS International Summary of Statistics. [online] Available from: https://www.elso.org/registry/internationalsummaryandreports/internationalsummary.aspx [Last accessed September, 2023].
8. Peek GJ, Mugford M, Tiruvoipati R, Wilson A, Allen E, Thalanany MM, et al; CESAR trial collaboration. Efficacy and economic assessment of conventional ventilatory support versus extracorporeal membrane oxygenation for severe adult respiratory failure (CESAR): a multicentre randomised controlled trial. Lancet. 2009;374:1351-63.
9. Holzgraefe B, Broomé M, Kalzén H, Konrad D, Palmér K, Frenckner B. Extracorporeal membrane oxygenation for pandemic H1N1 2009 respiratory failure. Minerva Anestesiol. 2010;76(12):1043-51.
10. Makhoul M, Keizman E, Carmi U, Galante O, Ilgiyaev E, Matan M, et al. Outcomes of Extracorporeal Membrane Oxygenation (ECMO) for COVID-19 Patients: A Multi-Institutional Analysis. Vaccines (Basel). 2023;11(1):108.
11. Wagner PD. The physiological basis of pulmonary gas exchange: implications for clinical interpretation of arterial blood gases. Peter D. Wagner Eur Respir J. 2015;45(1):227-43.
12. Bartlett RH. Physiology of gas exchange during ECMO for respiratory failure. J Intensive Care Med. 2017;32(4):243-8.
13. Bartlett RH. Physiology of Extracorporeal Gas Exchange. Compr Physiol. 2020;10:879-91.
14. Lim H. The physiology of extracorporeal membrane oxygenation: The Fick principle. Perfusion. 2023;38(2):236-44.
15. Brogan TV, Thiagarajan RR, Rycus PT, Bartlett RH, Bratton SL. Extracorporeal membrane oxygenation in adults with severe respiratory failure: a multi-center database. Intensive Care Med. 2009;35(12):2105-14.
16. Mendiratta P, Wei JY, Gomez A, Podrazik P, Riggs AT, Rycus P, et al. Cardiopulmonary resuscitation requiring extracorporeal membrane oxygenation in the elderly: a review of the extracorporeal life support organization registry. ASAIO J. 2013;59(3):211-5.
17. Na SJ, Chung CR, Cho YH, Jeon K, Suh GY, Ahn JH, et al. Vasoactive inotropic score as a predictor of mortality in adult patients with cardiogenic shock: medical therapy versus ECMO. Rev Esp Cardiol (Engl Ed). 2019;72(1):40-7.
18. Weinberg A, Tapson VF, Ramzy D. Massive Pulmonary Embolism: Extracorporeal Membrane Oxygenation and Surgical Pulmonary Embolectomy. Semin Respir Crit Care Med. 2017;38(1):66-72.

19. Napp LC, Kühn C, Hoeper MM, Vogel-Claussen J, Haverich A, Schäfer A, et al. Cannulation strategies for percutaneous extracorporeal membrane oxygenation in adults. Clin Res Cardiol. 2016;105(4):283-96.
20. Thiele H, Zeymer U, Neumann FJ, Ferenc M, Olbrich HG, Hausleiter J, et al; IABP-SHOCK II Trial Investigators. Intraaortic balloon support for myocardial infarction with cardiogenic shock. N Engl J Med. 2012;367(14):1287-96.
21. Thompson JT, Molnar JA, Hines MH, Chang MC, Pranikoff T. Successful management of adult smoke inhalation with extracorporeal membrane oxygenation. J Burn Care Rehabil. 2005;26(1):62-6.
22. Cordell-Smith JA, Roberts N, Peek GJ, Firmin RK. Traumatic lung injury treated by extracorporeal membrane oxygenation (ECMO). Injury. 2006;37(1):29-32.
23. Toyoda Y, Bhama JK, Shigemura N, Zaldonis D, Pilewski J, Crespo M, et al. Efficacy of extracorporeal membrane oxygenation as a bridge to lung transplantation. J Thorac Cardiovasc Surg. 2013;145(4):1065-70.
24. Hartwig MG, Walczak R, Lin SS, Davis RD. Improved survival but marginal allograft function in patients treated with extracorporeal membrane oxygenation after lung transplantation. Ann Thorac Surg. 2012;93(2):366-71.
25. Hoetzenecker K, Klepetko W, Keshavjee S, Cypel M. Extracorporeal support in airway surgery. J Thorac Dis. 2017;9(7):2108-17.
26. D'Arrigo S, Cacciola M, Dennis M, Jung C, Kagawa E, Antonelli M, et al. Predictors of favourable outcome after in-hospital cardiac arrest treated with extracorporeal cardiopulmonary resuscitation: a systematic review and meta-analysis. Resuscitation. 2017;121:62-70.
27. Porhomayon J, El-Solh A, Papadakos P, Djalal ND. Cardiac output monitoring devices: an analytic review. Intern Emerg Med. 2012;7:163-71.
28. Schmidt M, Tachon G, Devilliers C, Muller G, Hekimian G, Bréchot N, et al. Blood oxygenation and decarboxylation determinants during venovenous ECMO for respiratory failure in adults. Intensive Care Med. 2013;39(5):838-46.
29. Tang J, Bergman J, Lam JM. Harlequin colour change: unilateral erythema in a newborn. CMAJ. 2010;182:E801.
30. Conrad SA, Broman LM, Taccone FS, Lorusso R, Malfertheiner MV, Pappalardo F, et al. The extracorporeal life support organization Maastricht treaty for nomenclature in extracorporeal life support. A position paper of the extracorporeal life support organization. Am J Respir Crit Care Med. 2018;198:447-51.
31. Choi JH, Kim SW, Kim YU, Kim SY, Kim KS, Joo SJ, et al. Application of veno-arterial-venous extracorporeal membrane oxygenation in differential hypoxia. Multidiscip Respir Med. 2014;9:55.
32. Slater JP, Guarino T, Stack J, Vinod K, Bustami RT, Brown JM 3rd, et al. Cerebral oxygen desaturation predicts cognitive decline and longer hospital stay after cardiac surgery. Ann Thorac Surg. 2009;87(1):36-44.
33. Kara A, Akin S, Dos Reis Miranda D, Struijs A, Caliskan K, van Thiel RJ, et al. Microcirculatory assessment of patients under VA-ECMO. Crit Care. 2016;20(1):344.
34. Dalton HJ, Garcia-Filion P, Holubkov R, Moler FW, Shanley T, Heidemann S, et al. Eunice Kennedy Shriver National Institute of Child Health and Human Development Collaborative Pediatric Critical Care Research Network. Association of bleeding and thrombosis with outcome in extracorporeal life support. Pediatr Crit Care Med. 2015;16(2):167-74.

35. Cho HJ, Kim DW, Kim GS, Jeong IS. Anticoagulation Therapy during Extracorporeal Membrane Oxygenator Support in Pediatric Patients. Chonnam Med J. 2017;53(2):110-7.
36. Esper SA, Welsby IJ, Subramaniam K, John Wallisch W, Levy JH, Waters JH, et al. Adult extracorporeal membrane oxygenation: an international survey of transfusion and anticoagulation techniques. Vox Sang. 2017;112:443-52.
37. Rychlíčková J, Šrámek V, Suk P. Use of fondaparinux in patients with heparin-induced thrombocytopenia on veno-venous extracorporeal membrane oxygenation: A three-patient case series report. Front Med (Lausanne). 2023;10:1112770.
38. Walker EA, Roberts AJ, Louie EL, Dager WE. Bivalirudin Dosing Requirements in Adult Patients on Extracorporeal Life Support With or Without Continuous Renal Replacement Therapy. ASAIO J. 2019;65:134-8.
39. Beiderlinden M, Treschan TA, Görlinger K, Peters J. Argatroban anticoagulation in critically ill patients. Ann Pharmacother. 2007;41:749-54.
40. Serpa Neto A, Schmidt M, Azevedo LC, Bein T, Brochard L, Beutel G, et al; ReVA Research Network and the PROVE Network Investigators. Associations between ventilator settings during extracorporeal membrane oxygenation for refractory hypoxemia and outcome in patients with acute respiratory distress syndrome: a pooled individual patient data analysis: Mechanical ventilation during ECMO. Intensive Care Med. 2016;42(11):1672-84.
41. Goncalves-Pereira J, Povoa P. Antibiotics in critically ill patients: a systematic review of the pharmacokinetics of beta-lactams. Crit Care. 2011;15:R206.
42. Shekar K, Roberts JA, McDonald CI, Fisquet S, Barnett AG, Mullany DV, et al. Sequestration of drugs in the circuit may lead to therapeutic failure during extracorporeal membrane oxygenation. Crit Care. 2012;16:R194.
43. Roberts JA, Ulldemolins M, Roberts MS, McWhinney B, Ungerer J, Paterson DL, et al. Therapeutic drug monitoring of beta-lactams in critically ill patients: proof of concept. Int J Antimicrob Agents. 2010;36:332-9.
44. DeGrado JR, Hohlfelder B, Ritchie BM, Anger KE, Reardon DP, Weinhouse GL. Evaluation of sedatives, analgesics, and neuromuscular blocking agents in adults receiving extracorporeal membrane oxygenation. J Crit Care. 2017; 37:1-6.
45. Aubron C, Cheng AC, Pilcher D, Leong T, Magrin G, Cooper DJ, et al. Factors associated with outcomes of patients on extracorporeal membrane oxygenation support: a 5-year cohort study. Crit Care. 2013;17:R73.
46. Aubron C, DePuydt J, Belon F, Bailey M, Schmidt M, Sheldrake J, et al. Predictive factors of bleeding events in adults undergoing extracorporeal membrane oxygenation. Ann Intensive Care. 2016;6(1):97.
47. Peek G, Wittenstein B, Harvey C, Machin D. Management of bleeding during ECLS. In: Van Meurs K, Lally KP, Peek, G, Zwischenberger JB (Eds). ECMO: Extracorporeal Cardiopulmonary Support in Critical Care, 3rd edition. Ann Arbor: Extracorporeal Life Support Organization; 2005.
48. Australia and New Zealand Extracorporeal Membrane Oxygenation (ANZ ECMO) Influenza Investigators; Davies A, Jones D, Bailey M, Beca J, Bellomo R, Blackwell N, et al. Extracorporeal Membrane Oxygenation for 2009 Influenza A(H1N1) Acute Respiratory Distress Syndrome. JAMA. 2009;302:1888-95.
49. Lamb KM, Cowan SW, Evans N, Pitcher H, Moritz T, Lazar M, et al. Successful management of bleeding complications in patients supported

with extracorporeal membrane oxygenation with primary respiratory failure. Perfusion. 2013;28(2):125-31.
50. Pavlushkov E, Berman M, Valchanov K. Cannulation techniques for extracorporeal life support. Ann Transl Med. 2017;5(4):70.
51. Tanaka D, Hirose H, Cavarocchi N, Entwistle JW. The Impact of Vascular Complications on Survival of Patients on Venoarterial Extracorporeal Membrane Oxygenation. Ann Thorac Surg. 2016;101:1729-34.
52. Hoeper MM, Tudorache I, Kühn C, Marsch G, Hartung D, Wiesner O, et al. Extracorporeal membrane oxygenation watershed. Circulation. 2014;130:864-5.
53. Aziz F, Brehm CE, El-Banyosy A, Han DC, Atnip RG, Reed AB. Arterial complications in patients undergoing extracorporeal membrane oxygenation via femoral cannulation. Ann Vasc Surg. 2014;28:178-83.
54. Roussel A, Al-Attar N, Alkhoder S, Radu C, Raffoul R, Alshammari M, et al. Outcomes of percutaneous femoral cannulation for venoarterial extracorporeal membrane oxygenation support. Eur Heart J Acute Cardiovasc Care. 2012;1:111-4.
55. Lin CY, Chen YC, Tsai FC, Tian YC, Jenq CC, Fang JT, et al. RIFLE classification is predictive of short-term prognosis in critically ill patients with acute renal failure supported by extracorporeal membrane oxygenation. Nephrol Dial Transplant 2006;21:2867-73.
56. Metra M, Nodari S, Parrinello G, Bordonali T, Bugatti S, Danesi R, et al. Worsening renal function in patients hospitalised for acute heart failure: clinical implications and prognostic significance. Eur J Heart Fail. 2008;10:188-95.
57. Fleming GM, Askenazi DJ, Bridges BC, Cooper DS, Paden ML, Selewski DT, et al. A multicenter international survey of renal supportive therapy during ECMO: the Kidney Intervention During Extracorporeal Membrane Oxygenation (KIDMO) group. ASAIO J. 2012;58(4):407-14.
58. Blijdorp K, Cransberg K, Wildschut ED, Gischler SJ, Jan Houmes R, Wolff ED, et al. Haemofiltration in newborns treated with extracorporeal membrane oxygenation: A case-comparison study. Crit Care. 13:R482009.
59. Bagshaw SM, Delaney A, Haase M, Ghali WA, Bellomo R. Loop diuretics in the management of acute renal failure: a systematic review and meta-analysis. Crit Care Resusc. 2007;9:60-8.
60. Lyu L, Long C, Hei F, Ji B, Liu J, Yu K, et al. Plasma free hemoglobin is a predictor of acute renal failure during adult venous-arterial extracorporeal membrane oxygenation support. J Cardiothorac Vasc Anesth. 2016;30:891-5.
61. Mateen FJ, Muralidharan R, Shinohara RT, Parisi JE, Schears GJ, Wijdicks EF. Neurological injury in adults treated with extracorporeal membrane oxygenation. Arch Neurol. 2011;68(12):1543-9.
62. Risnes I, Wagner K, Nome T, Sundet K, Jensen J, Hynås IA, et al. Cerebral outcome in adult patients treated with extracorporeal membrane oxygenation. Ann Thorac Surg. 2006;81(4):1401-6.
63. Xie A, Jayewardene ID, Dinale A, Macdonald PS, Pye R, Dhital K. Cerebral hypoxia during venoarterial extracorporeal membrane oxygenation: an in-vitro study. J Heart Lung Transplant. 2015;34(Suppl 4):S196-7.
64. Nasr DM, Rabinstein AA. Neurologic complications of extracorporeal membrane oxygenation. J Clin Neurol. 2015;11(4):383-9.
65. Schmidt M, Bréchot N, Hariri S, Guiguet M, Luyt CE, Makri R, et al. Nosocomial infections in adult cardiogenic shock patients supported by venoarterial extracorporeal membrane oxygenation. Clin Infect Dis. 2012;55:1633-41.

66. Kim GS, Lee KS, Park CK, Kang SK, Kim DW, Oh SG, et al. Nosocomial infection in adult patients undergoing veno-arterial extracorporeal membrane oxygenation. J Korean Med Sci. 2017;32:593-8.
67. O'Neill JM, Schutze GE, Heulitt MJ, Simpson PM, Taylor BJ. Nosocomial infections during extracorporeal membrane oxygenation. Intensive Care Med. 2001;27:1247-53.
68. Meyer DM, Jessen ME, Eberhart RC. Neonatal extracorporeal membrane oxygenation complicated by sepsis. Extracorporeal life support organization. Ann Thorac Surg. 1995;59:975-80.
69. Bizzarro MJ, Conrad SA, Kaufman DA, Rycus P; Extracorporeal Life Support Organization Task Force on Infections, Extracorporeal Membrane Oxygenation. Infections acquired during extracorporeal membrane oxygenation in neonates, children, and adults. Pediatr Crit Care Med. 2011;12:277-81.
70. Venkataraman R, Divatia JV, Ramakrishnan N, Chawla R, Amin P, Gopal P, et al. Multicenter observational study to evaluate epidemiology and resistance patterns of common intensive care unit-infections. Indian J Crit Care Med. 2018;22:20-6.
71. Rousse N, Robin E, Juthier F, Hysi I, Banfi C, Al Ibrahim M, et al. Extracorporeal life support in out-of-hospital refractory cardiac arrest. Artif Organs. 2016;40:904-9.
72. Shelton KT, Wiener-Kronish JP. Evolving Role of Anesthesiology Intensivists in Cardiothoracic Critical Care. Anesthesiology. 2020;133:1120-6.
73. Johnston L, Oldenburg G. Simulation for neonatal extracorporeal membrane oxygenation teams. Semin Perinatol. 2016;40:421-9.

CHAPTER 19

Delirium in Intensive Care

Prathamesh Milind Patwardhan, Sandeep Lakhani

ABSTRACT

Delirium is an acute confusional state diagnosed in critically ill patients, particularly the elderly. It is commonly encountered in the intensive care unit (ICU) in its hyperactive, hypoactive, or mixed form. It has a multifactorial etiology, and the diagnosis can often be challenging if not vigilant. The exact pathophysiology of delirium is incompletely understood and could involve neuroinflammation, altered neurotransmitter levels, abnormal stress response, or cortical/subcortical mechanisms. Various well-validated tools like Confusion Assessment Method for the ICU (CAM-ICU) and Intensive Care Delirium Screening Checklist (ICDSC) may aid in diagnosing delirium. A multicomponent approach with various nonpharmacological methods is recommended to prevent delirium. Treatment should focus on addressing the underlying causes and implementing reorientation methods, but pharmacological intervention may be necessary in severe cases of hyperactive delirium. Further research is needed to develop a robust diagnostic system, understand the pathophysiology, and explore new treatment modalities to significantly reduce delirium's associated morbidity, mortality, and healthcare costs.

Keywords: Delirium; Intensive care unit; CAM-ICU; ICDSC; Multicomponent interventions; Nonpharmacological prevention; Haloperidol

■ KEY POINTS

- It is crucial to always remain vigilant in the intensive care unit (ICU) as there is a high incidence of delirium in admitted patients.
- Regular screening with various available screening tools is indicated for early diagnosis.
- Nonpharmacological multicomponent prevention methods should be tried first for all at-risk patients, and pharmacological alternatives should be carefully chosen on a case-by-case basis to safeguard the well-being of patients and carers.

INTRODUCTION

Delirium is a preventable and treatable clinical syndrome characterized by a disturbance of consciousness and cognitive function (perception, judgment, reasoning, evaluation, and learning). It has an acute onset (usually over 1-2 days), a fluctuating course, and is associated with poor outcomes if not dealt with urgently.[1]

Many terms are used interchangeably to describe patients with delirium, such as encephalopathy, acute brain failure, acute confusional state, and postoperative or ICU psychosis.

It is a clinical diagnosis made only at the bedside and has a multifactorial association. Despite increased efforts targeting awareness of this condition, delirium often goes unrecognized in the face of evidence that it is usually the cognitive manifestation of serious underlying medical or neurologic illness.[2]

The anesthetist/intensivist needs to try and understand the various features, risk factors, presentation, diagnosis, and management of this condition to reduce associated morbidity, mortality, and healthcare costs significantly.

INCIDENCE AND PREVALENCE

Generally, delirium can be found wherever there are sick patients. Nearly 30% of elderly medical patients experience delirium at some time during hospitalization.[2,3]

It is often underreported either because of unawareness about the condition (hypoactive and mixed delirium are especially difficult to diagnose), unavailability of robust reporting procedures in place[1] and/or it usually presents as the cognitive manifestation of serious underlying medical or neurologic illness.[4]

It has an average incidence rate of 29% during an ICU stay.[5] Still, with the correct use of standardized screening and diagnostic tools in the areas of interest for an intensivist, the incidence of delirium can be as high as 70%.[6] The average incidence has been reported as 10% in emergency departments[7] and 16% in post-acute care settings.[8]

RISK FACTORS

Among the multiple causative factors, certain factors make a patient more vulnerable to the development of delirium and are known as predisposing risk factors, while those that bring about the onset of delirium are referred to as precipitating risk factors.[9]

Some common examples include polypharmacy (particularly psychoactive drugs), infection, dehydration, immobility (including restraint use), malnutrition, and the use of bladder catheters.

BOX 1: Modifiable and nonmodifiable risk factors.

Modifiable risk factors:
- Medication-related[10]
- Benzodiazepines (dose-dependent manner)
- Anticholinergic drugs*
- Opioids*
- Corticosteroids*
- Blood transfusions[11]
- Environmental factors [increased noise, lack of daylight, disturbed or lack of diurnal sleep/wake patterns, poor sleep hygiene and admission to a ward (compared with a personal room)] increase the risk of delirium
- History of alcohol excess/psychoactive medication/nicotine use

Non-modifiable risk factors:
- Elderly (age 65 or more),
- Preexisting sensory impairment
- Cognitive impairment (past or present) and/or dementia/prior coma/stroke or Parkinson's disease
- Pre-ICU emergency surgery or trauma (current hip fracture/postoperative patients)
- History of hypertension
- High severity of illness at admission (any clinical condition that is deteriorating or is at risk of deterioration) [graded using (APACHE) scores]
- Sepsis
- Systemic organ failure
- Long-term care patients
- Many triggering factors can be modified, whereas predisposing risk factors cannot be changed

* They are probably associated with the development of delirium, but some studies do not support this.
(APACHE: acute physiology and chronic health evaluation; ICU: intensive care unit)

Various risk factors can be divided into modifiable and nonmodifiable risk factors as shown in **Box 1**.

PATHOPHYSIOLOGY

The pathophysiology of delirium needs to be better understood, and existing hypotheses are based on a combination of observations, investigations, and animal study data (animal studies are still new and need validation). These suggest that even though there is no single common mechanism for the development of delirium, there could be a final common neural pathway.

Possible mechanisms for delirium could be due to the following:
- *Neuroinflammation:* Increased concentration of proinflammatory cytokines like interleukins and tumor necrosis factor-alpha (TNF-α) in the peripheral circulation and eventually in the central nervous system (CNS) can lead to prolonged neuroinflammation (even for months)

and has been linked with delirium (particularly hyperactive form) in many critical illnesses such as sepsis (where mental changes may precede fever), trauma, e.g., acute hip fracture[12] and cardiopulmonary bypass.[13]

It has been proposed from some preclinical studies that the high levels of these proinflammatory markers affect the structural and functional integrity of the blood-brain barrier facilitating their entry into CNS. This has been supported by a few studies in patients with preoperative peripheral injuries, such as fractures, which are associated with increased inflammatory mediators in the cerebrospinal fluid (CSF).[14,15]

These inflammatory mediators result in the loss of synaptic plasticity,[16] neuroapoptosis,[17] and impaired neurogenesis.[18]

There appears to be a correlation between postoperative delirium and elevated levels of peripheral C-reactive protein (CRP) and interleukin 6 concentrations as well.[19]

There appears to be varying findings in studies regarding the potential association between recurrent exposure to general anesthesia (GA) among older individuals and a heightened probability of experiencing delirium. Even though there is a high risk of abnormal cortical thickening[20] with repeated surgeries under GA, it has not shown increased deposition of β-amyloid due to neuroinflammation, which is suspected to be one of the causative factors for delirium.

- *Neurotransmitter-related:* Neurotransmitter abnormalities, e.g., acetylcholine and dopamine, are proposed in the pathogenesis of delirium. Acetylcholine is thought to be involved in neuroplasticity; plays a central role in attention, memory, and consciousness; and is considered one of the most critical factors in the pathogenesis of delirium.[21,22]

  Their abnormal levels put patients with Alzheimer's disease, dementia with Lewy bodies, and Parkinson's disease dementia at risk for developing delirium because of cholinergic deficiency resulting due to degeneration of acetylcholine-producing neurons in the basal forebrain.

  Also, increases in dopamine can lead to delirium, and patients with Parkinson's disease who are getting treated with dopaminergic medications can develop a delirium-like state that features visual hallucinations, fluctuations, and confusion.

  The elderly population with dementia can have delirium even with a smaller dose of anticholinergic medication (e.g., reversal of neuromuscular blockade) compared to young adults. Still, even healthy young individuals can develop delirium with very high doses of anticholinergic medications.

- *Aberrant stress response:* The aberrant stress response hypothesis suggests that on experiencing stress, the limbic-hypothalamic-pituitary-adrenal axis is activated, resulting in elevated cortisol levels. The response in

healthy individuals is adaptive and has effective feedback regulation. However, with impaired feedback regulation in the at-risk population, sustained high cortisol levels can contribute to the development of delirium.
- *Cortical versus subcortical mechanisms:* Attention has a diffuse localization within the brain stem, thalamus, prefrontal cortex, and parietal lobes. Electroencephalography (EEG) in acutely ill patients established that delirium was a disturbance of global cortical function, characterized by slowing of the dominant posterior alpha rhythm and the appearance of abnormal slow wave activity[23] except in delirium accompanying alcohol and sedative drug withdrawal, in which low-voltage, fast wave activity predominated.

    Sometimes focal lesions such as subcortical ischemic strokes have led to delirium in otherwise healthy persons. Based on the results of brainstem auditory evoked potential, somatosensory evoked potentials right parietal and medial dorsal thalamic lesions, the basal ganglia, and pontine reticular formation have been reported to get most commonly involved.[24]
- Neuroimaging studies have also shown cerebral atrophy, white matter hyperintensities, and cortical infarcts. These structural changes affect neural network function and may thus predispose to delirium.[25,26]
- Additionally, delirium may be associated with the production of a random and loose brain network and reduced concomitant activity of brain regions.[27]

CLINICAL PRESENTATION

Delirium can present with various features **(Box 2)** and can be classified as: (1) hypoactive, (2) hyperactive, and (3) mixed (most common).

It is common for this condition to develop rapidly and fluctuate throughout the day, leading to feelings of restlessness in the evening and nighttime (known as "sundowning") and drowsiness during the day.

The hypoactive subtype is particularly underdiagnosed and is characterized by reduced alertness, motor activity, and speech. Patients are often misdiagnosed as having depression, although a decreased level of consciousness does not characterize depression.

BOX 2: Common features of delirium.

- Disturbance of consciousness
- Altered cognition (worsened concentration, slow responses, confusion)
- Altered perception (visual or auditory hallucinations)
- Changes in physical function (reduced mobility, reduced movement, restlessness, agitation, changes in appetite, sleep disturbance)
- Changes in social behavior (difficulty engaging with or following requests, withdrawal or alterations in communication mood and/or attitude)

The hyperactive subtype is characterized by restlessness, increased and inappropriate motor activity, and sometimes agitation, and is usually seen in patients in withdrawal from alcohol or other drugs and is easier to diagnose but is rarely observed in severely ill patients as they may be sedated and ventilated.

Most patients would fluctuate between hypoactive and hyperactive delirium symptoms in the mixed subtype.

Further evidence is needed to establish a firm relationship between clinical symptoms and outcomes. Patients with more severe delirium, including psychomotor agitation, had higher mortality rates, and nursing home placement.[28] Delirium that does not resolve before discharge is also a risk factor for nursing home placement.[29]

■ DIAGNOSIS AND EVALUATION

The diagnosis of delirium is clinical and is made at the bedside and hence needs a thorough evaluation of patients with history, general examination, and systemic examination. The patient admitted to the ICU might already be experiencing delirium, and hence a high index of suspicion is needed **(Table 1)**.

Several screening tools like Confusion Assessment Method for the ICU (CAM-ICU), the Intensive Care Delirium Screening Checklist (ICDSC), the

TABLE 1: Approach to diagnosis of delirium.

Elements	Salient points
History	• Past medical history, drug history, addictions can help identify at-risk patients • Relatives'/carers' input can help to get to a diagnosis • Nearly impossible to obtain from a confused patient
General examination	• A focused assessment is needed as it may not be allowed by an uncooperative patient • Focus on vital signs, the state of hydration, skin condition, and potential infectious foci • Nonspecific findings like multifocal myoclonus and asterixis are usually seen in metabolic/toxic delirium and do not help establish any particular medical etiology within the metabolic/toxic category
Systemic examination	• Emphasis on systems suspected of involvement based on presentation • Neurological examination focusing on the level of consciousness, degree of attention or inattention, visual fields, and unambiguous cranial nerve and motor deficits → important to identify individuals with a higher likelihood of focal neurologic disease • In the absence of an obvious cause for delirium, further testing

A2F bundle, the 4AT tool, and Nursing Delirium Screening Scale (Nu-DESC) can aid physicians and nurses in identifying patients with delirium.

While the 4AT is the best-validated delirium tool in literature with >25 diagnostic test accuracy studies involving >5,000 patients and is highly sensitive and specific, CAM-ICU and ICDSC are the most used in the ICU and postsurgical scenarios.

Using the also well-validated CAM-ICU,[30-32] a diagnosis of delirium should be considered if there is:
- Acute onset and fluctuating course
- Inattention, accompanied by either
- Disorganized thinking
- An altered level of consciousness.

It also considers mechanically ventilated patients and has scored observed behaviors, nonverbal responses to simple questions, and visual and auditory recognition tasks. It is also valid for patients in neuro-ICU, patients with alcohol withdrawal, and dementia and is available in 20 languages.

The PADIS (Pain, Agitation/sedation, Delirium, Immobility, and Sleep Disruption in adult patients in the ICU) clinical practice guidelines recommend routine delirium monitoring in all adult ICU patients during every shift (every 8–12 hours) and as needed.[33]

Patients are considered delirium-free when they are CAM-ICU-negative for 24 hours.

There are prediction tools available as well. While E-PRE-DELIRIC (Early Prediction of Delirium in ICU patients) predicts delirium at the time of admission to the ICU with an accuracy of 68%, the PRE-DELIRIC tool predicts delirium 24 hours after admission to ICU.

In addition to the aforementioned risk factors, patients in neurocritical care units with focal neurological signs (e.g., stroke)/traumatic brain injury pose a unique diagnostic challenge considering their background pathology and its associated compilations [e.g., subarachnoid hemorrhage, seizures (convulsive as well as nonconvulsive), and the need for prolonged sedation to keep intracranial pressure (ICP) in check].

INVESTIGATIONS

The history and physical examination guide the investigations. A cost-effective workup for delirium focuses upon the most likely possibilities, which may include:
- Fluid and electrolyte disturbances (dehydration, hyponatremia, and hypernatremia)
- Infections (urinary tract, respiratory tract, skin, and soft tissue)
- Drug or alcohol toxicity
- Withdrawal from alcohol

- Withdrawal from barbiturates, benzodiazepines, and selective serotonin reuptake inhibitors
- Metabolic disorders (hypoglycemia, hypercalcemia, uremia, liver failure, thyrotoxicosis)
- Low perfusion states (shock, heart failure)
- Postoperative states, especially in older adults.

Less common causes that should be considered include hypoxemia, hypercarbia, Wernicke encephalopathy, adrenal failure, primary CNS infection, seizures, trauma, and paraneoplastic syndromes.

Imaging is not routinely required for diagnosing delirium and is usually considered when a structural cause is suspected. EEG is a very sensitive but nonspecific investigation;[34] however it can be used to resolve uncertainty in patients in whom the diagnosis of delirium is in doubt.

■ PREVENTION

Tailored, multicomponent interventions by a multidisciplinary team should be delivered to the at-risk population after assessment within 24 hours of admission to the ICU. Prevention can be pharmacological and nonpharmacological.

Nonpharmacological Prevention

This mainly involves modifying the risk factors.

All these interventions reduce delirium, even though well-powered and well-designed studies do not strongly support the evidence. PADIS guidelines have recommended their practice **(Table 2)**.

Pharmacological Prevention

Haloperidol does not have beneficial effects on either prevention or early treatment of delirium according to a large randomized controlled trial (RCT), and similar is the case with statins and cholinesterase inhibitors, but preventive dexmedetomidine has shown the reduction in the incidence of delirium.[33]

Ramelteon (melatonin receptor agonist) had an exceptionally strong effect on the prevention of delirium in a small RCT in nonintubated patients in the ICU or the acute ward.[35]

Minimizing exposure to drugs that cause delirium, like benzodiazepines, reduces delirium. Even though opioids can cause delirium, pain relief should be the priority if they are essential, and a multimodal analgesic technique will help to reduce their dose. The available evidence on the impact of drugs with anticholinergic effects and corticosteroids is limited and contradictory. Consequently, making definitive recommendations is not feasible.

TABLE 2: Nonpharmacological methods of delirium prevention.

Intervention	Examples
Orientation protocols	Appropriate lighting and clear signage, a clock and a calendar, windows with outside views, verbal reorientation
Cognitive stimulation	Regular visits from family and friends, avoiding sensory overstimulation
Address dehydration and/or constipation	Fluid resuscitation, bowel protocols
Prevent and treat hypoxia	Oxygen delivery systems, pulse oximeters
Address infection	Screen and treat with appropriate antimicrobials, avoid unnecessary catheterization, following infection control procedures
Immobility or limited mobility	Early mobilization postsurgery and minimized use of physical restraints for patients with limited mobility, carrying out active range-of-motion exercises
Address pain	Assess for pain, look for nonverbal signs of pain, and start and review pain relief daily
Medication review	Type and number of medications
Address poor nutrition	Dietician consultation, provide dentures
Address sensory impairment	Ensure hearing and visual aids are available and functioning, removing reversible causes (e.g., ear wax)
Promote good sleep patterns and sleep hygiene	Avoiding nursing or medical procedures/reduce noise to a minimum/avoid scheduling medication rounds during sleep time

▪ TREATMENT

Initial Management

- Identify and treat the underlying cause/causes.
- Ensure effective communication and reorientation and provide reassurance for people diagnosed with delirium.
- Consider involving family, friends, and carers to help with this; provide a suitable care environment.

Agitated Patient

If a person with delirium is distressed or considered a risk to themselves or others, verbal and nonverbal de-escalation techniques are ineffective or inappropriate; symptom control is occasionally necessary to prevent harm or to allow evaluation and treatment.

Consider giving short-term haloperidol (usually for 1 week or less), but it should be restricted to delirium with agitation and psychosis.[33]

Dexmedetomidine and clonidine are highly promising alternatives when exploring other options.

In Unresolving Delirium

- Re-evaluate for underlying causes.
- Follow up and assess for dementia.

Anxiety in these patients can be challenging to assess and could be due to hallucinations and delusions. Starting benzodiazepines can be tricky and may prolong delirium in such cases. Centrally acting alpha-2 agonists, dexmedetomidine/clonidine, also have anxiolytic properties.

Disturbances in sleep can be treated with benzodiazepines but with delirium risk, as mentioned above.

Patients receiving antipsychotic treatment may be switched to quetiapine (25–50 mg at night). It has sedative effects and does not induce natural sleep. The newer atypical antipsychotic agents, quetiapine, risperidone, ziprasidone, and olanzapine, have fewer side effects in other clinical settings, and in small studies, they appear to have similar efficacy to haloperidol.[36-38]

Theoretically, alpha-2 agonist drugs may promote sleep, but this has yet to be studied extensively.

Alcohol Withdrawal

Mechanically Ventilated Patients

- Prescribe chlordiazepoxide regime via nasogastric (NG) route as per local hospital policy.
- Avoid chlordiazepoxide if the patient is on midazolam infusion.
- Intravenous (IV) clonidine or dexmedetomidine may be considered if agitation prevents extubation.

Nonventilated Patients

- Prescribe chlordiazepoxide regime NG/PO.
- Lorazepam 0.5–1 mg IV/intramuscular (IM) QDS and 0.5–1 mg IV/IM PRN if no enteral route; max dose 4 mg in first 6 hours
- Clonidine 50–150 μg QDS NG/PO may be added if an additional sedative is indicated.

▰ WAY FORWARD

There are still various aspects of delirium that need to be explored. We need to focus on developing an easy-to-use, reliable, accurate assessment tool that applies to most care areas and not restricted by language.

Further research also needs to be done in the areas like multicomponent nonpharmacological intervention for prevention and treatment of delirium, the impact of education programs to train people for identifying delirium, and the role of atypical antipsychotics, typical antipsychotics, benzodiazepines, or acetylcholinesterase inhibitors for prevention and treatment of delirium in high-risk patients.

CONCLUSION

Delirium is a disturbance of consciousness and cognitive function. Although it can be seen very commonly in the ICU in its hyperactive, hypoactive, or mixed forms; it can often be missed; especially the hypoactive subtype. The etiology of delirium is multifactorial, with some modifiable and some nonmodifiable factors. These may either lead to delirium or increase a patient's susceptibility. The pathophysiology of delirium is still incompletely understood and could be due to a combination of neuroinflammation, altered neurotransmitter levels, abnormal stress response, or cortical/subcortical mechanisms. The diagnosis is made clinically at the bedside with the help of history, detailed examination, investigations, and various well-validated tools like CAM-ICU and ICDSC. It can be potentially prevented with the help of a multicomponent approach and a high index of suspicion in all patients admitted to the ICU. Implementation of nonpharmacological interventions could lead to delirium prevention. Pharmacological methods have not shown promising results yet. Delirium treatment centers around identifying and treating causes and reorientation methods first. Pharmacological intervention takes precedence depending upon the state of delirium, where patient and staff safety would be a priority. Various aspects of delirium need to be probed further to develop a robust diagnostic system, understanding the pathophysiology, and newer treatment modalities to significantly reduce its associated morbidity, mortality, and healthcare costs.

REFERENCES

1. National Institute for Health and Care Excellence. (2023). Delirium: prevention, diagnosis, and management in hospital and long-term care. Clinical guideline [CG103]. [online] Available from: https://www.nice.org.uk/guidance/cg103 [Last accessed September, 2023].
2. Francis J. Delirium in older patients. J Am Geriatr Soc. 1992;40:829.
3. Inouye SK, Rushing JT, Foreman MD, Palmer RM, Pompei P. Does delirium contribute to poor hospital outcomes? A three-site epidemiologic study. J Gen Intern Med. 1998;13:234.
4. Josephson SA, Miller BL. Confusion and delirium. In: Jameson JL, Fauci AS, Kasper DL, Hauser SL, Longo DL, Loscalzo J (Eds). Harrison's Principles of Internal Medicine, 20th edition. New York: McGraw Hill, Health Professions Division; 2018. pp. 147-51.
5. Rood P, Huisman-de Waal G, Vermeulen H, Schoonhoven L, Pickkers P, van den Boogaard M. Effect of organisational factors on the variation in incidence of delirium in intensive care unit patients: a systematic review and meta-regression analysis. Aust Crit Care. 2018;31:180-7.

6. McNicoll L, Pisani MA, Zhang Y, Ely EW, Siegel MD, Inouye SK. Delirium in the intensive care unit: occurrence and clinical course in older patients. J Am Geriatr Soc. 2003;51:591-8.
7. Elie M, Rousseau F, Cole M, Primeau F, McCusker J, Bellavance F. Prevalence and detection of delirium in elderly emergency department patients. CMAJ. 2000;163:977-81.
8. Lawlor PG, Gagnon B, Mancini IL, Pereira JL, Hanson J, Suarez-Almazor ME, et al. Occurrence, causes, and outcome of delirium in patients with advanced cancer: a prospective study. Arch Intern Med. 2000;160:786-94.
9. Elie M, Cole MG, Primeau FJ, Bellavance F. Delirium risk factors in elderly hospitalized patients. J Gen Intern Med. 1998;13:204-12.
10. Zaal IJ, Devlin JW, Peelen LM, Slooter AJ. A systematic review of risk factors for delirium in the ICU. Crit Care Med. 2015;43:40-7.
11. Rudiger A, Begdeda H, Babic D, Krüger B, Seifert B, Schubert M, et al. Intraoperative events during cardiac surgery are risk factors for the development of delirium in the ICU. Crit Care. 2016;20:264.
12. van Munster BC, Korevaar JC, Zwinderman AH, Levi M, Wiersinga WJ, De Rooij SE. Time-course of cytokines during delirium in elderly patients with hip fractures. J Am Geriatr Soc. 2008;56:1704-9.
13. Stefano GB, Bilfinger TV, Fricchione GL. The immune-neuro-link and the macrophage: postcardiotomy delirium, HIV-associated dementia and psychiatry. Prog Neurobiol. 1994;42:475-88.
14. Cape E, Hall RJ, van Munster BC, de Vries A, Howie SE, Pearson A, et al. Cerebrospinal fluid markers of neuroinflammation in delirium: a role for interleukin-1β in delirium after hip fracture. J Psychosom Res. 2014;77:219-25.
15. Neerland BE, Hall RJ, Seljeflot I, Frihagen F, MacLullich AM, Raeder J, et al. Associations between delirium and preoperative cerebrospinal fluid C-reactive protein, interleukin-6, and interleukin-6 receptor in individuals with acute hip fracture. J Am Geriatr Soc. 2016;64:1456-63.
16. Prieto GA, Tong L, Smith ED, Cotman CW. TNFα and IL-1β but not IL-18 suppresses hippocampal long-term potentiation directly at the synapse. Neurochem Res. 2019;44:49-60.
17. Tian Y, Chen KY, Liu LD, Dong YX, Zhao P, Guo SB. Sevoflurane exacerbates cognitive impairment induced by A $β_{1-40}$ in rats through initiating neurotoxicity, neuroinflammation, and neuronal apoptosis in rat hippocampus. Mediators Inflamm. 2018;2018:3802324.
18. Ekdahl CT, Claasen JH, Bonde S, Kokaia Z, Lindvall O. Inflammation is detrimental for neurogenesis in adult brain. Proc Natl Acad Sci U S A. 2003;100:13632-7.
19. Liu X, Yu Y, Zhu S. Inflammatory markers in postoperative delirium (POD) and cognitive dysfunction (POCD): a meta-analysis of observational studies. PLoS One. 2018;13:e0195659.
20. Sprung J, Warner DO, Knopman DS, Petersen RC, Mielke MM, Jack CR Jr, et al. Exposure to surgery with general anaesthesia during adult life is not associated with increased brain amyloid deposition in older adults. Br J Anaesth. 2020;124:594-602.
21. Mach JR Jr, Dysken MW, Kuskowski M, Richelson E, Holden L, Jilk KM. Serum anticholinergic activity in hospitalized older persons with delirium: a preliminary study. J Am Geriatr Soc. 1995;43:491-5.
22. Campbell N, Boustani M, Limbil T, Ott C, Fox C, Maidment I, et al. The cognitive impact of anticholinergics: a clinical review. Clin Interv Aging. 2009;4:225-33.

23. Romano J, Engel GL. Delirium: I. Electroencephalographic data. Arch Neurol Psychiatr. 1944;51:356-77.
24. Trzepacz PT. The neuropathogenesis of delirium. A need to focus our research. Psychosomatics. 1994;35:374-91.
25. Shioiri A, Kurumaji A, Takeuchi T, Matsuda H, Arai H, Nishikawa T. White matter abnormalities as a risk factor for postoperative delirium revealed by diffusion tensor imaging. Am J Geriatr Psychiatry. 2010;18:743-53.
26. Omiya H, Yoshitani K, Yamada N, Kubota Y, Takahashi K, Kobayashi J, et al. Preoperative brain magnetic resonance imaging and postoperative delirium after off-pump coronary artery bypass grafting: a prospective cohort study. Can J Anaesth. 2015;62:595-602.
27. van Dellen E, van der Kooi AW, Numan T, Koek HL, Klijn FA, Buijsrogge MP, et al. Decreased functional connectivity and disturbed directionality of information flow in the electroencephalography of intensive care unit patients with delirium after cardiac surgery. Anesthesiology. 2014;121:328-35.
28. Marcantonio E, Ta T, Duthie E, Resnick NM. Delirium severity and psychomotor types: their relationship with outcomes after hip fracture repair. J Am Geriatr Soc. 2002;50:850-7.
29. McAvay GJ, Van Ness PH, Bogardus ST Jr, Zhang Y, Leslie DL, Leo-Summers LS, et al. Older adults discharged from the hospital with delirium: 1-year outcomes. J Am Geriatr Soc. 2006;54:1245.
30. Ely EW, Inouye SK, Bernard GR, Gordon S, Francis J, May L, et al. Delirium in mechanically ventilated patients: validity and reliability of the confusion assessment method for the intensive care unit (CAM-ICU). JAMA. 2001;286:2703-10.
31. Luetz A, Heymann A, Radtke FM, Chenitir C, Neuhaus U, Nachtigall I, et al. Different assessment tools for intensive care unit delirium: which score to use? Crit Care Med. 2010;38:409.
32. Mitasova A, Kostalova M, Bednarik J, Michalcakova R, Kasparek T, Balabanova P, et al. Poststroke delirium incidence and outcomes: validation of the Confusion Assessment Method for the Intensive Care Unit (CAM-ICU). Crit Care Med. 2012;40:484-90.
33. Devlin JW, Skrobik Y, Gélinas C, Needham DM, Slooter AJC, Pandharipande PP, et al. Clinical practice guidelines for the prevention and management of pain, agitation/sedation, delirium, immobility, and sleep disruption in adult patients in the ICU. Crit Care Med. 2018;46:e825-e73.
34. van der Kooi AW, Leijten FS, van der Wekken RJ, Slooter AJ. What are the opportunities for EEG-based monitoring of delirium in the ICU? J Neuropsychiatry Clin Neurosci. 2012;24:472-7.
35. Hatta K, Kishi Y, Wada K, Takeuchi T, Odawara T, Usui C, et al. Preventive effects of ramelteon on delirium: a randomized placebo-controlled trial. JAMA Psychiatry. 2014;71:397-403.
36. Parellada E, Baeza I, de Pablo J, Martínez G. Risperidone in the treatment of patients with delirium. J Clin Psychiatry. 2004;65:348-53.
37. Skrobik YK, Bergeron N, Dumont M, Gottfried SB. Olanzapine vs haloperidol: treating delirium in a critical care setting. Intensive Care Med. 2004;30:444-9.
38. Hawkins SB, Bucklin M, Muzyk AJ. Quetiapine for the treatment of delirium. J Hosp Med. 2013;8:215-20.

CHAPTER 20

Objective Pain Monitoring: A Gift from Artificial Intelligence

Rajesh Bhavsar, Laima M, Thomas Stroem

ABSTRACT

Nociception management is a fundamental part of general anesthesia (GA). Despite noteworthy technological advancements, intraoperative analgesic delivery is still at the discretion of treating anesthesiologists. The dose of the analgesics is built on the judgment of the severity of nociception by the anesthesiologist, typically based on basic vital parameters. Here, the clinician must correlate the values of vital parameters to different physiological situations before making their logical connection to nociception which may result in apparent subjective variation with consequent over- or under-antinociceptive treatment.

Over the last decades, various objective nociception monitors have yet to be developed without appreciable global acceptance. Artificial intelligence (AI), i.e., machine learning, has been increasingly integrated into medical equipment. These machine learning algorithms learn patients' behavior and responses to the treatments and make suitable adjustments in the subsequent delivery of the therapy. The latest objective pain monitor incorporates supervised machine learning and deep learning (through the neural network) software, which identifies the severity of nociception based on presaved data and derives an index. It further learns patients' behavior in different situations, outlines a response profile specific to the patient, and then adjusts the index. With this monitor, intraoperative analgesic management has been optimized and offered to encourage intraoperative and postoperative conditions.

Keywords: Nociception; Machine learning; Artificial intelligence

▌ KEY POINTS

- Intraoperative pain management is based on assessing vital parameters about various physiological situations and their logical connection to pain.
- Analgesic drug delivery shows considerable variation with the risk of under- or overtreatment, which may have short-term or long-term consequences.

- There is a need for a universally acceptable objective pain assessment and monitoring strategy.
- The assessment of vital parameters and their logical connection to pain can be outsourced to artificial intelligence (AI) and software algorithms.
- Advancement software algorithms can further learn the patients' responses and prompt therapy adjustment.

■ INTRODUCTION

The role of anesthesiologists, apart from performing procedures, is to make several intraoperative vital decisions urgently to avoid life-threatening situations and unwanted complications. This warrants continuous close vigilance, instant and constant analysis of data derived from monitors and clinical observations, logical thinking, and arriving at appropriate conclusions based on previous experience, memory, and knowledge. This intelligent decision-making drill is subjective and carries the potential for variation. Furthermore, even though humans possess remarkable cerebral talents, it has a tiny short-term working rapid access memory (RAM) which carries the risk of fatigability, leading to cognitive laziness that reflects as a tendency to shortcut mental work and slow and error-prone performance in even straightforward arithmetic or logical reasoning.[1] Although, through technological inventions, administration of anesthesia has become less stressful [automatic noninvasive blood pressure (NIBP), infusion pumps, patient-controlled analgesia (PCA) pumps], accurate [vaporizers, train of four (TOF), bispectral index (BIS), target-controlled infusion (TCI) pumps], easy (ventilator-integrated anesthesia machines), and safe (various alarm systems), due to complexity of assessment of pain especially in anesthetized patients, the mystery of objective pain monitoring is yet to be solved. Various efforts toward the development of reliable and accurate pain monitors were conducted. The recently introduced pain monitors showed promising results. It is interesting to be familiar with the latest objective nociception monitoring device based on advanced software technology.

■ PAIN: REVISITED

Pain is traditionally described as "an unpleasant sensory and emotional experience associated with actual or potential tissue damage," which motivates one to withdraw from damaging situations and protects a damaged body part. At the same time, it heals and avoids similar experiences in the future.[2] Pain and its treatment are highly subjective, and in awake, responsive patients, it entirely depends on its reporting. Analgesia therapy, in most situations, is a difficult task due to delays in optimal effect secondary to pharmacological properties and significant variations in reporting due to emotional components.

BOX 1: Objective pain monitoring.

- *CNS-based monitoring:*
  - Conox monitoring: qNOX
  - Entropy monitoring: Response entropy
- *ANS-based monitoring:*
  - Pupillometry
  - SPI
  - Nociception level index
  - Skin conductance
- *Spinal reflex-based monitoring:*
  - NFR

(ANS: autonomic nervous system; CNS: central nervous system; NFR: nociceptive flexor reflex; SPI: surgical pleth index)

Pain management is even more challenging without reporting in sedated or anesthetized patients. The treatment is traditionally based on the physiological manifestations (PM) of pain, like changes in heart rate, blood pressure, sweating, pupillary size, etc. As these surrogate parameters lack sensitivity and specificity, pain assessment during anesthesia needs logical reasoning, which is subjective and may result in the delivery of inappropriate doses of analgesics.

Opioids are the backbone of intraoperative analgesic therapy. Their inappropriate doses may lead to multiple adverse consequences such as intraoperative hemodynamic disturbances, acute or chronic postoperative pain,[3,4] postoperative respiratory depression,[5] cognitive disturbances, opioid-induced hyperalgesia (OIH),[6] postoperative urinary retention, postoperative ileus, nausea and vomiting, and shivering.[7] The opioid side effects lead to discomfort, morbidity, and prolonged hospital stay.[8]

Intraoperative pain, traditionally described as nociception, is the travel of noxious stimulus from its origin to cerebral centers leading to its PM. To increase the accuracy of intraoperative analgesic therapy, various objective pain monitors were introduced in the clinical practice in the last two decades, primarily based on single or multiple components of this nociception pathway **(Box 1)**.

OBJECTIVE PAIN MONITORING: OVERVIEW (TABLE 1)
Central Nervous System-based Monitoring
Entropy Monitoring: Response Entropy Index

Entropy monitor (GE Healthcare, USA) is based on the frequency of electroencephalographic (EEG) and electromyographic (EMG) waves. The software algorithm in the machine converts the frequencies into unitless indices (0–100). The state entropy (SE) index describes the depth of hypnosis. Response entropy (RE) index predicts the risk of motor response to a noxious

TABLE 1: Objective pain monitoring: Overview.

	Device	Score/unit	Measurement principle	Monitoring nociception	Comments
Central nervous system (CNS)-based monitoring	Entropy monitoring: Response entropy index	0–100 dimensionless	Electromyographic/ electroencephalographic patterns associated with nociception	May help to predict probability of sudden movement in response to stimulation[8]	To date, insufficient evidence to allow firm conclusions about perioperative use and its benefits
	qNOX	0–99 dimensionless	Electromyographic/ electroencephalographic patterns associated with nociception	May help to predict probability of sudden movement in response to stimulation[8]	"No published data to evaluate the score in this setting"
Autonomic nervous system (ANS)-based monitoring	Pupillometry	Absolute width or changes in pupillar width; pupillary pain index (PPI)	Sympathetic tone (pupillar innervation)	PPI correlate with remifentanil effect-site concentrations,[6] intraoperative nociception response predictions,[7-10] and postoperative pain assessments,[9,11,12] and demonstrate a faster response to stimuli than hemodynamic parameters for the prediction of the analgesic state before stimulation[6,13]	PPI influenced by the hypnotic level,[14] neostigmine, pupillary diseases (Horner and Holmes–Adie syndromes), blindness and ambient light conditions; discontinuous monitoring and need for careful corneal care, somewhat awkward method (requiring repeated access to open eye)

Contd...

Device	Score/unit	Measurement principle	Monitoring nociception	Comments
Analgesia nociception index (ANI)	0–100 dimensionless	Influence of ANS on heart rate variability observed on electrocardiography (ECG)	Superior at detecting painful stimulation compared with traditional hemodynamic parameters[16,17]	Well published; may be best for exclusion of significant nociception/pain; however, performance was attenuated by increasing remifentanil dosages,[16,17] limited interpretability;[19] ANI might be affected during apnea and after ephedrine and atropine[18]
Surgical pleth index (SPI)	0–100 dimensionless	Peripheral vascular and cardiac sympathetic tone	SPI-guided analgesia resulted in lower opioid[21] and propofol[22] consumption and shorter times to tracheal extubation[23]	Well researched, but guidelines for ideal range of SPI overall not well validated; only monitor which does not require consumables (but GE monitor); not reliable during inotropes, chronotropes, and vasoconstrictors use;[24] not recommended in pediatric population due to blood vessel distensibility and the higher heart rates at baseline[25]
Skin conductance	Number of peaks in skin conductance per second (PPS); can be interpreted after translating to visual analog scale (VAS) (n)	Peripheral (skin) sympathetic tone	PPS >0.2 may correlate with severe nociception and at the end of surgery, significant postoperative pain.[26,27] Unaffected by temperature, general hypoxia, low or high blood volume, beta blockers, or epinephrine, among other factors[22,25]	Easy to use, but PPS tends to react predominantly with higher levels of stress/nociception ("smoke detector")

Contd...

	Device	Score/unit	Measurement principle	Monitoring nociception	Comments
Spinal reflex-based monitoring	Nociceptive flexor reflex threshold monitor (NFRT)	mA	NFRT modification by level of analgesia	Higher predictive power of movement response to noxious stimulus than other indices; may aid the prediction of a response to a noxious stimulus;[33] depends on sex, age, weight (obesity), and distinct physiologic factors[29]	NFRT is a reasonably well-known instrument in pain research, but its perioperative use in clinical routine is not yet well-researched; limited predictive value for postoperative pain when measured at the end of surgery[34]
Multi-parameter scores	Nociception level (NOL) index	0–100 dimensionless	*Four parameters:* Skin galvanic response (sympathetic tone), plethysmographic pulse wave (sympathetic vascular tone), temperature, and accelerometry (association with nociception unclear)	May discriminate noxious stimuli slightly better than standard hemodynamics;[63,65] "ideal" intraoperative NOL may be 10–25[10]	Multiple parameters may increase accuracy, but to date, little evidence for clinical relevance

stimulus.[9] A high RE index before noxious stimulation predicted a higher risk of a motor response. However, lower values did not prevent a response when the opioid concentration is insufficient, despite adequate hypnosis, i.e., SE index.[10] Entropy-guided anesthesia during propofol–remifentanil general anesthesia (GA) has resulted in fewer unwanted patient responses compared to standard practice along with a reduction in opioid consumption.[11] However, no differences have been seen regarding recovery, hemodynamic parameters, or postoperative outcomes.

Conox Monitoring: qNOX Index

Similar to the entropy monitor, the Conox monitor (Fresenius Kabi AG, Germany) integrates two EEG-based unitless indices (0–100). Here, the level of consciousness is described by the qCON Index, which is better for predicting loss of consciousness, such as loss of verbal command and eyelash reflex.[12] The qNOX Index presents the probability for response to noxious stimuli and correlates with the intensity of noxious stimuli but not with the effect-site concentration of propofol and remifentanil.[9]

Autonomic Nervous System-based Monitoring

Pupillometry

Pupillometry is based on the absolute diameter or change in diameter of pupilar width. The pupillary pain index (PPI), derived from different infrared pupillometers, showed promising objective nociception monitoring properties. Pupil diameter reactivity has been shown to correlate with remifentanil effect-site concentrations,[13] intraoperative nociception response predictions,[14-16] and postoperative pain assessments.[17-19] Pupillometry has demonstrated a faster response to stimuli than heart rate and arterial pressure and allows for predicting the analgesic state before stimulation.[13,20] However, it was found that PPI values were influenced by the hypnotic level.[21] Further, the main drawbacks are the discontinuous monitoring and the need for careful corneal care, opening the eyelid in each of the multiple perioperative measurements required to follow patient changes. Measurements might also be affected by neostigmine, pupillary diseases (Horner and Holmes-Adie syndromes), and blindness. Additionally, care must be taken regarding ambient light conditions.

Analgesia Nociception Index Monitoring

The analgesia nociception index (ANI) is a dimensionless index that measures the influence of the parasympathetic system on heart rate variability observed on electrocardiography (ECG). ANI ranges from 0 (maximal nociception) to 100 (maximal analgesia).[22,23] Even though the ANI, pupillometry, and surgical pleth index (SPI) were found to be superior at detecting painful stimulation compared with traditional hemodynamic parameters, the performance was attenuated by increasing remifentanil dosages and baseline values showed significantly lower prediction probabilities for nociceptive responses.[23,24] Further, agents acting on the autonomic nervous system (ANS), such as ephedrine and atropine, may affect the index score.[25] The ANI is thus unreliable for approximately 10 minutes after ephedrine administration and 20 minutes after atropine administration. This raises concerns about other agents and drug combinations that affect the ANS, such as beta blockers.

While the ANI indicates noxious stimulations during GA anesthesia, its interpretability might be limited given the large associated interindividual variability and low reproducibility.[26] Finally, the ANI may also not be helpful during intubation when the patient is apneic.

Plethysmography-based Monitoring, i.e., Surgical Pleth Index

Plethysmography dynamics of peripheral vascular system secondary to noxious stimuli are analyzed and translated into a unitless index (SPI).[27] Which ranges from 0 to 100, where lower values indicate deeper analgesia and SPI >50 is considered inadequate analgesia. The SPI responds to remifentanil concentration changes and is higher at lower remifentanil concentrations. Additionally, the SPI reacts to surgical nociceptive stimuli and analgesic drug concentration changes during propofol-remifentanil anesthesia, where the SPI increases at skin incision and remains high during surgery than before surgery.[27] SPI-guided anesthesia has been reported to result in lower opioid[28] and propofol[29] consumption and shorter tracheal extubation[30] with more stable hemodynamics, a lower incidence of unwanted events, and shorter arousal times. SPI cannot be reliably used where inotropes, chronotropes, and vasoconstrictors are used.[31] Similarly, it cannot be used in the pediatric population due to blood vessel distensibility and the higher heart rates at baseline.[32]

Skin Conductance

Increments in sympathetic activity secondary to noxious stimuli result in the filling of the palmar and plantar sweat glands. The skin conductance increases transiently before the sweat evaporates, decreases again with sweat, and the consequent fluctuation is observed. The skin conductance algesimeter measures micro-fluctuations in skin conductance in peaks per second (PPS) from a delivered microcurrent in the palmar and plantar areas. The PPS can be interpreted by translating into the visual analog scale (VAS). PPS >0.2 may correlate with severe nociception and, at the end of the surgery, significant postoperative pain.[31,33-35] While PPS has shown moderate sensitivity and specificity at identified time points, with moderate-to-severe pain defined based on hormone plasma levels,[33] it does not reliably predict changes in stress hormone plasma levels during the intraoperative period.[33] Although clinically relevant benefits of using skin conductance are unclear, the advantages of skin conductance monitoring are as follows: it is unaffected by temperature (22–42°C), general hypoxia, low or high blood volume, beta blockers, or epinephrine, among other factors.[22,25] However, further research is needed to confirm these claims.

Spinal Reflex-based Monitoring

Nociceptive Flexor Reflex Threshold Monitoring

The analgesia level is quantified through the electrical intensity required to elicit a spinal polysynaptic withdrawal reflex.[36] The electrical stimulus is applied to the sural nerve, and its effect is measured using biceps femoris muscle EMG. The amount of current required increases with analgesia.[37-39] Under propofol/remifentanil GA, the nociceptive flexor reflex threshold (NFRT) increases with remifentanil,[29] with a higher predictive power of movement response to noxious stimulus (such as laryngeal mask airway insertion and skin incision) than other indices, such as the BIS, Noxious Stimulation Response Index, or Composite Variability Index.[30]

The nociceptive flexor reflex (NFR) may aid the prediction of a response to a noxious stimulus[40] and depends on sex, age, weight (obesity), and distinct physiologic factors.[27] Its limitations include the degree of neuromuscular blockade, skin impedance, peripheral nerve alterations, muscular diseases, and limited predictive value for postoperative pain when measured at the end of surgery.[4]

ARTIFICIAL INTELLIGENCE

All the monitoring systems derive conclusions after matching the information acquired through the different sensors with the prerecorded data in the device's memory. The prerecorded data is collected from the references in the literature or from the experimental subjects during the development of the device. Thus, the conclusions are ultimately based on reference values and need more specificity. All these systems are governed through the instructions delivered by the attending professional and have minimal data analysis, logical correlation, and decision-making abilities and may still carry the risk of variation and error.

In non-health-related industries, to increase accuracy and avoid errors, many components of similar decision-making drills have been outsourced to computer systems with special skills.[41,42] These skills are typically called artificial intelligence, defined as the study of algorithms that give machines the ability to reason and perform functions such as problem-solving, object, and word recognition, inference of world states, and decision-making.[43] It is nothing but the programming of computers to simulate cognitive functions of the human mind, such as pattern recognition and problem-solving. One important feature of AI is the ability to learn, that is, modification of actions based on previous experience.

The subsets of AI most relevant for healthcare include machine learning, neural network, deep learning, robotics, and computer vision.[44,45]

Machine Learning

Machine learning is one of the major subsets of AI relevant to healthcare. Traditional computers are incorporated with special programs/software or algorithms that elicit specific responses after receiving explicit instructions (e.g., the primary function of a word processing program is to display the text input by the user). Machine learning, on the other hand, allows the software to learn from and react to available or collected data without explicit instructions. Through machine learning, broad data can be analyzed, which include, but are not limited to, numerical data, images, text, and speech or sound.

Machine learning algorithms are used when it requires classification (i.e., dividing massive data into discrete groups) and regression (assessing data to understand better the relationship between two or more continuous or independent variables with the dependent variable).

Three standard machine learning algorithms are used to solve problems: supervised, unsupervised, and reinforcement learning.[46]

Supervised Learning

In supervised learning, a pretrained algorithm(s) is incorporated into the machine to perform a specific task, such as to predict a prespecified output. The machine requires both training and test datasets. The machine learns the learning and analysis of associations between input and prespecified output through the training dataset. In contrast, the test dataset allows for the assessment of the performance of the algorithm on new data.[47] The supervised learning study on electronic health record data to identify patients who experienced postinduction hypotension presents an excellent example of supervised learning.[48] Some studies used external validation (i.e., a separate dataset) to assess the generalizability of the algorithm to other data sources.[49] Decision tree learning is a type of supervised learning algorithm that can be used to perform either classification (classification trees) or regression tasks (regression trees). Hu et al. used decision trees to predict total PCA consumption from features such as patient demographics, vital signs and aspects of their medical history, surgery type, and PCA doses delivered with the promise of using such approaches to optimize PCA dosing regimens.[50]

Unsupervised Learning

Unsupervised learning refers to algorithms identifying patterns or structures within a dataset and helps find novel ways of classifying patients, drugs, or other groups. It is effectively implemented to locate patients who could benefit most from certain drugs, such as asthmatics, and patients who would benefit most from glucocorticoid therapy, based on genomic analysis.[51]

Reinforced Learning

In reinforced learning, the software algorithm learns from its mistakes and successes while performing one task.[52] This technique has been used by Padmanabhan et al. to develop an anesthesia controller that used feedback from a patient's BIS and mean arterial pressure (MAP) to control the infusion rates of propofol (in a simulated patient model).[53]

Machine learning uses features within the data to perform its tasks. In classical machine learning, experts select the features (often referred to as handcrafted) to help guide the algorithms in analyzing complex data. This restricts these machines' usability to situations that do not adjust to the changes.

Neural Network and Deep Learning

To overcome the shortcomings of classical machine learning, several advanced automatic algorithm selection and processing systems are developed. The most popular system is the neural network, inspired by biological nervous systems. It has multiple layers of computational units (neurons) with multiple connections between neurons.[54] While a neural network with a single layer can still make approximate predictions, additional hidden layers can help to optimize and refine for accuracy. Thus, neural networks are a framework within which different machine learning algorithms work freely between layers duplicating the behavior of the human brain—albeit far from matching its ability—allowing it to "learn" from large amounts of data (e.g., image recognition, data classification).

The collection, reorganization, and logical analysis process through various algorithms of a large data pool using a neural network with three or more layers essentially is described as a "deep learning".[55] It is the most advanced subset of machine learning and drives many AI applications and services that improve automation, complex analysis, and physical tasks without human intervention.[44] Unlike in classical machine learning, where features are handcrafted, deep learning self-learns and analyzes all available features within the training set to determine which features allow for the optimal achievement of the deep neural network's given task (e.g., object recognition from an image). Deep learning technology lies behind everyday products and services (such as digital assistants, voice-enabled TV remotes, and credit card fraud detection) as well as emerging technologies (such as self-driving cars).[56] Given their flexibility in analyzing various types of data, deep learning through neural networks is a technique that has now been applied to other subfields of AI, including natural language processing, robotics, and computer vision.[57] Within the field of anesthesia, multiple examples of the applications of neural networks exist, including depth of anesthesia monitoring and control of anesthesia delivery.[58] The latest addition to the list is the nociception level monitor.

■ NOCICEPTION LEVEL INDEX MONITOR

Nociception level (NOL) index monitor is the latest multiparameter objective pain monitor, which displays the severity of pain through a unitless index called NOL which ranges from 0 to 100, where lower values indicate lower nociception and more profound analgesia. The machine derives the index through different parameters from multiple biosignals, reported as a function of heart rate variability (at 0.15–0.4 Hz band power), plethysmograph wave amplitude, and skin conductance.[59,60] All biosignals are collected with a finger probe containing photoplethysmographic and galvanic skin sensors, a skin temperature sensor, and a three-axis accelerometer (ACC). The NOL is updated every 5 seconds, and recommended values are between 10 and 25 for maintenance.

NOL Software

The NOL monitor uses both supervised machine learning and deep learning (through neural network) software. A random forest algorithm (RFA) generates the NOL index in the initial monitoring phase. The RFA, introduced by Breiman in 2001,[61] is a powerful method that predicts by aggregating results from an ensemble of randomized regression trees **(Fig. 1)**.

During the development of the monitor, controlled surgical scenarios were simulated on study subjects under GA, where increasing intensities of noxious stimuli were delivered to trigger sympathetic responses seen through PM. The PM were captured through the four sensors (described further) and indexed (NOL index) by clinicians into 0–100 depending on the severity of

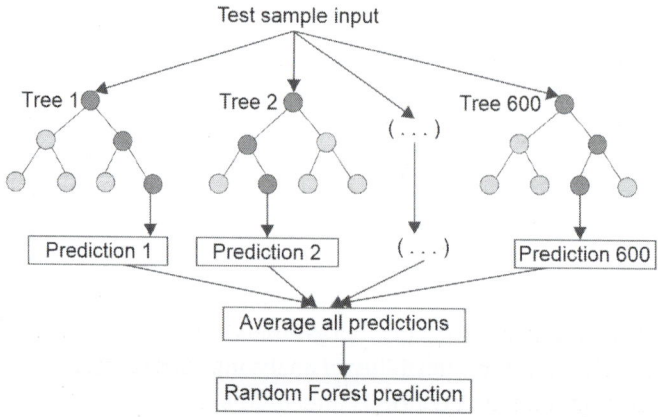

Fig. 1: Random rorest algorithm.

the delivered noxious stimulus, where 0 is a non-nociceptive state while 100 is severe nociception. A collection of thousands of data points of nociception patterns regarding physiological response, interactions, and correlations between different variables, including multiple mathematical derivatives, consists of several pairs of input, i.e., PM and NOL index. This collected data is used as a training dataset for the RFA for supervised machine learning.

During the initial phases of intraoperative monitoring, the captured PM of the patient is matched with the preloaded database to locate the corresponding predefined NOL index.

Further, the algorithm personalizes the NOL index to the individual patient by implementing an adaptive weighting mechanism between the static model and the patient's unique physiologic responses during the surgical procedure. As more data is gathered for the currently monitored patient, the influence of the preloaded population data decreases, and the weighting of the patient's unique physiological response increases, and thus the NOL output is personalized to the patient.

This personalization confers benefits in clinical practice as patients vary widely in their response to nociceptive stimuli and analgesia. NOL does not only treat the "average" patient since wide interpatient variability is associated with the response to the nociceptive stimulus and the analgesia, but using a personalized measure, NOL can also objectively assess patients with extreme responses (outliers) who do not match the typical population models on which drug dose–response curves are based, and therefore treat outlier cases requiring less or more analgesia than predicted.

Hardware: Probe, Sensor, and Display (Fig. 2)

The monitor comprises a display and processing unit, a reusable finger probe, and a single-use sensor **(Fig. 3)**. The finger probe and the single-use sensor acquire physiological signals and carry them to the processing unit to derive the corresponding NOL index and various derivatives, which are then displayed on the screen. The finger probe and single-use sensor continuously acquire four physiological signals through the following four sensors **(Fig. 4)**:

1. *Photoplethysmography (PPG):* Photoplethysmography, known most commonly as PPG, utilizes the same principles as SPI where infrared light is used to measure the volumetric variations of blood circulation. This measurement provides valuable information about the cardiovascular system.
2. *Galvanic skin response (GSR):* Based on the principles similar to skin conductance monitor, GSR, or sometimes referred to as electrodermal activity (EDA) or skin conductance, is a method to measure the electrical conductivity of the skin in response to sympathetic stimuli.
3. Peripheral temperature (Temp)
4. ACC

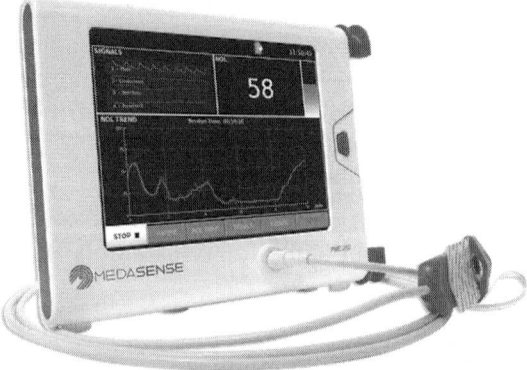

Fig. 2: Nociception level (NOL) index monitor and probe.
Courtesy: Reproduced with permission of Medtronic Danmark AS.

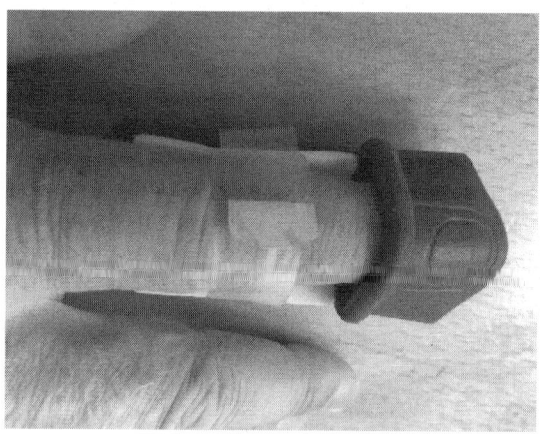

Fig. 3: Finger with single-use sensor.
Courtesy: Reproduced with permission of Medtronic Danmark AS.

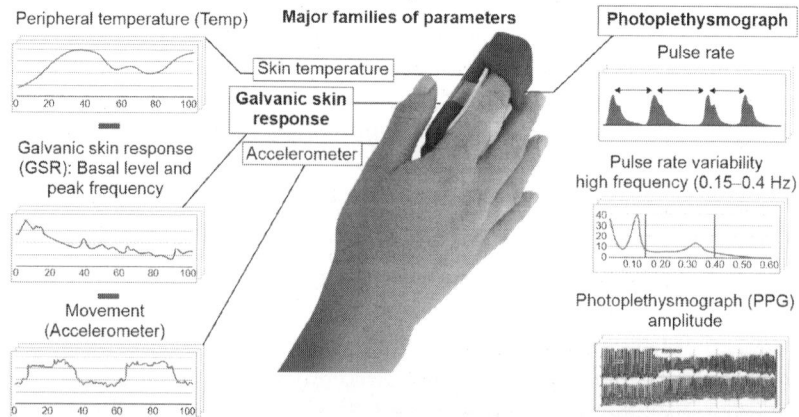

Fig. 4: Physiological signals through the following four sensors.
Courtesy: Reproduced with permission of Medtronic Danmark AS.

From these four signals, the NOL algorithm extracts and analyses nociception-related physiological parameters and derivatives: pulse rate, pulse rate variability, pulse wave amplitude, skin conductance level, peripheral temperature, movement, and various other derivatives.

Peripheral temperature and movement are guardrails supporting algorithm validity and do not contribute directly to the algorithm calculation.

■ CLINICAL APPLICABILITY

Under GA, the NOL index has been reported to have a higher intraoperative sensitivity and specificity than heart rate and MAP in predicting responses to noxious stimuli, such as intubation, incision, and tetanic stimulation.[44,62] NOL-guided analgesia during major abdominal surgery has been reported to result in 30% less remifentanil consumption.[63] Peristimulus changes in the NOL have also been reported to correlate with the remifentanil dosage.[64] In abdominal surgery with fentanyl/sevoflurane, despite the nonsignificant differences in fentanyl and morphine consumption after surgery, an improvement in the postoperative pain scores has been seen in patients receiving NOL-guided fentanyl administration compared to patients receiving the standard heart rate and MAP-guided fentanyl administration.[65] However, in this study, no clear differences were observed between the NOL values during NOL-guided administration and standard care,[65] as essentially all were within or below the recommended maintenance values of 10–25. This suggests that the NOL index scale definition is not well adjusted for NOL-guided administration because the recommended value range (10–25) is relatively narrow and large—not centered within the whole dynamic range (0–100). Thus, the NOL index should be rescaled for greater sensitivity and dynamics.

■ VALIDITY

Various researchers worked to investigate the reliability of the NOL monitor. Through an interventional study Edry et al., revealed that, NOL index responded progressively to increased stimulus intensity and remained unchanged in response to non-noxious stimuli validating its efficacy in detecting noxious stimuli at various intensity and differentiating from non-noxious stimuli.[62]

Similarly, apart from superiority and reliability of NOL over HR and MAP, Martini et al., further revealed that, in contrast to HR and MAP, the NOL was not affected by hemodynamic effects of remifentanil.[60]

Likewise, Stöckle et al.,[67] published a supportive evidence that the NOL monitoring is a promising index to assess the level of nociception in patients under general anesthesia. Here, they found that area under the ROC curve (AUC) for the NOL during standardized stimulation was larger than for all other parameters at the exception of ANI and the AUC of NOL for nociception during tracheal intubation was greater.

PITFALLS

The PMD-200 monitor cannot anticipate or predict the application of nociceptive stimuli during surgery. The clinician is the only person who can anticipate applying such nociceptive stimuli. Suppose the patient's requirements for opioid doses/concentrations upon tracheal intubation were used to calibrate the individual patient's requirements. In that case, that information can be used subsequently to guide the nociception–antinociception balance (NANB). Furthermore, NOL should not be used to guide preemptive analgesia before emergence since it cannot predict the PK/PD (pharmacokinetics/pharmacodynamics) effects of the drugs postsurgery. During emergence, NOL values may be high due to sympathetic arousal unrelated to nociception and, therefore, should not be used to guide the analgesia dosing. The NOL monitor must be used by anesthesia personnel trained in GA, with all the best practices and procedures implicit therein, including dosing analgesics in anticipation of noxious stimuli. Limiting the intended users and providing education and training mitigates this risk.

Conditions interfering with correctly acquiring the photoplethysmography signal, skin conductance, and various artifacts may temporarily lead to difficulty interpreting NOL values. These include cardiac arrhythmias, electrocautery, severe hypothermia, excessive motion, and impediments to blood flow, such as arterial catheters, blood pressure cuffs, infusion lines, and some vasoactive drugs. Alerts on the screen mitigate this and do not display an NOL value if the signal quality is inadequate. Evidence suggests that the clinical performance of NOL in patients receiving chronic beta blockers as part of their care was equivalent to that of ordinarily normotensive patients.[66]

Conditions affecting the ANS and the volemic state of the patient may temporarily lead to difficulty in interpreting NOL values. These conditions include administering vasoactive drugs, extremes of patient positioning (i.e., steep Trendelenburg), and hypovolemia. However, the algorithm recognizes Trendelenburg's positioning and adjusts using the ACC. In addition, the NOL is constantly normalized to the patient's earlier data. The influence of a bolus of short-acting vasoactive drugs such as phenylephrine and ephedrine on NOL values (moderate increase) is short-lived,[68] and should be expected to fade within 2–3 minutes.

CONCLUSION

One of the more straightforward ways a computer can be used in anesthesia is to design a servo system, for instance, to maintain BIS within a specified range by continuous assessment and adjustment of the anesthetic agent(s) infusion rate. If the program is designed to learn from its experience, this will come under machine learning.

REFERENCES

1. Kahneman D. Thinking, Fast and Slow. New York: Macmillan; 2011.
2. Raja SN, Carr DB, Cohen M, Finnerup NB, Flor H, Gibson S, et al. The revised International Association for the Study of Pain definition of pain: concepts, challenges, and compromises. Pain. 2020;161(9):1976-82.
3. Kehlet H: Multimodal approach to control postoperative pathophysiology and rehabilitation. Br J Anaesth. 1997;78(5):606-17.
4. Jakuscheit A, Weth J, Lichtner G, Jurth C, Rehberg B, von Dincklage F. Intraoperative monitoring of analgesia using nociceptive reflexes correlates with delayed extubation and immediate postoperative pain: a prospective observational study. Eur J Anaesthesiol. 2017;34(5):297-305.
5. Lee LA, Caplan RA, Stephens LS, Posner KL, Terman GW, Voepel-Lewis T, et al. Postoperative opioid-induced respiratory depression: a closed claims analysis. Anesthesiology. 2015;122(3):659-65.
6. Fletcher D, Martinez V. Opioid-induced hyperalgesia in patients after surgery: a systematic review and a meta-analysis. Br J Anaesth. 2014;112(6):991-1004.
7. Berardino K, Carroll AH, Popovsky D, Ricotti R, Civilette MD, Sherman WF, et al. Opioid use consequences, governmental strategies, and alternative pain control techniques following total hip arthroplasties. Orthop Rev (Pavia). 2022;14(4):35318.
8. Frauenknecht J, Kirkham KR, Jacot-Guillarmod A, Albrecht E. Analgesic impact of intra-operative opioids vs. opioid-free anaesthesia: a systematic review and meta-analysis. Anaesthesia. 2019;74(5):651-62.
9. Jensen EW, Valencia JF, López A, Anglada T, Agustí M, Ramos Y, et al. Monitoring hypnotic effect and nociception with two EEG-derived indices, qCON and qNOX, during general anaesthesia. Acta Anaesthesiol Scand. 2014;58(8):933-41.
10. Weil G, Passot S, Servin F, Billard V. Does spectral entropy reflect the response to intubation or incision during propofol-remifentanil anesthesia? Anesth Analg. 2008;106(1):152-9.
11. Gruenewald M, Zhou J, Schloemerkemper N, Meybohm P, Weiler N, Tonner PH, et al. M-Entropy guidance vs standard practice during propofol-remifentanil anaesthesia: a randomised controlled trial. Anaesthesia. 2007;62(12):1224-9.
12. Melia U, Gabarron E, Agustí M, Souto N, Pineda P, Fontanet J, et al. Comparison of the qCON and qNOX indices for the assessment of unconsciousness level and noxious stimulation response during surgery. J Clin Monit Comput. 2017;31(6):1273-81.
13. Barvais L, Engelman E, Eba JM, Coussaert E, Cantraine F, Kenny GN. Effect site concentrations of remifentanil and pupil response to noxious stimulation. Br J Anaesth. 2003;91(3):347-52.
14. Sabourdin N, Barrois J, Louvet N, Rigouzzo A, Guye ML, Dadure C, et al. Pupillometry-guided intraoperative remifentanil administration versus standard practice influences opioid use: a randomized study. Anesthesiology. 2017;127(2):284-92.
15. Neice AE, Behrends M, Bokoch MP, Seligman KM, Conrad NM, Larson MD. Prediction of opioid analgesic efficacy by measurement of pupillary unrest. Anesth Analg. 2017;124(3):915-21.

16. Duceau B, Baubillier M, Bouroche G, Albi-Feldzer A, Jayr C. Pupillary reflex for evaluation of thoracic paravertebral block: a prospective observational feasibility study. Anesth Analg. 2017;125(4):1342-7.
17. Paulus J, Roquilly A, Beloeil H, Théraud J, Asehnoune K, Lejus C. Pupillary reflex measurement predicts insufficient analgesia before endotracheal suctioning in critically ill patients. Crit Care. 2013;17(4):R161.
18. Kantor E, Montravers P, Longrois D, Guglielminotti J. Pain assessment in the postanaesthesia care unit using pupillometry: a cross-sectional study after standard anaesthetic care. Eur J Anaesthesiol. 2014;31(2):91-7.
19. Dualé C, Julien H, Pereira B, Abbal B, Baud C, Schoeffler P. Pupil diameter during postanesthetic recovery is not influenced by postoperative pain, but by the intraoperative opioid treatment. J Clin Anesth. 2015;27(1):23-32.
20. Aissou M, Snauwaert A, Dupuis C, Atchabahian A, Aubrun F, Beaussier M. Objective assessment of the immediate postoperative analgesia using pupillary reflex measurement: a prospective and observational study. Anesthesiology. 2012;116(5):1006-12.
21. Sabourdin N, Peretout JB, Khalil E, Guye ML, Louvet N, Constant I. Influence of depth of hypnosis on pupillary reactivity to a standardized tetanic stimulus in patients under propofol-remifentanil target–controlled infusion: a crossover randomized pilot study. Anesth Analg. 2018;126(1):70-7.
22. Jeanne M, Clément C, De Jonckheere J, Logier R, Tavernier B. Variations of the analgesia nociception index during general anaesthesia for laparoscopic abdominal surgery. J Clin Monit Comput. 2012;26(4):289-94.
23. Boselli E, Bouvet L, Bégou G, Dabouz R, Davidson J, Deloste JY, et al. Prediction of immediate postoperative pain using the analgesia/nociception index: a prospective observational study. Br J Anaesth. 2014;112(4):715-21.
24. Funcke S, Sauerlaender S, Pinnschmidt HO, Saugel B, Bremer K, Reuter DA, et al. Validation of Innovative Techniques for monitoring nociception during general anesthesia: a clinical study using tetanic and intracutaneous electrical stimulation. Anesthesiology. 2017;127(2):272-83.
25. Graça R, Lobo FA. Analgesia Nociception Index (ANI) and ephedrine: a dangerous liasion. J Clin Monit Comput. 2021;35(4):953-4.
26. Gruenewald M, Ilies C, Herz J, Schoenherr T, Fudickar A, Höcker J, et al. Influence of nociceptive stimulation on analgesia nociception index (ANI) during propofol-remifentanil anaesthesia. Br J Anaesth. 2013;110(6):1024-30.
27. Huiku M, Uutela K, van Gils M, Korhonen I, Kymäläinen M, Meriläinen P, et al. Assessment of surgical stress during general anaesthesia. Br J Anaesth. 2007;98(4):447-55.
28. Chen X, Thee C, Gruenewald M, Wnent J, Illies C, Hoecker J, et al. Comparison of surgical stress index-guided analgesia with standard clinical practice during routine general anesthesia: a pilot study. Anesthesiology. 2010;112(5):1175-83.
29. Bergmann I, Göhner A, Crozier TA, Hesjedal B, Wiese CH, Popov AF, et al. Surgical pleth index-guided remifentanil administration reduces remifentanil and propofol consumption and shortens recovery times in outpatient anaesthesia. Br J Anaesth. 2013;110(4):622-8.
30. Won YJ, Lim BG, Kim YS, Lee M, Kim H. Usefulness of surgical pleth index-guided analgesia during general anesthesia: a systematic review and meta-analysis of randomized controlled trials. J Int Med Res. 2018;46(11):4386-98.

31. Ledowski T, Ang B, Schmarbeck T, Rhodes J. Monitoring of sympathetic tone to assess postoperative pain: skin conductance vs surgical stress index. Anaesthesia. 2009;64(7):727-31.
32. Park JH, Lim BG, Kim H, Lee IO, Kong MH, Kim NS. Comparison of surgical pleth index-guided analgesia with conventional analgesia practices in children: a randomized controlled trial. Anesthesiology. 2015;122(6):1280-7.
33. Ledowski T, Pascoe E, Ang B, Schmarbeck T, Clarke MW, Fuller C, et al. Monitoring of intra-operative nociception: skin conductance and surgical stress index versus stress hormone plasma levels. Anaesthesia. 2010;65(10):1001-6.
34. Storm H, Myre K, Rostrup M, Stokland O, Lien MD, Raeder JC. Skin conductance correlates with perioperative stress. Acta Anaesthesiol Scand. 2002;46(7):887-95.
35. Gjerstad AC, Storm H, Hagen R, Huiku M, Qvigstad E, Raeder J. Comparison of skin conductance with entropy during intubation, tetanic stimulation and emergence from general anaesthesia. Acta Anaesthesiol Scand. 2007;51(1):8-15.
36. Skljarevski V, Ramadan NM. The nociceptive flexion reflex in humans—review article. Pain. 2002;96(1):3-8.
37. Rhudy JL, France CR. Defining the nociceptive flexion reflex (NFR) threshold in human participants: a comparison of different scoring criteria. Pain. 2007;128(3):244-53.
38. von Dincklage F, Hackbarth M, Mager R, Rehberg B, Baars JH. Monitoring of the responsiveness to noxious stimuli during anaesthesia with propofol and remifentanil by using RIII reflex threshold and bispectral index. Br J Anaesth. 2010;104(2):201-8.
39. von Dincklage F, Correll C, Schneider MH, Rehberg B, Baars JH. Utility of nociceptive flexion reflex threshold, bispectral index, composite variability index and noxious stimulation response index as measures for nociception during general anaesthesia. Anaesthesia. 2012;67(8):899-905.
40. Jakuscheit A, Posch MJ, Gkaitatzis S, Neumark L, Hackbarth M, Schneider M, et al. Utility of nociceptive flexion reflex threshold and bispectral index to predict movement responses under propofol anaesthesia. Somatosens Mot Res. 2017;34(2):139-44.
41. Tajmir SH, Lee H, Shailam R, Gale HI, Nguyen JC, Westra SJ, et al. Artificial intelligence-assisted interpretation of bone age radiographs improves accuracy and decreases variability. Skeletal Radiol. 2019;48(2):275-83.
42. Ampadi Ramachandran R, Chi SW, Srinivasa Pai P, Foucher K, Ozevin D, Mathew MT. Artificial intelligence and machine learning as a viable solution for hip implant failure diagnosis-Review of literature and in vitro case study. Med Biol Eng Comput. 2023;61(6):1239-55.
43. Bellman R. An Introduction to Artificial Intelligence: Can Computers Think? San Francisco: Boyd & Fraser Publishing Company; 1978.
44. Davenport T, Kalakota R. The potential for artificial intelligence in healthcare. Future Healthc J. 2019;6(2):94-8.
45. Hashimoto DA, Witkowski E, Gao L, Meireles O, Rosman G. Artificial Intelligence in anesthesiology: current techniques, clinical applications, and limitations. Anesthesiology. 2020;132(2):379-94.
46. Russell S, Norvig P. Artificial Intelligence: A Modern Approach, 3rd edition. Upper Saddle River, NJ: Prentice Hall; 2009.

47. Bisgin H, Liu Z, Fang H, Xu X, Tong W. Mining FDA drug labels using an unsupervised learning technique—topic modeling. BMC Bioinformatics. 2011;12 Suppl 10(Suppl 10):S11.
48. Kendale S, Kulkarni P, Rosenberg AD, Wang J. Supervised Machine-learning predictive analytics for prediction of postinduction hypotension. Anesthesiology. 2018;129(4):675-88.
49. Machine Learning for Anesthesiologists: A Primer: Erratum. Anesthesiology. 2019;130(6):1098.
50. Hu YJ, Ku TH, Jan RH, Wang K, Tseng YC, Yang SF. Decision tree-based learning to predict patient controlled analgesia consumption and readjustment. BMC Med Inform Decis Mak. 2012;12:131.
51. Hakonarson H, Bjornsdottir US, Halapi E, Bradfield J, Zink F, Mouy M, et al. Profiling of genes expressed in peripheral blood mononuclear cells predicts glucocorticoid sensitivity in asthma patients. Proc Natl Acad Sci USA. 2005;102(41):14789-94.
52. Sutton R, Barto A. Reinforcement Learning: An Introduction. Cambridge: MIT Press; 1998.
53. Padmanabhan R, Meskin N, Haddad WM. Closed-loop control of anesthesia and mean arterial pressure using reinforcement learning. 2014 IEEE Symposium on Adaptive Dynamic Programming and Reinforcement Learning (ADPRL), Orlando, FL. 2014;1-8.
54. McCulloch WS, Pitts W. A logical calculus of the ideas immanent in nervous activity. 1943. Bull Math Biol. 1990;52(1-2):99-115; discussion 73-97.
55. LeCun Y, Bengio Y, Hinton G. Deep learning. Nature. 2015;521(7553):436-44.
56. Hashimoto DA, Witkowski ER, Gao L, Meireles OR, Rosman G. Artificial intelligence in anesthesiology: current techniques, clinical applications, and limitations. Anesthesiology. 2020;132(2):379-94.
57. Benzy VK, Jasmin EA, Koshy RC, Amal F. Wavelet Entropy based classification of depth of anesthesia. 2016 International Conference on Computational Techniques in Information and Communication Technologies (ICCTICT). 2016:521-4.
58. Ortolani O, Conti A, Di Filippo A, Adembri C, Moraldi E, Evangelisti A, et al. EEG signal processing in anaesthesia. Use of a neural network technique for monitoring depth of anaesthesia. Br J Anaesth. 2002;88(5):644-8.
59. Ben-Israel N, Kliger M, Zuckerman G, Katz Y, Edry R. Monitoring the nociception level: a multi-parameter approach. J Clin Monit Comput. 2013;27(6):659-68.
60. Martini CH, Boon M, Broens SJ, Hekkelman EF, Oudhoff LA, Buddeke AW, et al. Ability of the nociception level, a multiparameter composite of autonomic signals, to detect noxious stimuli during propofol–remifentanil anesthesia. Anesthesiology. 2015;123(3):524-34.
61. Breiman L. Random Forests. Machine Learning. 2001;45(1):5-32.
62. Edry R, Recea V, Dikust Y, Sessler DI. Preliminary intraoperative validation of the nociception level index: a noninvasive nociception monitor. Anesthesiology. 2016;125(1):193-203.
63. Meijer FS, Martini CH, Broens S, Boon M, Niesters M, Aarts L, et al. Nociception-guided versus standard care during remifentanil–propofol anesthesia: a randomized controlled trial. Anesthesiology. 2019;130(5):745-55.

64. Renaud-Roy E, Stöckle PA, Maximos S, Brulotte V, Sideris L, Dubé P, et al. Correlation between incremental remifentanil doses and the Nociception Level (NOL) index response after intraoperative noxious stimuli. Can J Anesth. 2019;66(9):1049-61.
65. Meijer F, Honing M, Roor T, Toet S, Calis P, Olofsen E, et al. Reduced postoperative pain using Nociception Level-guided fentanyl dosing during sevoflurane anaesthesia: a randomised controlled trial. Br J Anaesth. 2020;125(6):1070-8.
66. Bergeron C, Brulotte V, Pelen F, Clairoux A, Bélanger ME, Issa R, et al. Impact of chronic treatment by β1-adrenergic antagonists on Nociceptive-Level (NOL) index variation after a standardized noxious stimulus under general anesthesia: a cohort study. J Clin Monit Comput. 2022;36(1):109-20.
67. Stöckle PA, Julien M, Issa R, Décary E, Brulotte V, Drolet P, et al. Validation of the PMD100 and its NOL Index to detect nociception at different infusion regimen of remifentanil in patients under general anesthesia. Minerva Anestesiol. 2018;84(10):1160-8.
68. Raft J, Coulombe MA, Renaud-Roy E, Tanoubi I, Verdonck O, Fortier LP, et al. Impact of intravenous phenylephrine bolus administration on the nociceptive level index (NOL). J Clin Monit Comput. 2020;34(5):1079-86.

CHAPTER 21

Methadone for Perioperative Pain

Skule Bakke, Rajesh Bhavsar, Thomas Stroem

ABSTRACT

Methadone is a long-acting opioid with rapid onset of action. It has a potent μ opioid receptor agonist and N-methyl-D-aspartate (NMDA) receptor antagonist activity, which helps to attenuate the development of hyperalgesia and tolerance. Its characteristic mechanism and distinctive pharmacological features make it most preferred in treating chronic and neuropathic pain and in replacement therapy for opiate abusers. Although it has been previously used as a perioperative analgesic, it did not receive global acceptance due to apprehension of respiratory depression and QT prolongation.

With the global rise in average life expectancy, comorbidities requiring anticoagulant therapy have also exponentially increased, making perioperative pain management challenging in these patients, as central and peripheral nerve blockade is advised with caution. However, a review of recent investigations reveals that intraoperative methadone may be an exciting alternative, especially under these circumstances.

Keywords: QT prolongation; Respiratory depression; NMDA antagonist

■ KEY POINTS

- Methadone is potent μ receptor agonist with a rapid onset and prolonged duration of action.
- Traditionally used in chronic and neuropathic pain and replacement therapy for opiate abusers.
- Respiratory depression, QT prolongation, and serotonin syndrome are well-known concerns.
- It has been used in various perioperative situations without alarming complications.
- Recommended doses vary and depend on the surgical procedure. The general recommendation is 0.25-0.3 mg/kg (or a fixed dose of 20 mg).
- Methadone administered at the induction of anesthesia is most beneficial.
- For postoperative respiratory depression, naloxone infusion is recommended.

INTRODUCTION

Average life expectancy in the world has increased secondary to developments in medical diagnostics and therapeutics along with general health awareness.[1] Age-related comorbidities such as ischemic heart disease (IHD), cerebrovascular disease, and peripheral vascular disease requiring anticoagulant therapy have also increased with increasing age.

Postoperative pain management in patients on anticoagulant therapy subjected to emergency operations is challenging as central neural blockade is not recommended due to inadequate pause of anticoagulant medicine. As an alternative, peripheral nerve blocks (PNB) have been suggested as postoperative analgesic therapy despite a lack of robust data on clinical impact beyond its well-acknowledged beneficial effects, such as reducing pain and opioid consumption along with improved quality of early recovery and possible risk of metastasis after cancer surgery.[2]

When performed correctly, PNB is overall safe. However, regardless of technique or location, there are rare but serious risks such as failure, bleeding, short duration of action, infection, damage to surrounding structures, permanent nerve injury, and systemic toxicity. Further, there are some difficult situations and contraindications, such as uncooperative patients (pediatric patients, combative patients, or those with severe dementia), preexistent neurologic deficit, systemic or active local infection at the site of the block, body habitus, or obesity obscuring optimal ultrasonographic visualization and presence of coagulopathy.[3,4]

Traditionally, weaker analgesics such as paracetamol and nonsteroidal anti-inflammatory drugs (NSAIDs), shorter-acting opioids,[5] including fentanyl, hydromorphone, morphine, and sufentanil, have been administered as intravenous boluses for postoperative analgesia. However, this strategy causes fluctuating serum levels, leading to periods of inadequate pain relief alternating with periods of excessive sedation.[6,7]

It is well-known that suboptimal pain control is accompanied by an array of adverse outcomes, including increased morbidity, worse physical function, impaired quality of life, diminished sleep, and prolonged opioid use during and after hospitalization.[8] Moreover, inadequate postoperative analgesia may also be associated with adverse consequences in multiple organ systems, including cardiovascular (coronary ischemia and arrhythmias), pulmonary (hypoventilation and pulmonary infection), gastrointestinal (ileus, nausea, and vomiting), renal (urinary retention and oliguria), and neurological (delirium) systems.[8-12] Importantly, poorly controlled pain in the early postoperative period may trigger the development of chronic postsurgical pain.[8-12]

Therefore, there has long been a demand for an ideal analgesic medication that would provide a steady constant level of pain control over long latency time intervals without many side effects.

METHADONE: AN INTERESTING ALTERNATIVE

Methadone is a unique and potent μ opioid receptor agonist with a rapid onset of action. Its unique mechanism and distinctive pharmacological features play an essential role in the treatment of chronic,[7,13] neuropathic,[8,14] cancer pain[9,15] and as replacement therapy for opiate abusers.[10,16] As methadone slowly clears from the bloodstream, an abrupt offset of analgesia is less likely to occur.

With this distinctive drug profile, methadone was found to be an exciting option in the treatment of perioperative pain and has been investigated in pediatric,[11,16] cardiac,[12,17,18] complex spine,[7,19] and abdominal surgery.[20] Further, few published studies have compared intraoperative methadone to fentanyl or sufentanil in cardiac surgery,[17,18] spine surgery,[19] laparoscopy,[19] hysterectomy,[20] abdominal surgery,[21] and major surgery in children.[22]

HISTORY AND PHARMACOLOGY OF METHADONE

During the second world war, the supply of morphine was plummeting. German leader (*Führer*)—Adolf Hitler ordered the development of an alternative to morphine, which resulted in the invention of methadone in 1938 by Max Bockmuhl and Gustav Erhart. It had a trade name of Dolophine, after the first name of Hitler.[23] However, this information is controversial since Dolophine originates in Latin, where *Dolor* means pain and *Fin* means end.[24] Methadone, however, had poor acceptance by German soldiers due to its adverse effects.

The name methadone is derived from fragments of its chemical name (6-dimethylamine-4,4-diphenyl-3-heptanone)[25] and is currently accepted to designate its racemic mixture.

Methadone is administered as a racemic mixture of two enantiomers: R-methadone and S-methadone. It is an alkaline liposoluble drug with pKa of 9.2.[26] It has fast and almost complete absorption after oral consumption and has bioavailability between 67 and 95%.[27] It can be located in plasma 30 minutes after oral ingestion, while peak plasma concentration reaches within 2.5–3 hours.

Methadone has a long half-life of approximately 24 hours and has a significant interindividual variation of 8–90 hours. This makes it far superior to other opioid analgesics, such as morphine ($t_{1/2}$ = 2–4 hours), hydromorphone ($t_{1/2}$ = 2–3 hours), or fentanyl ($t_{1/2}$ = 4 hours)[28] **(Table 1)**.

Single intravenous bolus initiates pain relief approximately within 10–20 minutes, lasting from 4 to 8 hours. The duration of action is less than excretion time and increases accumulation risk after repeated doses.[28] The minimum effective blood concentration of methadone was determined to be 57.9 ± 15.2 ng/mL, which was higher than that determined in their earlier investigation (31.6 ± 11.1 ng/mL),[29] suggesting that the minimal effective concentration may vary with surgical procedure.

TABLE 1: Pharmacokinetic properties of methadone and morphine.

Parameters	Methadone	Morphine
Bioavailability	80%	30%
Plasma binding	60–90%	35%
Half-life	30 hours	3–4 hours
Active metabolites	No	Yes
Influence by kidney failure	+	+++
Influence by liver failure	+++	+

TABLE 2: Interactions of concern: Methadone.

CYP3A4	CYP2B6		
Induction	Inhibition	Inhibition	Alpha glycoprotein inhibitors
Thiopental	Fluconazole	Chlorpromazine	Actiomicin
Carbamazepine	Fluoxetine	Fluoxetine	Doxarubecin
Glucocorticoids	Vanlafaxine	Haloperidol	Sertaline
Barbiturates	Macrolides	Levopromazine	Paroxetine
Phenytoin	Ciprofloxacin	Paroxetine	Vinblastine
	Grape juice	Fluvoxamine	

Methadone has a large volume of distribution, which can be explained by its lipophilic nature.[30] The drug gets saturated throughout tissues such as the brain, intestine, kidney, liver, muscles, and lungs. Clinically, this property may lead to building up of methadone in tissues after administering repeated doses, thus increasing the risk of overdose. And when the consumption is stopped, the drug gets gradually redistributed, maintaining a small plasma concentration. This also explains why methadone is less prone to induce withdrawal syndrome.

It is metabolized in the liver, and its metabolites are excreted by urine (20–50%) and feces (10–45%). In the liver, methadone is metabolized by several isoforms of P450 cytochromes (e.g., CYP3A4, CYP2B6) which degrade it to its inactive metabolites (2-ethyl-1.5-dimethyl-3.3-diphenyl pyrrolidine and 2-ethyl-5-methyl-3.3-diphenyl-pyrroline)[31] **(Table 2)**.

A wide variability of responses have been observed among individuals exposed to methadone, which may be attributed to genetic polymorphism in the encoding of cytochromes involved with its metabolism, in addition to the polymorphism of carrier proteins and opioid receptors along with various drug interactions (*see* **Table 2**).[32]

As methadone has basic pH, the urinary excretion depends on urinary pH, i.e., only 4% gets excreted at a pH above 6, while >30% gets excreted when the pH is below 6.[33]

In the presence of renal failure, methadone can be eliminated through feces[34] and thus may be considered safe for patients with kidney failure and undergoing dialysis. But some authors still recommend dose reduction when the glomerular filtration rate is below 10 mL/min.[34]

Methadone acts by binding to µ, κ, and δ opioid receptors where the activities such as analgesia, respiratory depression, dependence, and tolerance are primarily triggered by µ activation.[27] In contrast to the usual observation that opioids show tolerance and cross-tolerance, an experimental study has shown that methadone is less sensitive to tolerance since its ED_{50} was not altered after previous exposure to morphine.[35]

Methadone crosses the placental barrier and may induce withdrawal syndrome in the neonate.[36,37]

It can be found in breast milk in low concentrations, which are harmless to the infant.

■ CLINICAL APPLICABILITY: PREVIOUS EXPERIENCE

Methadone was investigated against morphine in upper abdominal procedures,[21] where the time from initial pain control until the first supplemental dose of opioid needed was significantly longer in the methadone group (21 hours) compared to the morphine group (6 hours) and total requirements for opioids, were lower in the patients given methadone (12 vs. 41 mg in the morphine group).

Similarly, in hysterectomy patients, methadone showed significantly less postoperative opioid requirement and lower pain scores than morphine group.[38] Correspondingly, in cesarean deliveries, methadone at the mean dose of 0.17 mg/kg showed 40% less requirement of opioids in the first 48 hours postoperative and showed significantly lower pain scores as compared to fentanyl, morphine, or both.[39]

In cardiac surgical patients, methadone administered at 20 mg after induction showed significantly less postoperative analgesic requirement (45% less) and lower pain scores than morphine.[18] Similar findings were observed when methadone (0.1 mg/kg) was administered at the end of cardiac surgery.[40]

Further, a large intraoperative clinical trial comparing methadone (0.3 mg/kg) and fentanyl (12 µg/kg) given before cardiopulmonary bypass showed that postoperative opioid requirements and pain scores were reduced by approximately 40% during the first 3 postoperative days in the methadone group[17] and patient satisfaction with pain management on a 100-mm verbal analog scale was higher as compared to the fentanyl group. These findings demonstrated that despite an extended period between anesthetic induction and tracheal extubation in the intensive care unit, a dose of methadone given before surgery provided a prolonged analgesia benefit.[41]

Similar to cardiac surgery, methadone was also tried in major spine surgery. With a 0.2 mg/kg dose at induction compared to continuous sufentanil infusion, Gottschalk et al.[19] found that opioid requirements and pain scores were approximately 50% lower in the methadone group, even 48 hours after surgery. Analogous observations were noted in a larger randomized trial comparing methadone (0.2 mg/kg) and hydromorphone (2 mg)[7] during the first 3 postoperative days.

In elective total hip replacement surgery randomized to receive 10 mg of methadone at induction of anesthesia or at the end of the procedure[41] on postoperative day 1, the requirements for opioid pain medication were approximately twofold higher in the group given methadone at the end of the surgery, suggesting that dosing before the procedure is beneficial.

Methadone has also been investigated in ambulatory surgical patients (most undergoing laparoscopic cholecystectomy, tubal ligation, salpingectomy, oophorectomy, or salpingectomy with oophorectomy) through randomized, double-blinded, dose-finding study.[5] Here, opioid consumption, pain intensity, and opioid side effects were assessed in the hospital and for 30 days postoperatively using home diaries. In-hospital non-methadone opioid use (morphine equivalents) was less in patients given methadone compared to the control group. In the first 30 postoperative days, patients administered 0.15 mg/kg methadone reported less pain at rest ($p = 0.02$) and used fewer opioid pills than controls.

Relatively limited investigations were observed in the literature on using methadone in the pediatric population. A randomized double-blinded comparative study of similar doses of methadone (0.2 mg/kg) and morphine in children (ages 3–7 years) undergoing major surgical procedures[22] showed that during the first 3 postoperative days, fewer patients in the methadone group had severe pain scores (18%) compared to the morphine group (35%), and analgesic requirements were less in the methadone cohort.

■ METHADONE: MAJOR CONCERNS

Respiratory Depression

Clinically alarming respiratory depression and QT prolongation are two major concerns about using methadone. However, various randomized, observational, or retrospective trials showed no differences in the incidence of respiratory depression (respiratory rates <8–12 breaths/min), hypoxemic events (oxygen saturations <92–90%), and level of postoperative sedation between methadone and control groups during the postanesthesia care unit (PACU) admission, on the surgical wards, or in the intensive care unit.[5,7,17,18,20–22,29,40,42,43] Further, no patients from the methadone group required naloxone infusions for prolonged respiratory depression.

If naloxone is required in the PACU for methadone-induced respiratory depression, an infusion should be considered. The half-life of naloxone (approximately 90 minutes) is considerably shorter than that of methadone (35 hours with a dose of 20 mg). Recurrent respiratory depression has been reported in patients given a single dose of naloxone after cardiac surgery.[44]

Postoperative nausea and vomiting (PONV) are significant side effects of opioids that contribute to the delay in discharge from PACU. Methadone, being a potent opioid, carries these side effects. However, the incidences of PONV did not differ between the methadone and control groups, except for higher-risk patients in the PACU (but not on the wards)[38] and lower-risk in methadone patients in the intensive care unit.[18]

Here, it is essential to note that most clinical trials were small and not powered to assess safety outcome measures, particularly rare events such as significant respiratory depression. In addition, high-risk patients were excluded from enrollment in many studies. Although limited data from randomized studies suggest that the risks of methadone do not exceed conventional shorter-acting opioids, additional information from larger-scale investigations is needed (mainly related to respiratory depression).

QT Prolongation

An increased risk of QT prolongation, torsade de pointes, and cardiac death[45] has been observed in patients receiving methadone maintenance therapy for opioid dependence disorder. The dose and chronicity of consumption directly influence the potential for QT prolongation and the development of arrhythmias.[45] Various factors, including drugs (such as methadone), stress, hypothermia, and electrolyte disturbances, were found to be associated with QTc (QT interval corrected for heart rate) prolongation in patients undergoing major noncardiac surgery.[46] Here, a QTc interval defined as >440 ms for men or >460 ms for women was observed in >51% of patients, which resolved in all subjects by the first postoperative day.[43] Torsade de pointes was not observed in any patients. However, none of the randomized trials specifically mention the effect of a single intravenous dose of methadone on the QT interval and the risk of arrhythmias.

Similarly, no higher incidence of adverse cardiac events has been observed in patients administered perioperative methadone in clinical studies. Additionally, a systematic review of torsade de pointes case reports described no such event after intraoperative methadone use.[47]

Serotonin Syndrome

Methadone, being a synthetic opioid, inhibits serotonin transport at clinically relevant concentrations, which may result in increases in intrasynaptic levels of serotonin.[48] This may, theoretically, result in the development of "serotonin syndrome", which is manifested as altered mental status, autonomic instability (fever, tachycardia), or neuromuscular abnormalities (rigidity, tremor, clonus) in the perioperative period. This is predominantly seen in patients on chronic methadone maintenance therapy who receive other serotonergic medications, including monoamine oxidase inhibitors, selective serotonin reuptake inhibitors, serotonin-norepinephrine reuptake inhibitors, and tricyclic antidepressants.[48] However, serotonin syndrome has not been reported in patients administered intravenous methadone perioperatively.

Safety in High-risk Population

The observation by Gourlay et al.[49] revealed that the terminal half-life of methadone was positively correlated with age, which suggests that more careful dosing of methadone is required in the elderly. However, as the majority of critical clinical trials excluded the high-risk patient groups, limited experience exists regarding the use of methadone in high-risk, elderly, and morbidly obese patients, except for studies performed in cardiac surgical patients. There exists particular concern about the use of methadone in morbidly obese patients. Although these patients were not excluded from many clinical trials, the efficacy and safety of methadone has not been specifically assessed.

■ DOSE

Despite various dose-response studies,[5,42] an appropriate and accurate dose of methadone that may offer prolonged analgesia without respiratory depression has not been identified yet. However, specific facts were revealed, such as the minimal effective concentration of methadone required for pain relief may vary dependent upon the surgical procedure.[29,49] Therefore, it is likely that more painful operations (major spine surgery) may require larger doses of methadone, and the administration of 0.25-0.3 mg/kg may be insufficient.[42,50]

On the other hand, in laparoscopic surgical patients, doses of 0.1-0.15 mg/kg ideal body weight may provide sufficient analgesia with no side effects (median dose of 9 mg in the higher-dose group).[5]

There is no clarity about whether ideal or actual body weight should be used to calculate the accurate dose of methadone. Only three studies reported whether methadone was dosed on actual or ideal body weight.[5,7,40] Using ideal body weight may minimize interpatient variability in dosing, resulting in minimal effective blood concentrations below the threshold for analgesia in some patients. On the other hand, using actual body weight, especially in obese patients, may result in high blood concentrations of methadone, causing prolonged respiratory depression.

Various doses have been used in clinical trials, ranging from 0.1 to 0.3 mg/kg, with most studies using a dose of either 0.2 mg/kg or a fixed dose of 20 mg. It is advised through a recent review that the administration of methadone may be simplified by giving a standard dose at induction (10–20 mg), dependent upon the expected degree of postoperative pain.[51]

Estimation of appropriate doses of methadone for opioid-dependent and tolerant patients is challenging. Patients presenting for specific complex orthopedic procedures, such as complicated spinal surgery, may already receive potent opioids for preexisting neuropathic pain. Although it can be logically assumed that these patients may benefit from larger doses of intraoperative methadone, inadequate and inaccurate information on the degree of tolerance at the time of surgery makes the dose estimation challenging. Therefore, it is suggested that titration of additional methadone in the PACU may benefit this patient population based on the degree of sedation and respiratory rate.[21,49]

METHADONE ADVANTAGES

Chronic postsurgical pain is frequently observed in 10–50% of patients. It is attributed to the perception of acute pain in the immediate postoperative period. Acute pain perception activates the N-methyl-D-aspartate (NMDA) receptors, which results in an extended rise in the transmission of nociception.[52] The consequent hyperalgesia and allodynia may contribute to transitioning from acute to chronic pain.[53] Even though it is speculated that ketamine, which is a potent NMDA receptor antagonist and can reduce the development of chronic postsurgical pain 3 and 6 months after surgery, there is only limited evidence documenting that any perioperative agent can consistently reduce the risk of chronic pain after surgery.[54]

As methadone is also an NMDA antagonist like ketamine[55,56] and has the potential to reduce the intensity of postoperative pain, a single dose of intraoperative methadone may offer a preventive analgesic effect and decrease the risk of the development of chronic postsurgical pain.

Further, it has been shown that chronic opioid exposure, predominantly to methadone, decreases coronary disease extension, as compared to nonexposed patients.[57] This finding was confirmed by an experimental study where exposure to morphine has decreased the area of myocardial infarction when administered before ischemia and reperfusion.[58,59] Like this observation, it is documented that methadone and morphine produce similar myocardial infarct size-sparing effects that are δ opioid receptor-mediated and dependent on the duration of myocardial ischemia.[60]

CONCLUSION

Methadone is a long-acting opioid with a unique pharmacokinetic profile. It has additional central nervous system effects (NMDA receptor antagonism and inhibition of serotonin and norepinephrine uptake) that may enhance recovery by attenuating the development of hyperalgesia and tolerance and improving mood state. Randomized clinical trials in patients undergoing various surgical procedures have documented that using methadone in the operating room is associated with significant reductions in postoperative analgesic requirements compared to patients administered shorter-acting intraoperative opioids. In addition, most studies also demonstrated that pain scores were significantly lower in patients given methadone. The risk of opioid-related side effects was not increased in the methadone groups in any randomized clinical investigations.

For procedures associated with higher levels of postoperative pain (major spine or open abdominal or thoracic), a dose of 20 mg at induction of anesthesia has been demonstrated to provide long-lasting analgesia with minimal risk of postoperative respiratory depression. Smaller doses (10-15 mg) have been administered in the elderly or those with limited physiologic reserve due to existent comorbidities. The careful titration of additional methadone in the PACU (3-5 mg with at least 20 minutes between doses) can further prolong the duration of postoperative analgesia. For procedures associated with moderate levels of postoperative pain (laparoscopic procedures), a dose of 10 mg before surgical incision may provide sufficient postoperative analgesia in most patients.

Most studies have used a single dose of methadone at anesthesia induction and avoided using other intraoperative opioids. The investigation by Porter et al. documented that the administration of methadone before surgery was more effective in reducing postoperative analgesic requirements than a dose given at surgical closure. Furthermore, the peak respiratory depressant effect of methadone occurs approximately 8-10 minutes after administration. When an appropriate dose is given at induction of anesthesia, the peak respiratory depressant effect occurs when the airway is controlled, and the duration of the surgery will allow sufficient time for spontaneous ventilation recovery. Due to the long half-life of methadone, there are limited data to suggest that repeat dosing is required in the operating room. If opioid-induced respiratory depression is suspected after the administration of methadone, a naloxone infusion may be required, and careful respiratory monitoring is indicated for the first 24-48 hours.

The reasons why methadone is not more commonly administered to surgical patients (outside of complex spine surgery) are uncertain. Still, they may be related to misconceptions about the agent's pharmacokinetics and duration of action, concerns about prolonged respiratory depression after its administration, or limited published literature supporting its use in the perioperative setting. Currently, most investigations have been relatively small in size and should be considered "pilot studies". Further, larger-scale, randomized trials are required to more clearly define the efficacy and safety of methadone use in the perioperative period. Data from such trials are needed before the routine use of methadone in surgical patients can be recommended. Optimal dosing regimens in various surgical procedures and appropriate use in high-risk patient populations have yet to be determined. In addition, the risk of postoperative respiratory depression, compared to shorter-acting opioids, has not been definitively established. Finally, studies to determine the potential beneficial effects of a dose of intraoperative methadone on quality of recovery variables, bowel function, and hospital length of stay in enhanced recovery after surgery protocols, as well as the development of chronic postsurgical pain, are required.

REFERENCES

1. Macrotrends. World Life Expectancy 1950-2023. [online] Available from: [https://www.macrotrends.net/countries/WLD/world/life-expectancy#:~:text=The%20life%20expectancy%20for%20World,a%200.24%25%20increase%20from%202019 [Last accessed September, 2023].
2. Jakobsson J, Johnson MZ. Perioperative regional anaesthesia and postoperative longer-term outcomes. F1000Res. 2016;5:F1000 Faculty Rev-2501.
3. Wiederhold BD, Garmon EH, Peterson E, Stevens JB, O'Rourke MC. Nerve Block Anesthesia. In: StatPearls [Internet] Treasure Island (FL): StatPearls Publishing; 2023.
4. Joshi G, Gandhi K, Shah N, Gadsden J, Corman SL. Peripheral nerve blocks in the management of postoperative pain: challenges and opportunities. J Clin Anesth. 2016;35:524-9.
5. Komen H, Brunt LM, Deych E, Blood J, Kharasch ED. Intraoperative Methadone in Same-Day Ambulatory Surgery: A Randomized, Double-Blinded, Dose-Finding Pilot Study. Anesth Analg. 2019;128(4):802-10.
6. Kharasch ED, Hoffer C, Whittington D, Sheffels P. Role of hepatic and intestinal cytochrome P450 3A and 2B6 in the metabolism, disposition, and miotic effects of methadone. Clin Pharmacol Ther. 2004;76(3):250-69.
7. Murphy GS, Szokol JW, Avram MJ, Greenberg SB, Shear TD, Deshur MA, et al. Clinical Effectiveness and Safety of Intraoperative Methadone in Patients Undergoing Posterior Spinal Fusion Surgery: A Randomized, Double-blinded, Controlled Trial. Anesthesiology. 2017;126(5):822-33.
8. Beattie WS, Badner NH, Choi PT. Meta-analysis demonstrates statistically significant reduction in postoperative myocardial infarction with the use of thoracic epidural analgesia. Anesth Analg. 2003;97(3):919-20.
9. Pöpping DM, Elia N, Marret E, Remy C, Tramèr MR. Protective effects of epidural analgesia on pulmonary complications after abdominal and thoracic surgery: a meta-analysis. Arch Surg. 2008;143(10):990-9; discussion 1000.
10. Singh N, Sidawy AN, Dezee K, Neville RF, Weiswasser J, Arora S, et al. The effects of the type of anesthesia on outcomes of lower extremity infrainguinal bypass. J Vasc Surg. 2006;44(5):964-8; discussion 968-70.
11. Wu R, Haggar F, Porte N, Eipe N, Raiche I, Neville A, et al. Assessing the feasibility of a randomised, double-blinded, placebo-controlled trial to investigate the role of intraperitoneal ropivacaine in gastric bypass surgery: a protocol. BMJ Open. 2014;4(8):e005823.

12. Agarwal R, Hecht TE, Lazo MC, Umscheid CA. Venous thromboembolism prophylaxis for patients undergoing bariatric surgery: a systematic review. Surg Obes Relat Dis. 2010;6(2):213-20.
13. Haroutiunian S, McNicol ED, Lipman AG. Methadone for chronic non-cancer pain in adults. Cochrane Database Syst Rev. 2012;11(11):CD008025.
14. McNicol ED, Ferguson MC, Schumann R. Methadone for neuropathic pain in adults. Cochrane Database Syst Rev. 2017;5(5):CD012499.
15. Nicholson AB, Watson GR, Derry S, Wiffen PJ. Methadone for cancer pain. Cochrane Database Syst Rev. 2017;2(2):CD003971.
16. Mattick RP, Breen C, Kimber J, Davoli M. Methadone maintenance therapy versus no opioid replacement therapy for opioid dependence. Cochrane Database Syst Rev. 2009;2009(3):CD002209.
17. Murphy GS, Szokol JW, Avram MJ, Greenberg SB, Marymont JH, Shear T, et al. Intraoperative Methadone for the Prevention of Postoperative Pain: A Randomized, Double-blinded Clinical Trial in Cardiac Surgical Patients. Anesthesiology. 2015;122(5):1112-22.
18. Udelsmann A, Maciel FG, Servian DC, Reis E, de Azevedo TM, Melo Mde S. Methadone and morphine during anesthesia induction for cardiac surgery. Repercussion in postoperative analgesia and prevalence of nausea and vomiting. Rev Bras Anestesiol. 2011;61(6):695-701.
19. Gottschalk A, Durieux ME, Nemergut EC. Intraoperative methadone improves postoperative pain control in patients undergoing complex spine surgery. Anesth Analg. 2011;112(1):218-23.
20. Richlin DM, Reuben SS. Postoperative pain control with methadone following lower abdominal surgery. J Clin Anesth. 1991;3(2):112-6.
21. Gourlay GK, Willis RJ, Lamberty J. A double-blind comparison of the efficacy of methadone and morphine in postoperative pain control. Anesthesiology. 1986;64(3):322-7.
22. Berde CB, Beyer JE, Bournaki MC, Levin CR, Sethna NF. Comparison of morphine and methadone for prevention of postoperative pain in 3- to 7-year-old children. J Pediatr. 1991;119(1 Pt 1):136-41.
23. Payte JT. A brief history of methadone in the treatment of opioid dependence: a personal perspective. J Psychoactive Drugs. 1991;23(2):103-7.
24. Shah S, Diwan S. Methadone: does stigma play a role as a barrier to treatment of chronic pain? Pain Physician. 2010;13(3):289-93.
25. Fishman SM, Wilsey B, Mahajan G, Molina P. Methadone reincarnated: novel clinical applications with related concerns. Pain Med. 2002;3(4):339-48.
26. Nilsson MI, Widerlöv E, Meresaar U, Anggård E. Effect of urinary pH on the disposition of methadone in man. Eur J Clin Pharmacol. 1982;22(4):337-42.
27. Garrido MJ, Tróconiz IF. Methadone: a review of its pharmacokinetic/pharmacodynamic properties. J Pharmacol Toxicol Methods. 1999;42(2):61-6.
28. Payne R, Inturrisi CE. CSF distribution of morphine, methadone and sucrose after intrathecal injection. Life Sci. 1985;37(12):1137-44.
29. Gourlay GK, Wilson PR, Glynn CJ. Pharmacodynamics and pharmacokinetics of methadone during the perioperative period. Anesthesiology. 1982;57(6):458-67.
30. Gabrielsson JL, Johansson P, Bondesson U, Paalzow LK. Analysis of methadone disposition in the pregnant rat by means of a physiological flow model. J Pharmacokinet Biopharm. 1985;13(4):355-72.

31. Sporkert F, Pragst F. Determination of methadone and its metabolites EDDP and EMDP in human hair by headspace solid-phase microextraction and gas chromatography-mass spectrometry. J Chromatogr B Biomed Sci Appl. 2000;746(2):255-64.
32. Li Y, Kantelip JP, Gerritsen-van Schieveen P, Davani S. Interindividual variability of methadone response: impact of genetic polymorphism. Mol Diagn Ther. 2008;12(2):109-24.
33. Anggård E, Gunne LM, Homstrand J, McMahon RE, Sandberg CG, Sullivan HR. Disposition of methadone in methadone maintenance. Clin Pharmacol Ther. 1975;17(3):258-66.
34. Dean M. Opioids in renal failure and dialysis patients. J Pain Symptom Manage. 2004;28(5):497-504.
35. Angst MS, Clark JD. Opioid-induced hyperalgesia: a qualitative systematic review. Anesthesiology. 2006;104(3):570-87.
36. Wojnar-Horton RE, Kristensen JH, Yapp P, Ilett KF, Dusci LJ, Hackett LP. Methadone distribution and excretion into breast milk of clients in a methadone maintenance programme. Br J Clin Pharmacol. 1997;44(6):543-7.
37. Wang EC. Methadone treatment during pregnancy. J Obstet Gynecol Neonatal Nurs. 1999;28(6):615-22.
38. Chui PT, Gin T. A double-blind randomised trial comparing postoperative analgesia after perioperative loading doses of methadone or morphine. Anaesth Intensive Care. 1992;20(1):46-51.
39. Russell T, Mitchell C, Paech MJ, Pavy T. Efficacy and safety of intraoperative intravenous methadone during general anaesthesia for caesarean delivery: a retrospective case-control study. Int J Obstet Anesth. 2013;22(1):47-51.
40. Carvalho AC, Sebold FJG, Calegari PMG, Oliveira BH, Schuelter-Trevisol F. Comparison of postoperative analgesia with methadone versus morphine in cardiac surgery. Braz J Anesthesiol. 2018;68(2):122-7.
41. Porter EJ, McQuay HJ, Bullingham RE, Weir L, Allen MC, Moore RA. Comparison of effects of intraoperative and postoperative methadone: acute tolerance to the postoperative dose? Br J Anaesth. 1983;55(4):325-32.
42. Sharma A, Tallchief D, Blood J, Kim T, London A, Kharasch ED. Perioperative pharmacokinetics of methadone in adolescents. Anesthesiology. 2011;115(6):1153-61.
43. Dunn LK, Yerra S, Fang S, Hanak MF, Leibowitz MK, Alpert SB, et al. Safety profile of intraoperative methadone for analgesia after major spine surgery: An observational study of 1,478 patients. J Opioid Manag. 2018;14(2):83-7.
44. Norris JV, Don HF. Prolonged depression of respiratory rate following methadone analgesia. Anesthesiology. 1976;45(3):361-2.
45. Alinejad S, Kazemi T, Zamani N, Hoffman RS, Mehrpour O. A systematic review of the cardiotoxicity of methadone. Excli J. 2015;14:577-600.
46. Nagele P, Pal S, Brown F, Blood J, Miller JP, Johnston J. Postoperative QT interval prolongation in patients undergoing noncardiac surgery under general anesthesia. Anesthesiology. 2012;117(2):321-8.
47. Johnston J, Pal S, Nagele P. Perioperative torsade de pointes: a systematic review of published case reports. Anesth Analg. 2013;117(3):559-64.
48. Baldo BA. Opioid analgesic drugs and serotonin toxicity (syndrome): mechanisms, animal models, and links to clinical effects. Arch Toxicol. 2018;92(8):2457-73.

49. Gourlay GK, Willis RJ, Wilson PR. Postoperative pain control with methadone: influence of supplementary methadone doses and blood concentration—response relationships. Anesthesiology. 1984;61(1):19-26.
50. Stemland CJ, Witte J, Colquhoun DA, Durieux ME, Langman LJ, Balireddy R, et al. The pharmacokinetics of methadone in adolescents undergoing posterior spinal fusion. Paediatr Anaesth. 2013;23(1):51-7.
51. Murphy GS, Szokol JW. Intraoperative methadone in surgical patients: a review of clinical investigations. Anesthesiology. 2019;131(3):678-92.
52. Kehlet H, Jensen TS, Woolf CJ. Persistent postsurgical pain: risk factors and prevention. Lancet. 2006;367(9522):1618-25.
53. Moyse DW, Kaye AD, Diaz JH, Qadri MY, Lindsay D, Pyati S. Perioperative ketamine administration for thoracotomy pain. Pain Physician. 2017;20(3):173-84.
54. McNicol ED, Schumann R, Haroutounian S. A systematic review and meta-analysis of ketamine for the prevention of persistent post-surgical pain. Acta Anaesthesiol Scand. 2014;58(10):1199-213.
55. Davis AM, Inturrisi CE. d-Methadone blocks morphine tolerance and N-methyl-D-aspartate-induced hyperalgesia. J Pharmacol Exp Ther. 1999;289(2):1048-53.
56. Sotgiu ML, Valente M, Storchi R, Caramenti G, Biella GE. Cooperative N-methyl-D-aspartate (NMDA) receptor antagonism and mu-opioid receptor agonism mediate the methadone inhibition of the spinal neuron pain-related hyperactivity in a rat model of neuropathic pain. Pharmacol Res. 2009;60(4):284-90.
57. Marmor M, Penn A, Widmer K, Levin RI, Maslansky R. Coronary artery disease and opioid use. Am J Cardiol. 2004;93(10):1295-7.
58. Schultz JJ, Hsu AK, Gross GJ. Ischemic preconditioning and morphine-induced cardioprotection involve the delta (delta)-opioid receptor in the intact rat heart. J Mol Cell Cardiol. 1997;29(8):2187-95.
59. Liang BT, Gross GJ. Direct preconditioning of cardiac myocytes via opioid receptors and KATP channels. Circ Res. 1999;84(12):1396-400.
60. Gross ER, Hsu AK, Gross GJ. Acute methadone treatment reduces myocardial infarct size via the delta-opioid receptor in rats during reperfusion. Anesth Analg. 2009;109(5):1395-402.

CHAPTER 22

Return to Intended Oncologic Therapy

Rajiv Chawla, Shagun Bhatia Shah, Uma Hariharan

ABSTRACT

Cancer is a disease in which some cells become abnormal, grow uncontrollably, and spread to other body parts through the blood and lymph systems.

The final goal of any cancer treatment is obtaining a complete cure. Establishing a complete cure requires individualized treatment, which is often multidisciplinary. Surgery is the *primary treatment* in most cases to remove as much of the cancer as possible. This is followed by adjuvant therapy which requires chemotherapy, radiotherapy, or a combination of both. In certain instances, chemotherapy or radiotherapy is given before reducing the tumor size, followed by surgery. This process is known as neoadjuvant therapy.

After cancer surgery, postoperative recovery, complications, and disability often prevent patients from receiving/resuming subsequent treatments (chemotherapy, radiotherapy). Thus, there is a disruption in the planned/intended therapy. It is opined (and observed) that the inability to complete all intended cancer therapies might negate the oncologic benefits of surgical therapy. The duration of delay in resuming the planned/intended therapy seems relevant.

Various strategies have been studied to reduce delays and facilitate *return to intended oncologic therapy* (RIOT). These include adopting minimally invasive surgery (MIS) instead of open surgery, utilizing enhanced recovery after surgery (ERAS) protocols, undertaking prehabilitation to improve and optimize the patients preoperatively, reduce rescheduling and postponement of planned cancer surgery for nonmedical reasons, and limit or avoid the use of opiates for pain relief. By adopting these techniques, quick/early recovery in the postoperative period is expected, enabling restoration of the intended therapy.

The relationship between RIOT and long-term oncologic outcomes suggests that RIOT rates can be reported as a quality indicator (QI). Further studies are underway to establish this.

Keywords: Chemotherapy; Gastric cancer; Oncologic treatment; Stomach neoplasms; Postoperative complications; Adjuvant therapy; Colorectal liver metastases; Minimally invasive surgery; Outcomes; Surgical oncology

Return to Intended Oncologic Therapy

■ KEY POINTS

- Cancer is a broad term. It describes the disease that results when cellular changes cause uncontrolled cell growth and division.
- The goal of any cancer treatment is obtaining a complete cure.
- Cancer treatment is often multimodal, requiring surgery, radiotherapy, chemotherapy, or all.
- Surgery is often the primary treatment to remove cancer cells, reducing cancer cell load. This is followed by radiotherapy or chemotherapy.
- Ideally, the treatment sequence: surgery-radiotherapy/chemotherapy should continue uninterrupted for an early cure from cancer.
- However, following surgery and radiotherapy/chemotherapy initiation, a "gap" often exists to allow for postoperative recovery. This gap tends to be variable depending upon the type of surgery: open/minimally invasive surgery (MIS), use of enhanced recovery after surgery (ERAS) protocols, postoperative complications, and rescheduling of surgery.
- The time interval between the end of surgery and the start of planned treatment for cancer is the topic of contention. The delay in returning to the intended oncological therapy has profound implications ranging from cancer recurrence, incomplete cure of cancer, increased hospital length of stay (LOS), and decreased overall survival.
- RIOT has been used as a quality indicator (QI) for cancer therapy.

> *"Anything worth doing is worth doing poorly–until you can learn to do it well."*
>
> —Zig Ziglar

■ INTRODUCTION

It was Hippocrates[1] who, in 400 BC, named the conglomeration or mass of cancerous cells *"karkinos,"* meaning "crab" in Greek. Interestingly, another Hippocratic term, *"oncos,"* also means "masses" in Greek. The World Health Organization (WHO) defines cancer[2] as "a large group of diseases that can start in almost any organ or tissue of the body when abnormal cells grow uncontrollably, go beyond their usual boundaries to invade adjoining parts of the body, and/or spread to other organs." Its synonyms include neoplasm and malignant tumor. Cancer can arise from any part of the body. Cells in the human body typically divide and grow into newer cells. When these cells grow old, they undergo cell death. Sometimes, abnormal or damaged cells grow and multiply, resulting in tumors (malignant or nonmalignant).

The origin of cancer is multifactorial,[3] and its effects can be multidimensional. Cancer is caused by genetic changes affecting the proto-oncogenes, tumor suppressor genes, and/or the DNA repair genes, which control our cell function and multiplication. Cells change from hyperplasia to

dysplasia to a precancerous state. Cancer-producing genetic changes occur due to the following:
- Errors of cell division
- DNA damage caused by harmful substances
- Inherited from parents/family.

CANCER TREATMENT

Goals of Cancer Treatment

The final aim of any oncotherapy is obtaining a complete cure for the disease.[4] The process of establishing these goals is individualized and dynamic. This is a multifaceted process with a multidisciplinary approach to ensure cancer-free survival and improved patient quality of life. The five primary goals of cancer therapy[5] include:
1. Cure
2. Prolongation of survival
3. Improvement in quality of life
4. Palliation of symptoms
5. Prevention and treatment of complication.

The determinants of the multitude of cancer treatments given rely on various aspects such as staging, cell type, patient tolerance, family support, and risk–benefit ratios.

The classification[6] of different oncological therapies can be done as follows:
- *Primary therapy:* This aims at destroying cancer cells and removing them from the body. The most common primary cancer treatment for solid tumors is surgery. For tumors that are either chemo- or radiosensitive, the patient may receive chemotherapy or radiation as the primary therapy.
- *Adjuvant therapy:* This aims at destroying any residual cancer cells to decrease the chances of recurrence. Chemotherapy, radiotherapy, and hormonal treatments can be part of adjuvant therapies. The term "neoadjuvant" is employed to describe treatment strategies before the primary therapy to increase efficacy.
- *Palliative therapy:* This addresses the adverse effects of various therapies and provides symptom control. They can be used for providing pain relief, oral care, lymphedema treatment, and chest optimization.

CANCER THERAPY OPTIONS

Treatment of cancer is multimodal, and the following are the various options[7] available for achieving the goals of cancer care:
- *Surgery:* Surgery aims to remove the cancer with a tumor-free margin.
- *Chemotherapeutic agents:* They are agents that destroy tumor cells.

- *Radiotherapy:* It also destroys tumor cells with the help of high-powered radiation beams. It can be in the form of external or internal beam radiotherapy.
- *Transplantation of the bone marrow:* This can be accomplished by using stem cells from a donor or the patient. It can be accompanied by immunosuppression as well as chemotherapeutic agents.
- *Immune treatment:* Biological therapy uses the body's immune system to fight cancer. Cancer can survive unchecked in the body because the immune system does not recognize it as an intruder. Immunotherapy can help the immune system "see" the cancer and attack it.
- *Hormone therapy:* The body's hormones fuel some types of cancer. Examples include breast cancer and prostate cancer. Removing those hormones from the body or blocking their effects may cause the cancer cells to stop growing.
- *Targeted drug therapy:* Targeted drug treatment focuses on specific abnormalities within cancer cells that allow them to survive. They are the building blocks of "precision medicine." Targeted therapies can be small-molecule drugs or monoclonal antibodies.
- *Cold-ablation therapy:* It is used to destroy cancer cells. During this, a cryoprobe is inserted into the cancer area, followed by tissue freezing and thawing. This process is repeated for cell destruction.
- *Radio-ablation:* It utilizes radiofrequency to destroy tumor cells. Cells near the needle are destroyed by the heat generated.
- Integrative medicine combines conventional/standard medical care with complementary and alternative medicine.
- Combination therapy, a treatment modality combining two or more therapeutic agents or methods, uses an amalgamation of anticancer drugs for additive or synergistic effects that target cancer-inducing or cell-sustaining pathways.

It has been found that sometimes, the vast paraphernalia of treatment options available falls short of the treatment goals as listed in abovementioned goals, even at the best of the centers. It is prudent to establish realistic goals for each cancer patient. The factors[8] influencing the choice of therapy include:
- Type and location of the cancer
- The extent of tumor spread
- Effectiveness and toxicity of available therapy
- Performance status of the patient
- Presence of symptoms
- Patient's preference.

WHAT IS "INTENDED THERAPY?"

The intention is the predecessor of the outcome, and intended therapy is the treatment plan for meeting the goal of managing any disease. In the case of cancer, the intended therapy would be to complete the course of all suggested treatment modalities for a complete cure. The earlier a cancer patient undergoes all the intended therapies, the earlier will he/she be free of cancer or obtain remission.

The term "Return to Intended Therapy" was coined by Aloia et al.[9] to understand the gaps in knowledge regarding the factors inhibiting or affecting any cancer patients' return to the suggested treatment modalities after undergoing any cancer therapy, as outlined above.

Precision Oncology: A Step Further in Intended Therapy

Precision oncology, defined as molecular profiling of tumors to identify targetable alterations, is rapidly developing and has entered the mainstream clinical practice.[10] Genomic testing involves stakeholders working in a coordinated fashion to deliver high-quality tissue samples to high-quality laboratories, where appropriate next-generation sequencing (NGS) molecular analysis leads to actionable results.[11] Clinicians should be familiar with the types of genomic variants reported by the laboratory and the technology used to determine the results, including limitations of current testing methodologies and reports. Genomic results are best interpreted with multidisciplinary input to reduce uncertainty in clinical recommendations relating to a documented variant.

Cancer Surgery: An "Intention–Action Gap" in Cancer Care[12]

Intent is the motivation or purpose behind our actions. Although our intent may be good, the outcome will not go as planned if it is not communicated well or the following behavior does not match it.

This "intention–action gap" is frequently seen in cancer treatment when combination therapy is used (**Fig. 1**). The goal of the treatment is CURE. After primary therapy (surgery), adjuvant therapy should be adopted at the earliest to eliminate the remaining cancer cells by chemotherapy or radiotherapy. However, surgery acts as a disruption/and delay to the planned management plans. In the postoperative recovery phase, the planned adjuvant therapy cannot be started immediately, and there could be delayed recovery due to postoperative complications: an ACTION GAP over good INTENTION (**Fig. 2**).

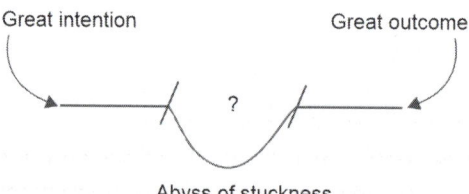

Fig. 1: The concept of "intention–action gap".

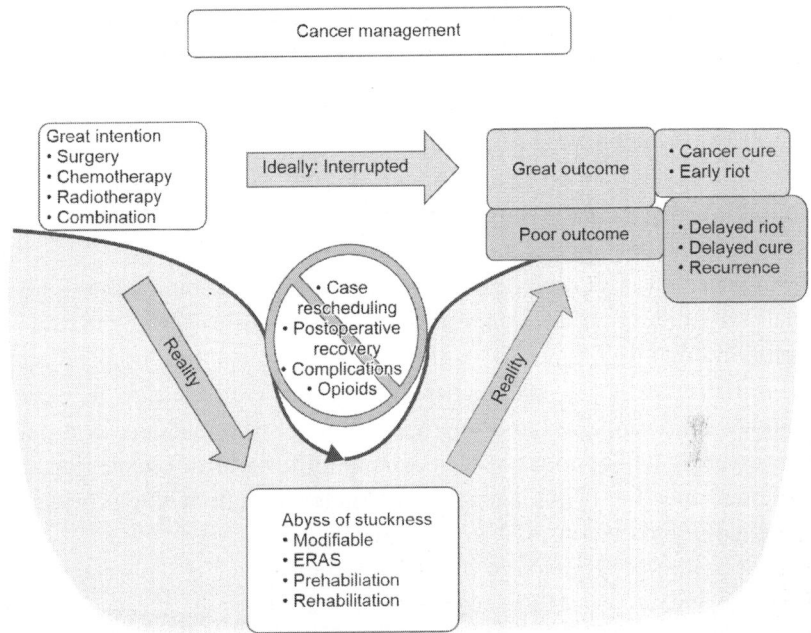

Fig. 2: "Intention–action gap" in cancer care. (ERAS: enhanced recovery after surgery)

We must pay special attention when our intent and actions do not match. The aim is to reduce this "action gap" to a minimum and restart the planned adjuvant therapy to enable early cancer cure. This phenomenon is called return to intended oncologic treatment (RIOT).

Return to Intended Oncologic Therapy : Bridging the "Intention–Action Gap" in Cancer Care

Surgery, chemotherapy, and radiotherapy comprise the three prongs of the multidisciplinary trident combating cancer. Modern cancer surgery will provide adequate tumor clearance with the lowest morbidity/invasiveness. Quality in surgery can be defined as "a surgical therapy offered to a patient for a specific condition, which cost-effectively improves the quality of life and is superior or equal to alternative nonsurgical therapies."[13] Any complications and/or general disability related to surgery that prevents patients from early RIOT may increase the risk of recurrence and partially or entirely negate the benefits of surgery **(Fig. 2)**. In this setting, the RIOT rate may serve as an essential QI for the combined oncosurgical treatment plan.

Several metrics exist to gauge the effect of oncosurgery, like 1-year mortality and 5-year survival rate. RIOT is a novel metric for evaluating the quality of oncosurgical therapy for malignancy.

The relationship between RIOT and long-term oncologic outcomes suggests that RIOT rates for both open- and MIS-approach cancer surgery should routinely be reported as a QI.[9]

Surgery: An Unavoidable Cause of Disruption in Intended Care

Surgical intervention, though regarded as the primary treatment for cancer, often disrupts the ongoing cancer treatment (chemotherapy, radiotherapy), either due to surgical complications or patient morbidity and disability. Minimally invasive cancer surgery[9] is purported to reduce the time to return to the intended oncological therapy.

Surgical complications and postoperative debility can hinder the ability of patients to undergo subsequent oncologic therapies and negate the value of surgical intervention. A new QI in surgical oncology can be envisaged in the time to RIOT. There are several challenges to quality assessment in surgical oncology, including the need for robust clinical trial evidence compared to medical oncology, inadequate coverage of long-term oncological and functional outcomes by QIs, and increasing heterogeneity of tumors impeding the development of uniform definitions of QIs.

Textbook oncologic outcome (TOO) is a comprehensive score comprising margin negative resection, appropriate lymph node assessment, no prolonged hospitalization, no 30-day readmission, no 90-day mortality, and timely administration of adjuvant chemotherapy. Being a valid hospital metric, TOO can be used to compare the overall quality of cancer care across institutions. Not only is it cumbersome, but it also does not include long-term oncological outcomes.

Cancer Recurrence and RIOT

Return to intended oncologic treatment involves postoperative treatment in chemotherapy, radiation, biological, or hormonal therapies after the surgery for specific types of malignancies. The timing of RIOT is usually 4-6 weeks after the surgical resection. When a patient undergoes a major oncological surgery and ends up with specific postoperative issues like surgical site infections (SSI), lung infection, sepsis, reexploration, paralytic ileus, etc., the hospital stay is increased, thereby delaying the discharge from the hospital. This also affects RIOT, as these patients cannot report for the proposed plan after surgery. It can also be used as a patient outcome parameter.[14] In this group of patients, recurrence is inevitable, regardless of the intraoperative anesthetic plan, as they could not undergo the adjuvant treatment due to specific unavoidable reasons. Delay in RIOT after major oncological surgeries due to medical and surgical causes and its association with a recurrence have not been validated in papers yet but is a severe issue that could solely or in association with other factors can be held responsible for recurrence. Enhanced recovery protocols by surgical teams and anesthesiologists are not enough to avoid adverse perioperative outcomes but can streamline patient management and have evidence-based protocols for better and enhanced recovery.

Return to Intended Oncologic Therapy: A Potentially Valuable End Point for Perioperative Research in Cancer Patients?[15]

Recently, initiatives such as ERAS, which minimizes surgical stress and facilitates a rapid return to normal function, have produced improved short-term outcomes (reduced LOS and complications) across various surgical procedures. *Shortened postsurgical recovery times facilitate earlier RIOT, maximizing the chances of successful treatment.* It is also postulated that reducing surgical stress and its consequent immunosuppression may reduce the likelihood of local tumor recurrence and distant metastases. Indeed, with evidence emerging for a positive correlation between RIOT rate and long-term oncological outcome in some cancers, it has been suggested that RIOT rate should be used as a quality metric for the surgical management of cancer. However, it is important to note that while evidence for the benefit of ERAS is growing, the impact on long-term mortality and disease-free survival in cancer surgery is yet to be shown conclusively.

LITERATURE REVIEW ON RIOT: EQUIVOCAL ROLE OF RIOT IN CANCER CURE AND CANCER RECURRENCE

The minimum important clinical difference for RIOT has not been identified so far and could be a function of the type of tumor, and whether any residual disease is present postsurgery. **Table 1** summarizes the impact of RIOT on overall survival, hospital LOS, and cancer recurrence in various types of cancer and the surgical interventions done. The impact of open versus MIS and the role of ERAS and anesthetic interventions like intraperitoneal ropivacaine are also informed in this table.[16-30]

PROSPECTS

Several studies have observed no association between RIOT and overall survival in ovarian cancer.[31-34] Indeed, commencing postoperative chemotherapy too early can be associated with adverse outcomes.[35-36]

Many of these studies are limited by their retrospective single-center design and inclusion of various grades and histological types of tumors. This variability raises the question of what defines the optimal interval between surgery and chemotherapy initiation. Prospective studies that randomize patients to different time intervals to provide more conclusive evidence are required. A minimum crucial clinical difference (MICD) has yet to be defined for RIOT and is likely to differ between tumors and the presence or absence

TABLE 1: Literature review on return to intended oncologic therapy (RIO⁻).

Authors (year); title	Method; sample size; patient population	Results	Remarks
Nurgalieva et al.[16] (2013) • Impact of timing of adjuvant chemotherapy (AC) initiation	• n = 14,380 • Breast cancer • Stage I–III	Patients were 1.8 times more likely to die from breast cancer when they initiated AC >3 m after surgery versus those who initiated AC <1 m after surgery	Early RIOT is advantageous in breast cancer patients
Hofstetter et al.[17] (2013) • Time interval from surgery to start of chemotherapy impacts prognosis in patients with advanced Ca ovary	• Retrospective study • Ovarian cancer • The association between RIOT interval and ensuing outcomes like disease-free and overall patient survival was studied	Early chemotherapy within 28 days of surgery (vs. delayed chemotherapy after 28 days) offered a survival benefit in patients in late stages of carcinoma ovary (hazard ratio 2.24; p value = 0.03)	Shorter RIOT interval provided survival benefit only in patients with residual tumor postsurgery
Mahner et al.[18] (2013) • Prognostic impact of the time interval between surgery and chemotherapy in advanced carcinoma ovary	• n = 3,326 • Carcinoma ovary • Individual patient data analysis of patients from three prospective randomized phase III trials conducted between 1995 and 2002 to investigate platinum–taxane-based chemotherapy regimens in advanced ovarian cancer	Early chemotherapy within 19 days of surgery provides survival benefits in patients without residual pathology; no benefit was observed in patients with residual pathology (hazard ratio 1.087; p value = 0.038)	The survival benefit results were not observed in patients with residual disease (contradicts Hofstetter et al.)

Contd...

Contd...

Authors (year): title	Method; sample size; patient population	Results	Remarks
• Aloia et al.[9] (2014) • Severe preoperative symptoms delay readiness to RIOT after liver resection	• n = 250 • Liver resection • A uniform 223-patient cohort posted for open liver metastatectomy/resection for colorectal carcinoma was compared with another cohort of 27 carcinoma liver patients who underwent minimally invasive hepatectomy	167/223 open hepatectomy patients received the planned postoperative chemotherapy/radiotherapy (RIOT rate = 75%); surgical complications (29/223 patients) and poor performance status (27/223 patients) precluded RIOT in the remaining 25% patients; high blood pressure [odds ratio (OR) 2.2, p value = 0.025], repeated chemotherapy instituted before surgery (OR 5.9, p value = 0.039), and postsurgical complications (OR 2.0, p value = 0.039) comprised the three major risk factors for failure to RIOT; reduced disease-free survival (DFS) (p value < 0.00) and overall patient survival (p = 0.005) stemmed from failure to RIOT; in contrast, 100% of minimally invasive hepatectomy patients successfully returned to intended therapy (p value = 0.038) within median 15 days versus 42 days for open surgery (p < 0.001)	The observed association between RIOT and DFS and overall patient survival suggests that RIOT rates are useful quality indicators for open as well as minimally invasive hepatectomy and hence should be consistently reported

Contd...

Contd...

Authors (year); title	Method; sample size; patient population	Results	Remarks
Tewari et al.[19] (2016) Early initiation of chemotherapy following complete resection of advanced ovarian cancer associated with improved survival: NRG oncology/ Gynecologic oncology Group study	• $n = 1,718$ • Ovarian cancer • Randomized, double-blind, placebo-controlled trial designed to study bevacizumab, in primary and maintenance therapy for patients with newly diagnosed advanced ovarian carcinoma; maximum attempt at debulking was an eligibility criterion; stage III patients, not stage IV, were required to have gross macroscopic or palpable residual disease following surgery; the survival impact of time to RIOT was studied using Cox regression models, stratified by treatment arm, residual disease and other clinical and pathologic factors	Patients were randomized, [stage III ($n = 1237$); stage IV ($n = 477$), including those with complete resection (stage IV only, $n = 81$), low-volume residual (≤ 1 cm, $n = 701$), and suboptimal (>1 cm, $n = 932$); on multivariate analysis, RIOT was predictive of overall survival (OS) ($p < 0.001$), with the complete resection group (stage IV) encountering an increased risk of death when time to initiation of chemotherapy exceeded 25 days [95% confidence interval (CI) 16.6–49.9 days]	Survival for advanced ovarian cancer may be adversely affected when RIOT occurs >25 days following surgery; results valid for stage IV only, as stage III patients with complete resection were not eligible; consistent with Gompertzian 1 kinetics where patients with microscopic residual are most vulnerable
Kim et al.[20] (2016) The impact of postoperative complications on a timely RIOT: The role of enhanced recovery in the cancer journey	• Review article • Breast cancer • Pancreatic cancer • Intraoperative ketorolac was associated with a decreased risk of breast cancer relapse versus other analgesics (sufentanil, ketamine, and clonidine) in breast cancer patients	Minimization of the physiological impact of surgery and anesthesia will prevent immune suppression and return more patients to adjuvant therapy, thereby reducing recurrence rates and prolonging survivals	Perioperative care techniques have the potential to impact cancer-specific survival (CSS)

Contd...

Authors (year): title	Method; sample size; patient population	Results	Remarks
• Timmermans et al.[21] (2018) • Interval between debulking surgery and adjuvant chemotherapy is associated with overall survival in patients with advanced ovarian cancer	• n = 4,097 • Ovarian cancer • Patients who received optimal/complete debulking surgery for primary Ca ovary (FIGO IIb–IV; 2008–2015) time to chemotherapy (TTC) was divided into three groups based on the interquartile range (IQR) [early (<25%)]; prolonged (>75%); intermediate TTC (25–75%); logistic regression was used to identify factors associated with a prolonged TTC and multivariable Cox regression to evaluate the independent effect of treatment interval on OS; primary debulking surgery (PDS) and interval debulking surgery (IDS) patients were analyzed separately	1,612 underwent PDS and 2,485 IDS; median TTC was 29 days; age ≥65, complete debulking surgery, postoperative complications (POC), and hospitalization ≥10 days were independently associated with a longer TTC for both PDS and IDS. TTC in the longest quartile was associated with poor OS after both PDS [hazard rate (HR) 1.43, 95% CI 1.09–1.88] and NACT-IDS [HR 1.22 (1.02–1.47)] when compared to the intermediate TTC, but only in patients with no macroscopic residual disease after surgery	Prolonged RIOT is an independent prognostic factor for worse OS after complete (interval) debulking surgery; advisable to start AC within 5–6 weeks after debulking surgery

Authors (year); title	Method; sample size; patient population	Results	Remarks
Lillemoe et al.[22] (2019) Detours on the road to recovery: What factors delay readiness to RIOT after liver resection for malignancy?	• n = 114 • Hepatic carcinoma • A prospectively maintained database was queried to identify data on consecutive hepatectomy patients for carcinoma liver and was retrieved from a database prospectively over 2 years; perioperative factors were compared between patients with early (≤28 postoperative days) vs. delayed (>28 postoperative days) clearance to RIOT; univariate analysis and multivariable logistic regression were performed	76 patients (67%) had an open surgical approach, 32 (28%) had a major hepatectomy, and 6 (5%) had a major complication, with no mortalities; 82 patients (72%) had early, while 32 patients (28%) had delayed RIOT readiness; patients with high preoperative symptom burden were more likely to have delayed RIOT readiness (OR 3.1, 95% CI 1.1–8.4, $p = 0.024$); on multivariable analysis, open surgical approach (OR 6.9, $p = 0.018$), length of stay (LOS) >5 days (OR 3.6, $p = 0.010$), any complication (OR 3.4, $p = 0.033$) postoperative nutritional and wound-healing parameters were associated with delayed RIOT readiness	This study highlights the importance of preoperative patient symptom burden on delayed postoperative recovery; as a cancer patient's RIOT after hepatectomy has a substantial impact on survival, it is critical to adhere to ERAS
Hayden et al.[23] (2020) Intraperitoneal ropivacaine reduces time to initiation of chemotherapy after surgery for advanced ovarian cancer	• n = 40 • Ovarian cancer • Prospective, double-blind, randomized, controlled • Open abdominal cytoreductive surgery patients were randomized to receive either intraperitoneal ropivacaine or saline; intraoperatively, ropivacaine 2 mg/mL or 0.9% saline was injected thrice intraperitoneally, and after operation via a catheter and analgesic pump into the peritoneal cavity for 72 hours	No ropivacaine-related complications recorded; pain intensity and rescue analgesic requirement was similar between groups; time to initiation of chemotherapy was significantly shorter in ropivacaine group (median 21 vs. 29 days; $p = 0.021$); time to home readiness, hospital discharge and incidence, and complexity of POC were similar between the groups	Intraperitoneal ropivacaine during and for 72 hours after cytoreductive surgery for ovarian cancer is safe and reduces the time interval to RIOT

Contd...

Authors (year); title	Method; sample size; patient population	Results	Remarks
• Tian et al.[25] (2020) • Short- and long-term outcomes associated with enhanced recovery after surgery protocol vs conventional management in patients undergoing laparoscopic gastrectomy	• n = 80 • Radical gastrectomy • Patients in the perioperative period with radical gastrectomy were enrolled and randomly divided into two groups: The ERAS group and the non-ERAS group; the differences between the two groups in terms of postoperative recoveries and complications rate were determined • According to the body mass index (BMI) level, the ERAS group was divided into two subgroups, namely, group A (BMI <28 kg/m², n = 16) and group B (BMI ≥28 kg/m², n = 24); the non-ERAS group was also divided into group C (BMI <28 kg/m², n = 18) and group D (BMI ≥28 kg/m², n = 22); the recovery and complications of each group were then determined	The postoperative LOS and visual analog scale pain score were less in the ERAS group than the non-ERAS group ($p < 0.05$); time to first postoperative exhaustion, first postoperative defecation, returning leukocyte count to normal, and stopping intravenous nutrition were significantly shorter in the ERAS group (n = 40), compared to the non-ERAS group (n = 40, all $p < 0.05$); the incidence of postoperative lower extremity intramuscular venous thrombosis was significantly higher in group D than in group B ($\chi^2 = 4.800$, $p = 0.028$); in addition, the incidence of lower extremity intermuscular venous thrombosis and lung infection in group D was higher than those in other groups	The perioperative ERAS program was associated with faster recovery in patients undergoing radical gastrectomy; for patients with higher BMI (BMI ≥28 kg/m²), the use of the perioperative ERAS program was more advantageous

Contd...

Authors (year): title	Method; sample size; patient population	Results	Remarks
• Ramos et al.[24] (2020) • Return to intended oncologic treatment in resected gastric cancer patients	• n = 313 • Retrospective study • Gastric cancer (GC) • Stage II/III GC patients treated with potentially curative gastrectomy; patients who could RIOT group and those who could not (inability to RIOT group) were analyzed	89 (28.4%) and 85 (27.2%) patients receive CRT and chemotherapy, respectively, representing a RIOT rate of 55.6%; reasons for inability to RIOT: General poor performance status (30.2%); surgical POC (20.1%); older age, higher ASA, D1 lymphadenectomy. Older age, neutrophil–lymphocyte ratio (NLR), and major POC were independent risk factors for inability to RIOT; 5-year DFS ($p = 0.008$) and OS ($p = 0.004$) were worse for the inability to RIOT group; absence of neoadjuvant therapy, total gastrectomy, pT3/T4, pN+, and inability to RIOT were associated with worse DFS; type of gastrectomy, lymphadenectomy, pN status, Rx resection, and RIOT group were associated with OS	Older age, high NLR, and major postoperative complications were risk factors for inability to RIOT; RIOT was an independent predictor of survival

Contd...

Authors (year); title	Method; sample size; patient population	Results	Remarks
• Yang et al.[26] (2020) • The effect of perioperative ERAS pathway management on short- and long-term outcomes of gastric cancer patients	• $n = 2,124$ • Single institute • Retrospective cohort study • All patients were pathologically proved to be gastric adenocarcinoma, and underwent standard radical gastrectomy with D2 lymphadenectomy during the period of 2007–2012; patients divided into ERAS and non-ERAS groups according to the different perioperative pathway protocol; propensity score matching method was used to balance the baseline characteristics; two groups were matched in a 1:1 ratio after matched; 521 cases per group after matched; the short-term clinical outcomes (POC, length of hospital stay, blood loss, 30-day readmission rate, etc.) and overall, 5-year survival rates were compared between the two groups	The incidence of overall POC was similar between the two groups (ERAS = 18.4%, non-ERAS = 19.4%, $p = 0.69$), including anastomotic leakage, abdominal hemorrhage; incidence of SSI, atelectasis, and venous thromboembolism in ERAS group was significantly lower than that in non-ERAS group; the number of lymph node harvested, operation time, intraoperative blood loss, and postoperative hospital cost in ERAS group were better than those in non-ERAS group; there were no significant differences in unplanned reoperation (ERAS = 3.1%, non-ERAS = 2.1%, $p = 0.33$), 30-day readmission rate (ERAS = 6.1%, non-ERAS = 5.6%, $p = 0.69$) and postoperative mortality (ERAS = 0.4%, non-ERAS = 0.2%, $p = 0.56$) between the two groups; the 5-year OS rates of non-ERAS and ERAS groups were 66.2% and 72.8% respectively ($p = 0.007$); on subgroup analysis, 5-year OS rates of stage I were 93.4 and 92.7% ($p = 0.73$), those of stage II and III were 82.2 vs. 75.2% ($p = 0.007$) and 47.6 vs. 35.7% ($p = 0.02$) in ERAS and non-ERAS group respectively	Perioperative ERAS pathway management is safe and feasible for patients with GC, without increasing the incidence of complications and 30-day readmission rate; this protocol can improve the prognosis of patients with GC

Contd...

Contd...

Authors (year); title	Method; sample size; patient population	Results	Remarks
Garcia-Nebreda et al.[27] (2022) Early return to RIOT after implementation of an ERAS pathway for GC surgery	• n = 70 • Gastric adenocarcinoma • Underwent surgery from January 2016 to 2021; (35 in pre-ERAS period and 35 in post-ERAS period)	14 of the pre-ERAS and 22 patients of the post-ERAS period received adjuvant therapy; time to RIOT was reduced in the post-ERAS period (median 39 days, IQR 31–49) by 12 days (95% CI 3–14 days, $p=0.01$) versus the pre-ERAS period (median 51 days, IQR 42–62); LOS was lower in the ERAS group (6 days, IQR 5–11 vs. 10 days, IQR 8–13, $p < 0.01$)	ERAS pathway for GC surgery was associated with earlier RIOT and shorter LOS
Kiong et al.[28] (2022) Enhanced recovery after surgery (ERAS) in head and neck oncologic surgery: Impact on RIOT and survival	• n = 200 • Head and neck oncosurgery patients on an ERAS pathway between March 1, 2016 and March 31, 2019 were matched to controls over the same interval; demographic, tumor-, and adjuvant therapy-related data were collected, including time to adjuvant therapy (TAT) and treatment package time (TPT); risk factors for TAT >42 days and TPT ≥85 days were assessed; OS was compared and risk factors for inferior OS determined	Baseline characteristics, comorbidities and tumor stage were similar; of 179 patients planned for adjuvant treatment, there was no difference in RIOT rate (89.0 vs. 87.5%, $p = 0.753$), proportion of TAT >42 days of surgery (55.6 vs. 59.7%, $p = 0.642$), or TPT ≥85 days (48.1 vs. 57.1%, $p = 0.258$), for the ERAS and control groups, respectively; alcohol use (OR 3.58) and recurrent disease status (OR 2.88) were independently associated with prolonged TAT; 3-year OS was similar between the ERAS and control groups (73 vs. 76%, $p = 0.521$)	ERAS protocol as practiced by the authors has not shown to hasten RIOT or reduce OS in head–neck oncosurgery

Contd...

Contd...

Authors (year): title	Method; sample size; patient population	Results	Remarks
• Li et al.[29] (2023) • The efficacy and timing of adjuvant chemotherapy in upper tract urothelial carcinoma	• n = 428 • Retrospective • Upper tract urothelial carcinoma (UTUC) • Patients with postoperatively confirmed pathological stages, muscle-invasive or greater-stage (pT2–4) disease, any nodal status, and metastasis-free (M0) disease were analyzed • Patients receiving AC were divided into the "<45 days" and "45–90 days" groups according to the time interval between surgery and AC initiation	• 132 patients underwent AC with platinum+ gemcitabine within 90 days after Sx, and 296 patients failed to initiate AC within 90 days • Median age = 68 years • Median follow-up = 25 months • No significant intergroup differences in age, sex, lymph node metastasis, tumor location, hydronephrosis, hematuria, or cancer grade • Patients undergoing AC initiated within 90 days of Sx showed a significantly ↓ mortality relative to patients who did not receive AC; shorter intervals between Sx and AC initiation <45 days versus 45–90 days did not improve patient OS and CSS and may have increased the incidence of adverse events	A platinum–gemcitabine regimen started postoperatively significantly improved OS and CSS in patients with UTUC at stages ≥pT2 (N0–3M0); no survival benefit seen in patients who started AC within 45 days post-Sx versus those who received AC within 45–90 days

Contd...

Contd...

Authors (year); title	Method; sample size; patient population	Results	Remarks
Thomas et al.[30] (2023) Enhanced recovery pathway in open and minimally invasive colorectal cancer surgery: A prospective study on feasibility, compliance, and outcomes in a high-volume resource limited tertiary cancer center	• n = 937 • Prospective observational audit of colorectal cancer surgery conducted from 2014 to 2019; compliance to ERAS protocol and its elements was recorded; impact of quantum of compliance (≥80 vs. <80%) to ERAS on postoperative morbidity, mortality, readmission, stay, reexploration, functional GI recovery, surgical-specific complications, and RIOT was evaluated for open and minimal invasive surgery (MIS)	Overall compliance with ERP was 73.3%; >80% compliance was observed in 332 (35.4%) patients in the entire cohort; patients with <80% compliance had significantly higher overall, minor and surgery-specific complications, longer postoperative stay, delayed functional gastrointestinal (GI) recovery for both open and MIS procedures; RIOT was observed in 96.5% patients; duration to RIOT was significantly shorter following open surgery with ≥80% compliance; compliance <80% was an independent predictor for POC	Beneficial impact of ↑ compliance to ERAS on postoperative outcomes after open and MIS for colorectal cancer seen; in a resource-limited setting, ERAS is feasible, safe, effective in both open and MIS for colorectal cancer

(ASA: American Society of Anesthesiologists; CRT: chemoradiotherapy; ERP: enhanced recovery program; NACT: neoadjuvant chemotherapy; SSI: surgical site infections) of residual disease. Varying definitions of early chemotherapy (15 days to 12 weeks postsurgery) by different studies detract from their comparability. This lack of agreement over what constitutes early chemotherapy adds to the complexity of determining if a short RIOT interval is clinically relevant in terms of overall or even disease-free survival. Future studies could focus on whether programs such as prehabilitation, including preoperative exercise training, nutrition, and psychological support, can influence RIOT.[14]

LIMITATIONS OF RETURN TO INTENDED ONCOLOGIC THERAPY

Various limitations of RIOT have been reported in clinical trials conducted to examine the impact of perioperative interventions. It needs to provide more information on whether the patient could tolerate only limited doses of chemotherapy, if further treatment was abandoned or postponed, or if a dose reduction was required, all of which regularly occur in clinical practice. Reduction in the intended chemotherapeutic dose and delays in further doses may also have a deleterious impact on overall survival, data not captured by the RIOT interval alone.

CONCLUSION

Return to intended oncologic therapy has emerged as a potentially viable parameter to benchmark postoperative recovery after cancer surgery. Time-to-surgery (TTS) after completion of neoadjuvant chemotherapy (NACT) and RIOT postoncosurgery are essential indicators of outcome in cancer care. Initially evaluated in hepatic resections for cancer, the inability to RIOT after surgery correlated with shorter disease-free and overall survival. RIOT may be viewed as a valid short-term surrogate marker of recovery after surgery, but its correlation with overall survival remains uncertain.

REFERENCES

1. Papavramidou N, Papavramidis T, Demetriou T. Ancient Greek and Greco-Roman methods in modern surgical treatment of cancer. Ann Surg Oncol. 2010;17(3):665-7.
2. Hausman DM. What Is Cancer? Perspect Biol Med. 2019;62(4):778-84.
3. Hanselmann RG, Welter C. Origin of cancer: an information, energy, and matter disease. Front Cell Dev Biol. 2016;4:1-12.
4. Balis FM. The goal of cancer treatment. Oncologist. 1998;3(4):210.
5. Khan FA, Akhtar SS, Sheikh MK. Cancer treatment—objectives and quality of life issues. Malays J Med Sci. 2005;12(1):3-5.
6. Debela DT, Muzazu SG, Heraro KD, Ndalama MT, Mesele BW, Haile DC, et al. New approaches and procedures for cancer treatment: current perspectives. SAGE Open Med. 2021;9:1-10.
7. Arruebo M, Vilaboa N, Sáez-Gutierrez B, Lambea J, Tres A, Valladares M, et al. Assessment of the evolution of cancer treatment therapies. Cancers (Basel). 2011;3(3):3279-330.

8. Kiebert GM, Stiggelbout AM, Kievit J, Leer JW, van de Velde CJ, de Haes HJ. Choices in oncology: factors that influence patients' treatment preference. Qual Life Res. 1994;3(3):175-82.
9. Aloia TA, Zimmitti G, Conrad C, Gottumukalla V, Kopetz S, Vauthey JN. Return to intended oncologic treatment (RIOT): a novel metric for evaluating the quality of oncosurgical therapy for malignancy. J Surg Oncol. 2014;110(2):107-14.
10. Lu CY, Terry V, Thomas DM. Precision medicine: affording the successes of science. NPJ Precis Onc. 2023;7(3):1-8.
11. Schwartzberg L, Kim ES, Liu D, Schrag D. Precision Oncology: Who, How, What, When, and When Not? Am Soc Clin Oncol Educ Book. 2017;37:160-9.
12. Andrew. (2010). Closing the intention-action gap. [online] Available from: https://itsunderstood.com/2010/09/closing-the-intention-action-gap/ [Last accessed September, 2023].
13. Clavien PA. Targeting quality in surgery. Ann Surg. 2013;258:659-68.
14. Finnerty DT, Buggy DJ. Return to intended oncologic therapy: a potentially valuable endpoint for perioperative research in cancer patients? Br J Anaesth. 2020;124:508-10.
15. Evans MT, Wigmore T, Kelliher LJS. The impact of anaesthetic technique upon outcome in oncological surgery. BJA Educ. 2019;19(1):14-20.
16. Nurgalieva ZZ, Franzini L, Morgan RO, Vernon SW, Liu CC, Du XL. Impact of timing of adjuvant chemotherapy initiation and completion after surgery on racial disparities in survival among women with breast cancer. Med Oncol. 2013;30:1-9.
17. Hofstetter G, Concin N, Braicu I, Chekerov R, Sehouli J, Cadron I, et al. The time interval from surgery to start of chemotherapy significantly impacts prognosis in patients with advanced serous ovarian carcinoma—analysis of patient data in the prospective OVCAD study. Gynecol Oncol. 2013;131(1):15-20.
18. Mahner S, Eulenburg C, Staehle A, Wegscheider K, Reuss A, Pujade-Lauraine E, et al. Prognostic impact of the time interval between surgery and chemotherapy in advanced ovarian cancer: analysis of prospective randomised phase III trials. Eur J Cancer. 2013;49(1):142-9.
19. Tewari KS, Java JJ, Eskander RN, Monk BJ, Burger RA. Early initiation of chemotherapy following complete resection of advanced ovarian cancer associated with improved survival: NRG Oncology/Gynecologic Oncology Group study. Ann Oncol. 2016;27(1):114-21.
20. Kim BJ, Caudle AS, Gottumukkala V, Aloia TA. The impact of postoperative complications on a timely return to intended oncologic therapy (RIOT): the role of enhanced recovery in the cancer journey. Int Anesthesiol Clin. 2016;54:33-46.
21. Timmermans M, van der Aa MA, Lalisang RI, Witteveen PO, Van de Vijver KK, Kruitwagen RF, et al. Interval between debulking surgery and adjuvant chemotherapy is associated with overall survival in patients with advanced ovarian cancer. Gynecol Oncol. 2018;150(3):446-50.
22. Lillemoe HA, Marcus RK, Kim BJ, Narula N, Davis CH, Aloia TA. Detours on the Road to Recovery: What Factors Delay Readiness to Return to Intended Oncologic Therapy (RIOT) After Liver Resection for Malignancy? J Gastrointest Surg. 2019;23(12):2362-71.
23. Hayden JM, Oras J, Block L, Thörn SE, Palmqvist C, Salehi S, et al. Intraperitoneal ropivacaine reduces time interval to initiation of chemotherapy after surgery for

advanced ovarian cancer: randomised controlled double-blind pilot study. Br J Anaesth. 2020;124(5):562-70.
24. Ramos MFKP, de Castria TB, Pereira MA, Dias AR, Antonacio FF, Zilberstein B, et al. Return to intended oncologic treatment (RIOT) in resected gastric cancer patients. J Gastrointest Surg. 2020;24:19-27.
25. Tian YL, Cao SG, Liu XD, Li ZQ, Liu G, Zhang XQ, et al. Short- and long-term outcomes associated with enhanced recovery after surgery protocol vs conventional management in patients undergoing laparoscopic gastrectomy. World J Gastroenterol. 2020;26:5646-60.
26. Yang FZ, Wang H, Wang DS, Niu ZJ, Li SK, Zhang J, et al. The effect of perioperative ERAS pathway management on short-and long-term outcomes of gastric cancer patients. Zhonghua Yi Xue Za Zhi. 2020;100:922-7.
27. Garcia-Nebreda M, Zorrilla-Vaca A, Ripollés-Melchor J, Abad-Motos A, Alvaro Cifuentes E, Abad-Gurumeta A, et al. Early return to intended oncologic therapy after implementation of an enhanced recovery after surgery pathway for gastric cancer surgery. Langenbecks Arch Surg. 2022;407(6):2293-300.
28. Kiong KL, Moreno A, Vu CN, Zheng G, Rosenthal DI, Weber RS, et al. Enhanced recovery after surgery (ERAS) in head and neck oncologic surgery: Impact on return to intended oncologic therapy (RIOT) and survival. Oral Oncol. 2022;130:1-8.
29. Li H, Zhou J, Chen R, Zhu J, Wang J, Wen R. The efficacy and timing of adjuvant chemotherapy in upper tract urothelial carcinoma. Urol Oncol. 2023;41(8):3561-9.
30. Thomas M, Agarwal V, DeSouza A, Joshi R, Mali M, Panhale K, et al. Enhanced recovery pathway in open and minimally invasive colorectal cancer surgery: a prospective study on feasibility, compliance, and outcomes in a high-volume resource limited tertiary cancer center. Langenbecks Arch Surg. 2023;408(1):99-118.
31. Rosa DD, Clamp A, Mullamitha S, Ton NC, Lau S, Byrd L, et al. The interval from surgery to chemotherapy in the treatment of advanced epithelial ovarian carcinoma. Eur J Surg Oncol. 2006;32:588-91.
32. Gadducci A, Sartori E, Landoni F, Zola P, Maggino T, Maggioni A, et al. Relationship between time interval from primary surgery to the start of taxane-plus platinum-based chemotherapy and clinical outcome of patients with advanced epithelial ovarian cancer: results of a multicenter retrospective Italian study. J Clin Oncol. 2005;23(4):751-8.
33. Aletti GD, Long HJ, Podratz KC, Cliby WA. Is time to chemotherapy a determinant of prognosis in advanced-stage ovarian cancer? Gynecol Oncol. 2007;104:212-6.
34. Paulsen T, Kaern J, Kaerheim K, Haldorsen T, Tropé C. Influence of interval between primary surgery and chemotherapy on short-term survival of patients with advanced ovarian, tubal or peritoneal cancer. Gynecol Oncol. 2006;102:447-52.
35. Flynn PM, Paul J, Cruickshank DJ; Scottish Gynaecological Cancer Trials Group. Does the interval from primary surgery to chemotherapy influence progression-free survival in ovarian cancer? Gynecol Oncol. 2002;86:354-7.
36. Sorbe B. Prognostic importance of the time interval from surgery to chemotherapy in treatment of ovarian carcinoma. Int J Gynecol Cancer. 2004;14:788-93.

CHAPTER 23

Nontechnical Skills in Anesthesiology

Pradeep Bhatia, Swati Chhabra

ABSTRACT

The aviation sector was the first to adopt training in nontechnical skills. In health care, anesthesiology was the first specialty to derive inspiration from the aviation sector. While many frameworks for nontechnical skills are available, a precise set of skills should be designed to cater to individual specialties and customized according to clinical tasks, workplace, and organizational environment. Training in nontechnical skills aims at the behavioral conditioning of the personnel to equip them with skills to prevent and manage errors. The anaesthetist's non-technical skills (ANTS) framework includes four main components: situation awareness, decision-making, teamwork, and task management. Many tools are available for measuring nontechnical skills in simulation or real-life scenarios. The anesthesia training curriculum should include nontechnical skills training, and the competency-based evaluation comprises all three paradigms, namely, medical knowledge and technical and nontechnical skills.

Keywords: Nontechnical skills; Anesthesia; Human factors; Situation awareness; Teamwork

■ KEY POINTS

- Anesthesia adopted nontechnical skills training from the aviation sector.
- Nontechnical skills aim at preventing and managing errors efficiently.
- The four essential components of the anaesthetist's non-technical skills (ANTS) framework are: (1) Situation awareness, (2) decision-making, (3) teamwork, and (4) task management.
- Many tools are available for measuring nontechnical skills in simulation or real-life scenarios.
- The anesthesia training curriculum should include nontechnical skills training, and the competency-based evaluation comprises all three paradigms, namely medical knowledge, technical and nontechnical skills.

INTRODUCTION

Nontechnical skills are a set of skills in the cognitive, social, and personal domains which, in conjunction with technical skills, lead to improved outcomes from the task at hand.[1] The aviation sector first adopted nontechnical skills. These were later incorporated into the training and workflow of other settings like the military, mining, and nuclear power plants, where errors and accidents could have dire consequences. For obvious reasons, the principles of nontechnical skills were adopted into health care and more so into specialties like anesthesiology, where crisis management is an inherent part of the practice. The majority of anesthesia-related adverse events, upon investigation, have been attributed to human errors like poor team dynamics, inadequate monitoring, suboptimal drug and equipment checks.[2,3] This created the need to adopt nontechnical skills and technical skills. Nontechnical skills are situational awareness, teamwork, decision-making, leadership, and stress management. Their adoption greatly enhances the technical skills for better task performance with lesser errors. Globally, the training and evaluation of nontechnical skills have been a part of the anesthesia curriculum, which complements the technical skills for improved patient safety. However, compliance varies, and the barriers are discussed later.

HISTORY OF NONTECHNICAL SKILLS

The aviation sector was the first to adopt training in nontechnical skills. In the 1970s, upon investigation, there were multiple aviation accidents that were found to be due to errors by pilots. This led to the conceptual development of Cockpit Resource Management Training with the aim of safer and more efficient flight services. Integrating all the involved resources, i.e., information, equipment, and personnel (pilots, cabin crew, ground staff, maintenance staff, dispatch crew), was the central concept behind an evolving program known as the crew resource management (CRM).[4] Over the years CRM has formulated NOTECHS, a system to measure the nontechnical skills of teams at their actual workplace rather than in a classroom setting.[5]

In health care, anesthesiology was the first specialty to derive inspiration from CRM. In 1990, Gaba et al. were the first to introduce anesthesia crisis resource management (ACRM). The principles gradually spread to other acute care settings like emergency medicine, critical care, neonatology, and even lesser acute care areas like wards.[6] While many frameworks for nontechnical skills are available, a precise set of skills should cater to individual specialties and customize according to clinical tasks, workplace, and organizational environment. Over the years, healthcare setups have adopted training and assessment modules for training and assessment of nontechnical skills in anesthesia, e.g., ANTS system and ACRM.[7]

PURPOSE OF NONTECHNICAL SKILLS

Training in nontechnical skills aims at the behavioral conditioning of the personnel to equip them with skills to prevent and manage errors. Error prevention and mitigation (upon error occurrence) would result in less damaging consequences. Robust skills, technical and nontechnical, help in efficient error management. Each system has inherent defense layers, which, in ideal conditions, should be foolproof. However, there could be dynamic holes in one or more layers of defense. The holes signify system deficiencies or active errors. Any action through these holes in one or two layers will not be hazardous if the other layers are intact. There could be adverse consequences in outcomes if these holes align. This has been popularly described with a Swiss cheese model of system accidents.[8]

The primary purpose of nontechnical skills in health care is to fill in as many holes in the defense layers of clinical practice while being beneficial to both the patient and the clinician.

APPLICATION OF NONTECHNICAL SKILLS IN ANESTHESIOLOGY

The ANTS framework includes four main components: (1) Situation awareness, (2) decision-making, (3) teamwork, and (4) task management.[9,10] These four components can be nested under cognitive or interpersonal skills and further categorized into elements for ease of training and evaluation **(Figs. 1 and 2)**. Other components such as communication, leadership/followership, and stress management are encompassed in the teamwork frame.[11] The application of nontechnical skills should not be reserved for a particular or demanding circumstance but should be followed daily, with consistency being the key. Conventionally, the components of nontechnical skills were said to be inherent to one's personality, which defined an anesthesiologist as a class apart from being an alert person or a team person. However, with the progress in behavioral sciences, we now know that the attributes can be taught and assessed objectively. Developing and maintaining good technical

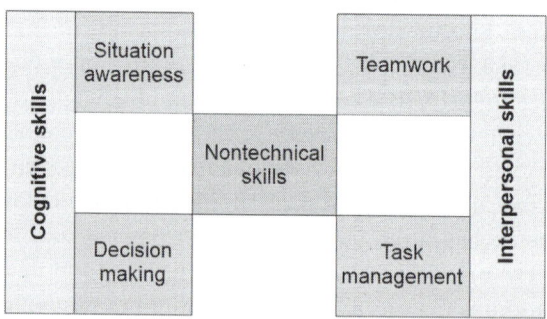

Fig. 1: The anaesthetist's non-technical skills (ANTS) system.

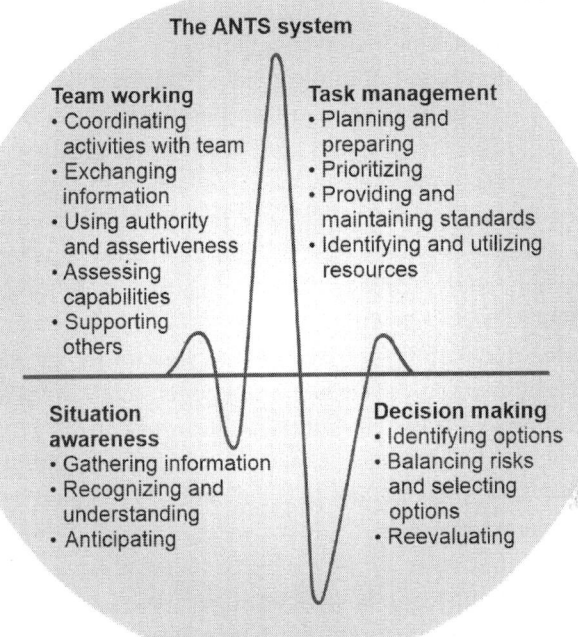

Fig. 2: Elements of anaesthetist's non-technical skills (ANTS) framework.
Source: Reproduced with permission from Flin et al.[9]

skills would free up mental space for learning nontechnical skills. Integrating the two sets of skills is scalable and results in safer and more effective patient care.

Situation Awareness

Situation awareness is the act of being aware of what is happening and involves thinking about what has happened and what is happening and thinking ahead. It involves gathering specific information by observing and continuously monitoring the work environment. This will help create a mental picture and to interpret if it is appropriate and expected for the current clinical scenario. Continuous monitoring will help update the mental picture and make a call for intervention (or omission of an intervention). Anticipating problems will help keep ahead in the event of adverse happenings and result in better patient outcomes. Thus, gathering information, recognizing, and anticipating are the three elements of situation awareness. The team leaders or team members can adopt different strategies to learn and practice the skill of situation awareness by adopting the principles of leadership and followership.[12] The team leader should lead a team briefing session which should be focused and inclusive.

Decision-making

The skill of decision-making involves diagnosing a situation and selecting the best course of action based on the clinical scenario, resources, knowledge, and technical skills. The three elements are identifying the options, balancing risk while selecting an option, and reevaluating and recourse if necessary. These are important in both electives as well as crises. Aviation uses a set sequence for decision-making with the help of tools like T-DODAR for in-flight decisions.[13] These are time at hand to decide (T); diagnosis of the problem (D); options (O) with their benefits, risks, and alternatives; decision (D); assignment of task (A); and review (R).

The nontechnical skill of decision-making can be supplemented by a clinical decision support system (CDSS) which might help in enhancing medical decisions with focused interpretation of clinical knowledge and patient information.[14] These systems are computerized programs that provide suggestions to the clinician at the point of care. These could be knowledge-based or non-knowledge-based. The knowledge-based CDSS generates rules on an "if-then" pattern and is directed by the literature, practice protocols, or patients. The non-knowledge-based CDSS collects data processed by artificial intelligence, machine learning, or pattern recognition. Cognitive aids, algorithms, and checklists can also be instrumental in decision-making.[15]

Teamwork

Anesthesia practice involves working in teams, and effective teamwork has five elements: (1) Coordination, (2) communication, (3) role adoption (leadership and followership) and graded assertiveness, (4) capability assessment, and (5) provision of support.[1,9] Coordination is essential to carry out the required technical and cognitive tasks. Communication is a way of exchanging information and is instrumental in better team coordination and task completion in routine and critical event scenarios. Closed-loop communication and standardized handover tools like SBAR (situation, background, assessment, recommendation) and SNAPPI (stop, notify, assessment, plan, prioritize, invite ideas)[16-18] have been recommended for seamless communication amongst the teams. The organizational culture and teams should work toward flattening the hierarchy since a steep team hierarchy could be detrimental to team coordination and communication, especially in a crisis.[19] For better team dynamics, some degree of authority gradient (hierarchy) is essential, and teams could utilize graded assertiveness tools to communicate when there is a risk to patient safety.[20]

Communication

Communication is an essential element of teamwork. Multiple strategies have been studied to find practical and effective ways of communication.

Systematized communication amongst the team members enhances teamwork. Calling a colleague by their first name (or as culturally acceptable) and making eye contact while communicating is as important as the message itself. The same can be applied while communicating with the patient and the family. Communication should be well structured by prioritizing critical information or adopting tools like SBAR and SNAPPI. Abbreviations and informal languages should not be used. Repetition can be done when appropriate to convey the message. For example, a bad example would be, *"umm...give 50 mics fenta, there is tachy"*. This information can be effectively shared as, "Neha, give 50, five zero micrograms of injection fentanyl intravenously, for the tachycardia". Additionally, the emphasis should be on the clarity, appropriate speed, and tone of the language. Thereafter, closed-loop communication would ensure that the correct message has been received (*"Sure, will draw 50 micrograms, five zero, of fentanyl for intravenous injection"*) and executed (*"50 micrograms of fentanyl given intravenously"*).

Task Management

These skills involve organizing the available resources and requisite activities to achieve a set goal for the task at hand. The four elements of effective task management are planning and preparing ahead, identifying and prioritizing the key points, maintaining standards of practice, and identifying and utilizing the available resources (requesting more resources, if needed).[9] Developing a primary plan, "plan B" strategies, and reviewing or updating the plan as required is a prerequisite for effective task management. Prioritizing time-sensitive issues and avoiding distractions will be beneficial, especially in crises. Adherence to good practices based on available evidence and guidelines ensures anesthetic care safety and quality. Judicious use of resources and adoption of all the components of nontechnical skills help in successful task completion and avoids stress and burnout in the team.

■ TRAINING IN NONTECHNICAL SKILLS

Organizations, trainers, and trainees should acknowledge that nontechnical skills are as necessary as clinical knowledge and technical skills. Training in nontechnical skills has been incorporated into the anesthesia curriculum. However, it must still be followed in letter and spirit in many places.[21]

Various propriety and free-to-use training programs in nontechnical skills are available, like ANTS, ACRM, MedTeams, and TeamStepps.[22-24] The training could be seminar-based, workshop-based, simulation-based, or at the bedside. It is still being determined if one form of training is better than the other. Training should be continuous, intensive, and spaced throughout the career. Additionally, there should be periodic evaluations of the program.

Nevertheless, training just the anesthesiologists in nontechnical skills would not result in the betterment of the system. Health care involves multiple teams working together or as a larger team for patient care. Multiple training programs are available for surgeons [Non-Technical Skills for Surgeons (NOTSS)] and scrub practitioners [Scrub Practitioner's List of Intraoperative Non-Technical Skills (SPLINTS)].[25,26] It will be worthwhile to bring these teams together for nontechnical skills training to build a favorable culture, translating into patient safety.[27] The team that works together should train in nontechnical skills to achieve common goals.

■ MEASURING THE NONTECHNICAL SKILLS

Measuring the performance of nontechnical skills is essential to ensure safe and quality perioperative care. An ideal tool for the purpose should be highly reliable and validated. Many such tools are available for measuring the nontechnical skills in simulation or real-life scenarios.[9,28-30] A systematic review identified and compared seven tools for assessing an anesthesiologist's nontechnical skills.[31] Fourteen studies were included to assess the reliability and validity of these tools. The ANTS rating system was found to be the most promising of all and had acceptable validity and reliability for the assessment of nontechnical skills of anesthetists in both simulated and clinical settings. The ANTS rating system is presented in **Tables 1 and 2**.

The evaluation of nontechnical skills should be linked to programs designed to evaluate performance, competency, and allow remediation, if required. Such programs could run in parallel with the assessment of technical skills and clinical knowledge.[32]

■ ROLE OF ORGANIZATIONS

Efficient and safe patient care is multidimensional and involves multiple bundles of care. Organizations, big or small, should identify the role of nontechnical skills in reducing the incidence and impact of errors. Apart

TABLE 1: Proforma for evaluation [anaesthetist's non-technical skills (ANTS) framework].

Rating	Description
4—Good	Performance was of a consistently high standard, enhancing patient safety; it could be used as a positive example for others
3—Acceptable	Performance was of a satisfactory standard but could be improved
2—Marginal	Performance indicated cause for concern, considerable improvement is needed
1—Poor	Performance endangered and potentially endangered patient safety, serious remediation is required
Not observed	Skill could not be observed in this situation

TABLE 2: A rating scale for the evaluation.

Category	Element	Rating*	Observation on performance	Category rating and debriefing notes
Task management	Planning and preparing			
	Prioritizing			
	Providing and maintaining status			
	Identifying and utilizing resources			
Team working	Coordinating activities with team			
	Exchanging information			
	Using authority and assertiveness			
	Assessing capabilities			
Situation awareness	Supporting others			
	Gathering information			
	Recognizing and understanding			
	Anticipating			
Decision-making	Identifying options			
	Balancing risks and selecting options			
	Reevaluating			

* According to **Table 1**.

from supporting continuous updates in clinical knowledge and technical skills, programs imparting training in nontechnical skills should also be encouraged. The work culture should be conducive to incident reporting without fearing administrative action. Any mishap should be empathetically approached, with support provided to the teams and individuals. Meanwhile, a system should be in place to identify the factors leading to the mishap and act to ameliorate the chances of recurrence in the future.

GLOBAL STATUS OF TRAINING IN NONTECHNICAL SKILLS

Institutions worldwide have developed or procured systems to train and evaluate nontechnical skills. While these systems might have differences in terminologies and modes of administration, the principles and essence of the programs are the same. The nontechnical skills training has been included in the anesthesia training curriculum, and the competency-based evaluation comprises all three paradigms, namely medical knowledge and technical and nontechnical skills.

In 2018, the Vital Anesthesia Simulation Training (VAST) course was a collaborative effort between Dalhousie University and the University of Rwanda. This is endorsed by the World Federation of Societies of Anesthesiologists (WFSA).[33] Gradually, VAST became a not-for-profit company registered in Australia. VAST offers a range of programs. The VAST course is a 3-day interdisciplinary simulation-based program to teach core perioperative practices and nontechnical skills. Learners from specialties like anesthesia, surgery, general medicine, nursing, and midwifery can enroll in the course. A recent study evaluated the role of VAST in promoting nontechnical skills in low-resource setting.[34] It was found that VAST significantly improved the participant's nontechnical skills immediately post course and at the 4-month follow-up, it was also noticed that the participants valued systematic frameworks and VAST cognitive aids. Improved teamwork facilitated behavior change, which is the crux of the nontechnical skills training. Other courses offered are VAST Facilitator Course (a 2–3-day workshop where participants are trained for design, delivery, and debriefing of interdisciplinary simulation scenarios); VAST Foundation Year (a 48-week simulation-based curriculum of weekly half-day active learning sessions for developing the fundamentals of anesthesia practice using simulation); and nontechnical skills find a significant place in the course curriculum. There are training sites worldwide, including one in Hyderabad, India.[35] Recent joint guidelines from the Difficult Airway Society and the Association of Anaesthetists have highlighted the role of nontechnical skills while providing guidance for clinicians, departments, and hospitals for the implementation of human factors in anesthesia.[12] It was emphasized in the guidelines that nontechnical skills can be learned and practiced daily to help the staff develop, maintain, and utilize the skills effectively.

The National Medical Commission (India) guidelines for competency-based postgraduate training programs in anesthesiology include training in cognitive, affective, and psychomotor domains.[36] The affective domain, as per the curriculum, includes the ability to function as a team, develop an attitude of cooperation with colleagues, and interact with the patient and the clinician or other colleagues to provide the best possible diagnosis or opinion. It also recommends developing communication skills to reports and professional opinions and interacting with patients, relatives, peers, and paramedical staff for effective teaching.

BARRIERS TO EFFECTIVE IMPLEMENTATION OF NONTECHNICAL SKILLS

While the importance of nontechnical skills in anesthesia was acknowledged in the 1990s, it is yet to achieve a cent percent application. Implementation is variable regarding inclusion in the anesthesia curriculum, simulated sessions, and actual work environment. Nontechnical skills are yet to see a complete integration with technical skills, majorly due to a lack of luster and thrill compared to the latter. Another barrier is inadequate training of the trainers. Widespread training of the staff should be ensured to the benefit of trainees. Nontechnical skills involve many terminologies from psychology, which anesthesiologists need to be more familiar with. Continuous training would be instrumental in making the terminologies related to nontechnical skills a shared understanding and a part of conversations.

Another barrier could be a need for dedicated and adequate time to include the components of nontechnical skills in day-to-day practice. The workday schedule could begin with a team brief, with each team member discussing the plan and a team debrief at the end. This provides ample time for assessing the challenges in the situation, delegating responsibilities, and identifying lacunae in the resources with actions taken toward fulfilling them. This makes patient care well-rounded and improves teamwork and task management.

CONCLUSION

Nontechnical skills are skills in the cognitive, social, and personal domains that lead to improved outcomes in conjunction with technical skills and clinical knowledge. Nontechnical skills help alleviate errors owing to their fundamental components of situation awareness, decision-making, teamwork, and task management. Incorporating nontechnical skills in anesthesia practice will significantly enhance patient safety and outcomes. The anesthesia curriculum should include training and evaluating trainees in nontechnical skills. Training of the trainers should also be prioritized. Multidisciplinary adoption of these skills should be encouraged by the organizations.

REFERENCES

1. Flin R, O'Connor P. Safety at the Sharp End: A Guide to Non-Technical Skills, 1st edition. Boca Raton: CRC Press; 2008.
2. Catchpole K, Mishra A, Handa A, McCulloch P. Teamwork and error in the operating room: analysis of skills and roles. Ann Surg. 2008;247:699-706.

3. Weller J, Boyd M. Making a difference through improving teamwork in the operating room: a systematic review of the evidence on what works. Curr Anesthesiol Rep. 2014;4:77-83.
4. Flin R. CRM (Nontechnical skills): A European perspective. In: Kanki B, Anca J, Chidester T (Eds). Crew Resource Management, 3rd edition. United States: Elsevier; 2019. pp. 185-206.
5. O'Connor P, Hoermann HJ, Flin R, Lodge M, Goeters KM; The Jartel Group. Developing a Method for Evaluating Crew Resource Management Skills: A European Perspective. Int J Aviat Psychol. 2002;12(3):263-85.
6. Gaba DM. Crisis resource management and teamwork training in anaesthesia. Br J Anaesth. 2010;105(1):3-6.
7. Radhakrishnan B, Katikar MD, Myatra SN, Gautam PL, Vinayagam S, Saroa R. Importance of non-technical skills in anaesthesia education. Indian J Anaesth. 2022;66:64-9.
8. Stein JE, Heiss K. The Swiss cheese model of adverse event occurrence—Closing the holes. Semin Pediatr Surg. 2015;24:278-82.
9. Flin R, Glavin R, Maran N, Patey R. (2012). Anaesthetists' Non-Technical Skills (ANTS) System Handbook v1.0. [online] Available from: https://research.abdn.ac.uk/wp-content/uploads/sites/14/2019/03/ANTS-Handbook-2012-1.pdf [Last accessed September, 2023].
10. Flin R, Patey R, Glavin R, Maran N. Anaesthetists' non-technical skills. Br J Anaesth. 2010;105:38-44.
11. Fadden S, Mercer S. Followership in complex trauma. Trauma. 2019;21:6-13.
12. Kelly FE, Frerk C, Bailey CR, Cook TM, Ferguson K, Flin R, et al. Implementing human factors in anaesthesia: guidance for clinicians, departments and hospitals: Guidelines from the Difficult Airway Society and the Association of Anaesthetists. Anaesthesia. 2023;78(4):458-78.
13. Network Team. (2020). Decision Making Models. The Pilot. [online] Available from: https://pilot-network.com/news/decision-making-models [Last accessed September, 2023].
14. Sutton RT, Pincock D, Baumgart DC, Sadowski DC, Fedorak RN, Kroeker KI. An overview of clinical decision support systems: benefits, risks, and strategies for success. NPJ Digit Med. 2020;3(1):17.
15. Lelaidier R, Balança B, Boet S, Faure A, Lilot M, Lecomte F, et al. Use of a hand-held digital cognitive aid in simulated crises: the MAX randomized controlled trial. Br J Anaesth. 2017;119:1015-21.
16. Weller JM, Torrie J, Boyd M, Frengley R, Garden A, Ng WL, et al. Improving team information sharing with a structured call-out in anaesthetic emergencies: a randomized controlled trial. Br J Anaesth. 2014;112(6):1042-9.
17. Boyd M, Cumin D, Lombard Boyd M, Torrie J, Civil N, Weller J. Read-back improves information transfer in simulated clinical crises. BMJ Qual Saf. 2014;23:989-93.
18. Lo L, Rotteau L, Shojania K. Can SBAR be implemented with high fidelity and does it improve communication between healthcare workers? A systematic review. BMJ Open. 2021;11:e055247.
19. Moppett IC, Shorrock ST. Working out wrong-side blocks. Anaesthesia. 2018;73:407-20.
20. Eppich W. "Speaking up" for patient safety in the pediatric emergency department. Clin Pediatr Emerg Med. 2015;16:83-9.

21. Pereira FSH, Garcia DB, Ribeiro ER. Identifying patient safety competences among anesthesiology residents: systematic review. Braz J Anesthesiol. 2022;72(5):657-65.
22. Morey JC, Simon R, Jay GD, Wears RL, Salisbury M, Dukes KA, et al. Error reduction and performance improvement in the emergency department through formal teamwork training: evaluation results of the MedTeams project. Health Serv Res. 2002;37(6):1553-81.
23. Clancy CM, Tornberg DN. TeamSTEPPS: assuring optimal teamwork in clinical settings. Am J Med Qual. 2007;22:214-7.
24. Dunn EJ, Mills PD, Neily J, Crittenden MD, Carmack AL, Bagian JP. Medical team training: applying crew resource management in the Veterans Health Administration. Jt Comm J Qual Patient Saf. 2007;33:317-25.
25. Yule S, Flin R, Maran N, Youngson G, Rowley D, Paterson-Brown S. Surgeons' non-technical skills in the operating room: reliability testing of the NOTSS behavior rating system. World J Surg. 2008;32:548-56.
26. Flin R, Mitchell L, McLeod B. Non-technical skills of the scrub practitioner: the SPLINTS system. ORNAC J. 2014;32(3):33-8.
27. Gaba DM, Howard SK, Fish KJ, Smith BE, Sowb YA. Simulation-based training in anesthesia crisis resource management (ACRM): a decade of experience. Simul Gaming. 2001;32(2):175-93.
28. Jirativanont T, Raksamani K, Aroonpruksakul N, Apidechakul P, Suraseranivongse S. Validity evidence of non-technical skills assessment instruments in simulated anaesthesia crisis management. Anaesth Intensive Care. 2017;45:469-75.
29. Hersey P, Laws D. Defining competence for workplace based assessment—a pragmatic and thorough method. Anaesthesia. 2009;64(12):1386.
30. Sharma B, Mishra A, Aggarwal R, Grantcharov TP. Non-technical skills assessment in surgery. Surg Oncol. 2011;20(3):169-77.
31. Boet S, Larrigan S, Martin L, Liu H, Sullivan KJ, Etherington C. Measuring non-technical skills of anaesthesiologists in the operating room: a systematic review of assessment tools and their measurement properties. Br J Anaesth. 2018;121(6):1218-26.
32. Riem N, Boet S, Bould MD, Tavares W, Naik VN. Do technical skills correlate with non-technical skills in crisis resource management: a simulation study. Br J Anaesth. 2012;109(5):723-8.
33. World Federation of Societies of Anaesthesiologists (WFSA). Vital Anaesthesia Simulation Training (VAST). World Federation of Societies of Anaesthesiologists (WFSA). [online] Available from: https://wfsahq.org/our-work/education-training/simulation-training-vast/ [Last accessed September, 2023].
34. Mossenson AI, Tuyishime E, Rawson D, Mukwesi C, Whynot S, Mackinnon SP, et al. Promoting anaesthetisia providers' non-technical skills through the Vital Anaesthesia Simulation Training (VAST) course in a low-resource setting. Br J Anaesth. 2020;124(2):206-13.
35. Vital Anaesthesia Simulation Training (VAST). [online] Available from: https://vastcourse.org [Last accessed September, 2023].
36. National Medical Commission. Guidelines for competency based postgraduate training programme for MD in Anaesthesiology. National Medical Commission. [online] Available from: https://www.nmc.org.in/wp-content/uploads/2019/09/MD-Anesthesia.pdf [Last accessed September, 2023].

CHAPTER 24

Advanced Features in the Modern Anesthesia Workstation

Bharti Wadhwa, Kiran Mahendru

ABSTRACT

Anesthesia workstations are pivotal in modern healthcare, facilitating the safe and efficient administration of anesthesia during surgical procedures. Recent years have witnessed significant advancements in anesthesia workstation technology, driven by a combination of research, engineering, and the integration of cutting-edge innovations. This chapter reviews the new technological additions in anesthesia workstations, exploring the latest developments in gas delivery systems, patient monitoring capabilities, ergonomic designs, and digital interfaces. By enhancing precision, safety, and patient outcomes, these advancements are reshaping the landscape of anesthesiology and fostering a more seamless surgical experience.

Keywords: Anesthesia machine; Low-flow anesthesia; Monitoring; Workstation

■ KEY POINTS

- New features in anesthesia workstations are designed to enhance patient safety, improve efficiency, and provide more advanced monitoring and control capabilities.
- Landmark features are enhanced gas delivery systems with increased precision, automated gas control (AGC) systems, artificial intelligence-based closed-loop systems, integrated decision support systems, remote monitoring, and telemedicine with integration of digital health technology.
- Modular designs and customization provide improved ergonomics. These promote user comfort and prevent fatigue during prolonged surgical procedures.
- Adopting new systems requires careful assessment of the benefits, usability, and training requirements.

■ INTRODUCTION

Anesthesia workstations form a crucial component of anesthesia delivery systems, ensuring precise and tailored administration of anesthetic agents to patients undergoing surgical procedures.

In 1917, Coxeter built the original HEG Boyle's machine. It has undergone multiple modifications since. While the primary anesthesia machine was a robust model, there was a high degree of wastage of anesthetic gases. The accuracy of the flowmeters could have been better, with a high chance of leakage, connection errors, and few feedback systems and alarms. Soon, the accuracy and efficiency of the anesthesia delivery system were recognized as paramount to patient safety, and the subsequent models of anesthesia machines incorporated additional features to improve the accuracy of gas flow with reduced leakage. The closed-loop circle breathing circuits provided the reuse of oxygen and anesthetic agents rather than complete waste as with an open circuit. Adding a mechanical ventilation system and incorporating multiple parameter monitors within the workstation made it more user-friendly and sophisticated.

Recently, the integration of artificial intelligence has made the anesthesia workstation "smarter" such that the machine can understand and perform tasks independently. They are constantly evolving to improve patient care, enhance safety, and provide more efficient workflow for anesthesiologists.

■ NEW FEATURES IN ANESTHESIA WORKSTATIONS

The recent technological additions aim to enhance the functionality and usability of anesthesia workstations. These additions include efficient and enhanced gas delivery systems, intelligent patient monitoring capabilities, ergonomic designs and user interfaces, drug delivery innovations, and remote wireless monitoring. We aim to explore these innovations and their potential impact on anesthesiology.

■ ENHANCED GAS DELIVERY SYSTEMS

The introduction of closed-loop anesthesia delivery systems, utilizing real-time feedback from patient monitoring, allows for automated adjustments to maintain the desired anesthetic depth. These techniques contribute to efficiently using anesthetic agents, reducing waste and the environmental impact. The most significant development is the application of low-flow anesthesia (LFA)/metabolic-flow anesthesia and AGC in the modern anesthesia workstation.

Low Flow and Metabolic Fresh Gas Flow

Low-flow anesthesia is the use of fresh gas flow (FGF) lower than the alveolar ventilation of a patient. The principle behind LFA is to remove the carbon dioxide and replenish the consumed gases with as little FGF as possible. The levels of LFA can be classified based on FGF requirements or the fraction of rebreathing **(Table 1)**.[1]

TABLE 1: Baker classification of fresh gas flow.

Baker classification[1]	Fresh gas flow
Medium flow	1–2 L/min
Low flow	500–1,000 mL/min
Minimal flow	250–500 mL/min
Metabolic flow	250 mL/min

For metabolic flow to be accurate, the system has to be leakage-free so that the FGF can be reduced to the gas volume which the patient absorbs and metabolizes while under anesthesia. Therefore, the minimal oxygen a normothermic patient requires for the metabolic process at rest is used as a sole carrier gas at a 250 mL/min flow. The basic requirements for the safe conduct of LFA/minimal-/metabolic-flow anesthesia are carbon dioxide absorbers. These mandatory gas analyzers display both the inspired and expired concentrations of oxygen, carbon dioxide, and inhalational agents, with vaporizers being able to deliver high and accurate concentrations at low FGF with minimal systemic leakage.

Advantages: The physiological benefits are the preservation of heat and humidity, enhanced flow dynamics augmenting the mucociliary clearance, improving the health of the airway epithelium, and reducing the effect of gas flows on drying up the airway secretions. The lower release of fluorocarbons and nitrous oxide contributes to the atmosphere's reduced greenhouse effect and photophysical properties.[2] Other advantages include decreased operation theater pollution, economic benefits with reduced anesthetic consumption, and savings of up to 75% regarding volatile agents.[3]

Concerns with LFA: Low-flow rates with a dilution of anesthetic gases and longer time constants result in slower induction and emergence, and rapid changes in concentrations may not be possible. Great care should be taken to ensure adequate oxygen is provided to meet the metabolic demands, and an oxygen analyzer will serve as a more sensitive monitor of oxygenation than a pulse oximeter with LFA. The gas flows need to be adjusted frequently to prevent the delivery of a hypoxic gas mixture and under-/overdosing of anesthetic agents. Further, more frequent exhaustion of the carbon dioxide absorber will require frequent changes and the possibility of accumulation of gases such as acetone, carbon monoxide, compound A, hydrogen, and ethanol. The United States Food and Drug Administration (US FDA) recommends keeping sevoflurane to <2 MAC (minimum alveolar concentration) hours with flow rates of 1–2 L/min. Flow rates <1 L/min are not recommended with sevoflurane and LFA.[4]

Minimal or metabolic flow is recommended as a "Green" anesthesia strategy.[2]

Automated Gas Control

Despite the obvious financial and environmental benefits of LFA/minimal-/metabolic-flow anesthesia, there is a reluctance to use it by many anesthesiologists. This reluctance is perhaps due to the associated ergonomic burden of multiple manual adjustments to maintain adequate depth of anesthesia and careful vigilance to prevent inadvertent delivery of a hypoxic gas mixture. In an exciting study by Avidan et al., the authors reported that with manual FGF and anesthetic agent concentration adjustment, anesthesia providers failed to maintain a MAC of >0.7 in 15% of the cases.[5] The other factors leading to resistance in daily use of low flows are an accumulation of toxic trace gases, risk of hypercapnia, variability in vaporizer dial setting increments, and the difference between the concentration of anesthetic agents inhaled by the patient and concentration in FGFs adjusted by the vaporizer.[6] To simplify low-flow techniques in day-to-day anesthesia practice, a propriety software algorithm has been introduced as AGC in some workstations. These include the Maquet Flow-i (Maquet, Solna, Sweden), the Aisys (GE, Madison, Wisconsin), and the Zeus (Dräger, Lubeck, Germany).[7]

Automated gas control provides control and precision for anesthetic agent administration with LFA during induction and emergence of anesthesia by simple presettings that specify the target-inspired oxygen, the end-tidal anesthetic agent, and the speed of induction required.

The target alveolar concentration or the end-expired concentration of potent inhalational anesthetic (F_A) and the target inspired oxygen concentration (FiO_2) are selected and set in the device before induction of anesthesia. The speed to achieve the desired target end-expired concentration of inhalational anesthetic can also be chosen (one out of nine different rates, with nine being the fastest).[8] The additional settings available are the lowest acceptable maintenance FGF, maximum concentration of the inspired agent, and carrier gas composition. The choice of speed with which the F_A of the concerned inhalational anesthetic will be achieved, along with the exponentially decreasing FGF, will determine the total amount of anesthetic agent used. It has been observed that the agent usage is also lower with slower speeds.[8]

Incorporation of AGC in anesthesia workstations can provide excellent safety and consistency to the use of low-flow techniques.[9,10] It will help reduce the number of interventions required during the induction phase of anesthesia, making the conduct of LFA ergonomically easier for the anesthesiologist. The additional advantages of the AGC software are the reduction in anesthesia waste, cost of potent inhalational agents, operating room pollution, and environmental burden in the form of the greenhouse effect. AGC will help ensure a better future for the coming generations by decreasing the ecological footprint and helping us move toward "Sustainable and Green Anesthesia".

■ DRUG DELIVERY INNOVATIONS

Advancements in drug delivery systems have led to the development of smart infusion pumps and automated drug libraries integrated with anesthesia workstations.

Drug delivery systems provide accurate and precise administration of anesthetic agents, muscle relaxants, analgesics, and other medications. Additionally, some workstations incorporate safety features like drug libraries, dose error reduction systems, and alerts for drug interactions or contraindications, reducing the risk of error and enhancing medication safety during anesthesia.

Automated drug delivery closed-loop systems optimize the delivery of anesthetic drugs for establishing adequate anesthetic depth and for sedation. A predetermined target is set, and the system decides to reach and maintain that anesthetic level. The components of an automated computer-based closed-loop anesthetic delivery system are the targeted therapeutic effect-controlled variable, a set point of this controlled variable that is clinically relevant, a control actuator, an infusion pump driving the drug, and an accurate, stable control algorithm. The system can have either a pharmacokinetic or a pharmacodynamic closed-loop controller. The pharmacokinetic model target is a specific drug dose, and the pharmacodynamic model is based on a specific therapeutic effect. These systems are intelligent computer closed-loop programs that facilitate better control of anesthesia with improved outcomes.

Artificial intelligence-based closed-loop systems such as iControl RP and McSleepy are being evaluated for routine clinical use.[11] In addition to the Bispectral Index (BIS) monitor, the iControl-RP monitors the vital signs of blood oxygen level, heart rate, respiratory rate, and blood pressure to determine how much anesthesia to deliver in the form of remifentanil and propofol infusions. The McSleepy is another pharmacologic robot that uses three syringe pumps to control the three components of general anesthesia (hypnosis, analgesia, and neuromuscular block) in an automated closed-loop anesthesia drug delivery system. Each component had specific monitoring: BIS; AnalgoScore (an-AL-go-score = a pain score derived from the heart rate and mean arterial pressure), which was used as the control variable to titrate the effective dose of remifentanil; and the train of four (TOF), which was a measure of the twitch strength of a muscle when its peripheral nerve was electrically stimulated.

Electroencephalogram-derived parameters BIS and entropy have been commonly used for anesthetic depth assessment in the anesthesia workstations BIS™ (Medtronic, Dublin, Ireland) and GE Entropy™ (GE Healthcare, Chicago IL, USA). However, they are unable to monitor nociception.[12] Additionally, diathermy may create artifacts influencing the validity of the anesthetic depth.

Reduced consumption of anesthetic drugs, better hemodynamic stability with decreased incidence of intraoperative hypotension, reduced postoperative complications, and increased intraoperative BIS and entropy values have been reported with advisory displays SmartPilot® View Dräger and Navigator® (GE Healthcare, Chicago IL, USA).[13,14]

Dräger SmartPilot View

The Dräger SmartPilot View (Dräger Medical, Lubeck, Germany) is another addition to better control of anesthetic drug demonstration. The depth of anesthesia is predicted using response surface models based on hypnotics and opioid interaction. It is a software designed to calculate and predict the effects of anesthetic drugs (hypnotics and analgesics) based on population models. It aims to guide drug delivery optimally and is patient-individualized to provide better hemodynamic stability and controlled perioperative conditions. It avoids over dosages to ensure faster and smoother recovery.

The software can be combined with Draeger workstations like Primus, Perseus A500, Zeus, and Atlan **(Fig. 1)**. These combinations can transfer data of measured ventilation and anesthetic gas concentration values. In combination with Zeus IE, it has the "what if" function that can show the calculated effect of an anesthetic agent setting before it is even confirmed. In the Perseus A500, the vapor view function can automatically transfer Vapor® 3000 and D-Vapor® 3000 hand dial settings and measure ventilation and gas concentration values.

Decision-making support: SmartPilot View can translate complex pharmacokinetic and pharmacodynamic algorithms into an easy-to-interpret visual display of anesthetic and hypnotic–analgesic levels.[15,16] It can display predicted anesthesia levels for up to 20 minutes and communicates with selected infusion pumps and vaporizer settings. It guides the anesthesiologist with the current status and the predicted anesthetic course in the next 10 minutes using a 2D pharmacodynamic diagram.[13,14] The anticipated effects of hypnotic and opioids are displayed on the x and y axes, respectively. The combined synergy is displayed as three different zones of isoboles in different grey tones **(Fig. 2)**. The three isoboles are as follows:
1. *Dark grey isobole:* Anesthetic depth to tolerate intubation and surgical incision
2. *Mid-grey isobole:* Anesthetic depth for the maintenance of surgery
3. *Light grey isobole:* Anesthetic depth for surgical closure.

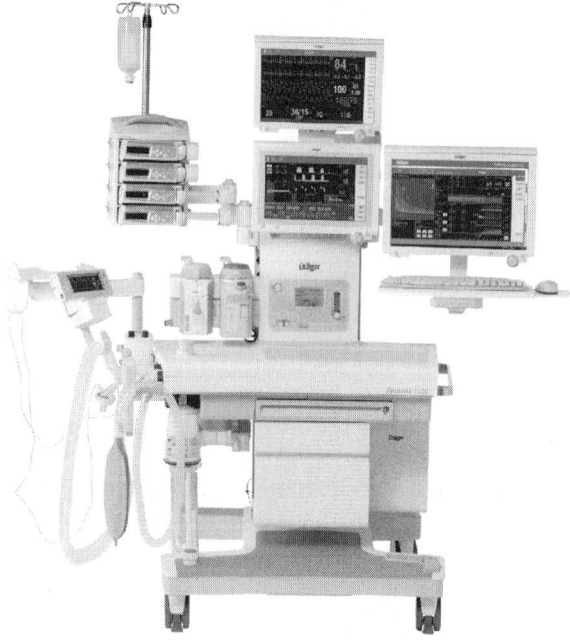

Fig. 1: Dräger workstation with integrated Dräger SmartPilot View.
Courtesy: Reproduced with permission of Draeger India Private Limited.

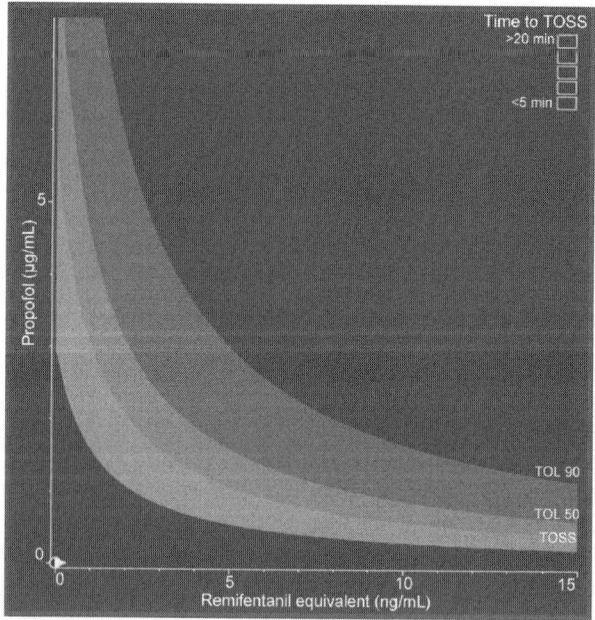

Fig. 2: The SmartPilot View display with three grey isoboles depicting the synergistic actions of hypnotics and analgesics.
Courtesy: Reproduced with permission of Draeger India Private Limited.

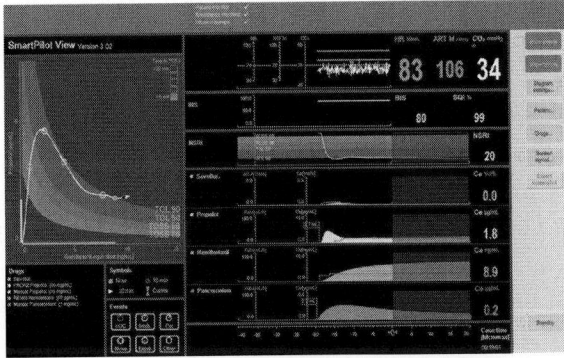

Fig. 3: Comprehensive data provided by the SmartPilot View.
Courtesy: Reproduced with permission of Draeger India Private Limited.

The actual anesthetic levels and the predicted (next 10 minutes) anesthetic levels are illustrated as dots on the isoboles **(Fig. 3)**. These isobole dots and lines represent how a patient will respond to a defined stimulus and indicate the level of anesthesia. This data can be utilized for the adjustment of the anesthetic depth by the anesthesiologist.

A new anesthetic depth index, "the Noxious Stimulation Response Index" (NSRI), with a range of 100–0, is also displayed quantitatively. The index helps to predict the intraoperative response to a noxious stimulus and is the probability of a patient tolerating the same.[17] Therefore, an NSRI of 100 means a 100% response probability, and an NSRI of 0 means a 0% probability of a response to a noxious stimulus.[18] It also shows the expected time of awakening a patient from anesthesia.

The drugs included in the pharmacokinetic model of Dräger SmartPilot View are hypnotics (propofol), opioids (fentanyl, remifentanil, alfentanil, sufentanil), volatile agents (desflurane, isoflurane, sevoflurane), and muscle relaxants (rocuronium, vecuronium, mivacurium, pancuronium). The demographic data supported by the software are patients aged 18–90 years, with height 150–200 cm, weight 40–140 kg, body mass index (BMI) ≤36, and the American Society of Anesthesiologists grading less than IV.

The patient-optimized titration of anesthetic drugs can lead to improved drug dosing, faster recovery,[19] better utilization of resources,[13] decision-making support systems, and comprehensive visualization. All these factors will improve workflow efficiency and optimize the operation room and postanesthesia care unit area utilization.

However, more research is required to ascertain the effectiveness and application of these devices. Strand et al. compared the SmartPilot View with standard anesthesia practice in low-risk gynecological surgery patients. The primary outcome was a higher mean arterial pressure and increased assessment precision in the SmartPilot View group. The authors reported no significant differences between the two groups.[20]

Integrated Decision Support Systems

Modern anesthesia workstations are now equipped with integrated decision support systems that provide real-time guidance and recommendations based on patient data. These systems use algorithms and evidence-based guidelines to assist anesthesiologists in making informed decisions about drug dosages, fluid management, ventilation parameters, and more. The features promote safer and more standardized anesthesia practices. An example is the Aisys CS[2] Anesthesia Delivery System with End-tidal (Et) Control from GE Healthcare. This feature automates end-tidal oxygen and end-tidal anesthetic agent delivery with Et Control software. The algorithm can make decisions, and gas flow, oxygen, anesthetic agent, and ventilator modes can all be adjusted in <3 seconds.

▪ REMOTE MONITORING AND TELEMEDICINE

Integrating telemedicine capabilities with anesthesia workstations enables remote monitoring and consultation, enhancing access to specialized expertise, and facilitating continuous support for patients in remote locations.

Wireless Connectivity and Remote Monitoring

This feature allows the anesthesiologist to monitor patients and adjust settings on the workstation from a separate location, such as a control room or a central monitoring station. Remote access can be particularly beneficial in critical care settings, highly infectious diseases like coronavirus disease 2019 (COVID-19) infection, or during complex procedures where close monitoring is required.

Remote access can be through a tablet or a smartphone. It can also be particularly useful when the anesthesiologist needs to move around the operating room or monitor multiple patients simultaneously.

The wireless console system uses Bluetooth or a light fidelity (Li-Fi) system to communicate with or control the anesthesia workstation. The wireless console can work with multiple devices, and the workstation acts as a Li-Fi router by connecting all devices within an operating room.

▪ INTEGRATION OF DIGITAL HEALTH TECHNOLOGIES

The digitalization of healthcare has paved the way for integrating anesthesia workstations with hospital information systems and electronic health records. Seamless data exchange facilitates real-time access to patient history, preoperative assessments, and medication profiles, streamlining the anesthesia workflow and promoting better-informed clinical decisions.

Electronic Record Integration with Anesthesia Workstation (AIMS)

Many modern anesthesia workstations are designed to integrate seamlessly with electronic medical record (EMR) systems.

An AIMS (Anesthesia Information Management System) installation is a hardware/software EMR solution integrated with the anesthesia workstation that interfaces with the patient and monitors. The record creation starts with documentation of the patient's name and demographic profile, scheduled procedure, preoperative assessment, and plan. The digital interface to the monitor helps capture the intraoperative period's real-time data. It can also retrieve data from the central data repository of the hospital in addition to the perioperative data. Thus, they can function as modules for storing pre- and postoperative patient information as well.[21]

This integration automatically documents anesthesia-related data such as drug administration, ventilation parameters, and monitoring data. This feature saves time, reduces errors, and facilitates comprehensive patient records by eliminating manual record-keeping. Apart from the improved workflow and data accuracy, all documentation and billing can be in a single record that helps preserve legally required documentation.

Electronic record keeping is much easier and more consistent than paper records due to the availability of prompts to the provider to enter the standard services. As the procedure ends, the provider can review the records and close the system. A significant concern with electronic records is the potential for artifacts. For example, leaning and pressure on the blood pressure cuff during the case would capture an increase in the patient's blood pressure in the automated records but would have been ignored in the manual records. The spurious record thus indicates a situation where the anesthesiologist should have responded. Despite the imperfections, the EMRs provide better, more efficient, and complete data management tools.

Data analytics and quality improvement: The collection and analysis of anesthesia-related data through anesthesia workstations contribute to quality improvement initiatives. Data analytics help identify trends, formulate anesthesia protocols, and enhance patient outcomes through evidence-based practices.

■ ERGONOMIC DESIGNS AND USER INTERFACES

The modern anesthesia workstation design focuses on user-centric interfaces and ergonomic considerations. These ergonomic designs promote user comfort and reduce fatigue during prolonged surgical procedures, ultimately enhancing patient safety.

Touchscreen interfaces: Many modern anesthesia workstations employ user-friendly interfaces that provide intuitive controls and easy access to various functions. These interfaces allow anesthesiologists to adjust settings, monitor patient data, and access additional features with minimal effort, enhancing efficiency and reducing the risk of errors.

Modular design and customization: Workstations are being designed with a modular approach, allowing customization and adaptation to individual anesthesiologist's preferences and specific clinical needs. Modular workstations enable adding or removing components, such as gas modules, monitoring modules, or additional storage, to create a tailored workstation setup.

SIMULATION AND TRAINING SOLUTIONS

Anesthesia workstations equipped with high-fidelity simulation capabilities allow for realistic training of anesthesia providers in controlled environments. Virtual reality simulations offer valuable practice scenarios, enhancing clinical competency and confidence in handling critical situations. The Virtual Anesthesia Machine (VAM) simulation designed by the University of Florida Health division is the flagship transparent reality simulation that led to the creation of the VAM website (link: http://vam.anest.ufl.edu/websims/VAM). The VAM simulates a generic anesthesia machine with an oxygen-driven bellows ventilator. The flow of gases is not only made visible but is also color-coded.

CONCLUSION

To err is human. Human factors and errors are firmly embedded as an essential cause of mishaps in clinical anesthetic practice. The modern anesthesiologist is overloaded with data, information, and multitasking necessities within a highly complex work environment.

The use of automation and technology to replace time-consuming and error-prone tasks holds substantial promise for improved safety. The continuous evolution of anesthesia workstations through new technological additions is revolutionizing the field of anesthesiology. From enhanced gas delivery systems and intelligent patient monitoring to ergonomic designs and digital interfaces, these innovations improve precision, safety, and efficiency in anesthesia care. Decision support systems can help make reliable and standardized decisions in complex environments, while automated closed-loop infusion systems reduce the anesthetic workload with reduced fatigue.

As technology advances, anesthesia workstations will play an increasingly integral role in shaping the future of surgical procedures and patient outcomes. Healthcare professionals must stay abreast of these developments and embrace the transformative potential they offer to benefit patients and providers.

However, while convenient with improved patient safety, the automated technology needs to be handled with caution as it can potentially introduce new and different errors. The new additions to the anesthesia workstation must be tested in actual operational settings to determine what, if any, unanticipated failures exist.

■ REFERENCES

1. Baker AB. Low flow and closed circuits. Anaesth Intensive Care. 1994;22(4):341-2.
2. Rübsam ML, Kruse P, Dietzler Y, Kropf M, Bette B, Zarbock A, et al. A call for immediate climate action in anesthesiology: routine use of minimal or metabolic fresh gas flow reduces our ecological footprint. Can J Anaesth. 2023;70(3):301-12.
3. Hönemann C, Hagemann O, Doll D. Inhalational anaesthesia with low fresh gas flow. Indian J Anaesth. 2013;57(4):345-50.
4. Food and Drug Administration. (2003). Ultane (Sevoflurane) volatile liquid for inhalation. [online] Available from: http://www.accessdata.fda.gov/drugsatfda_docs/label/2006/020478s016lbl.pdf [Last accessed September, 2023].
5. Avidan MS, Jacobsohn E, Glick D, Burnside BA, Zhang L, Villafranca A, et al; BAG-RECALL Research Group. Prevention of intraoperative awareness in a high-risk surgical population. N Engl J Med. 2011;365:591-600.
6. Colak YZ, Toprak HI. Feasibility, safety, and economic consequences of using minimal flow anaesthesia by Maquet FLOW-i equipped with automated gas control. Sci Rep. 2021;11(1):20074.
7. Upadya M, Saneesh PJ. Low-flow anaesthesia—underused mode towards "sustainable anaesthesia". Indian J Anaesth. 2018;62(3):166-72.
8. Carette R, De Wolf AM, Hendrickx JF. Automated gas control with the Maquet FLOW-i. J Clin Monit Comput. 2016;30(3):341-6.
9. Kennedy RR, French RA. A ten-year audit of fresh gas flows in a New Zealand hospital: the influence of the introduction of automated agent delivery and comparisons with other hospitals. Anaesth Intensive Care. 2014;42:65-72.
10. Singaravelu S, Barclay P. Automated control of end-tidal inhalation anaesthetic concentration using the GE Aisys Carestation™. Br J Anaesth. 2013;110:561-6.
11. Hemmerling TM, Arbeid E, Wehbe M, Cyr S, Taddei R, Zaouter C. Evaluation of a novel closed-loop total intravenous anaesthesia drug delivery system: A randomized controlled trial. Br J Anaesth. 2013;110:1031-9.
12. Constant I, Sabourdin N. Monitoring depth of anesthesia: from consciousness to nociception. A window on subcortical brain activity. Paediatr Anesth. 2015;25:73-82.
13. Cirillo V, Zito Marinosci G, De Robertis E, Iacono C, Romano GM, Desantis O, et al. Navigator® and SmartPilot® View are helpful in guiding anesthesia and reducing anesthetic drug dosing. Minerva Anestesiol. 2015;81:1163-9.
14. Leblanc D, Conté M, Masson G, Richard F, Jeanneteau A, Bouhours G, et al. SmartPilot® view-guided anaesthesia improves postoperative outcomes in hip fracture surgery: a randomized blinded controlled study. Br J Anaesth. 2017;119:1022-9.

15. Struys MM, Sahinovic M, Lichtenbelt BJ, Vereecke HE, Absalom AR. Optimizing intravenous drug administration by applying pharmacokinetic/pharmacodynamic concepts. Br J Anaesth. 2011;107:38-47.
16. Kennedy RR. Seeing the future of anesthesia drug dosing: moving the art of anesthesia from impressionism to realism. Anesth Analg. 2010;111:252-5.
17. Luginbühl M, Schumacher PM, Vuilleumier P, Vereecke H, Heyse B, Bouillon TW, et al. Noxious stimulation response index: a novel anesthetic state index based on hypnotic–opioid interaction. Anesthesiology. 2010;112(4):872-80.
18. Schumacher PM, Dossche J, Mortier EP, Luginbuehl M, Bouillon TW, Struys MM. Response surface modeling of the interaction between propofol and sevoflurane. Anesthesiology. 2009;111(4):790-804.
19. Morimoto Y, Shiramoto H, Yoshimura M. The usefulness of Smart Pilot View for fast recovery from desflurane general anesthesia. J Anesth. 2021;35(2):239-45.
20. Strand H, Elshaug AC, Bernersen Ø, Ballangrud R. Effectiveness of the advisory display SmartPilot® view in the assessment of anesthetic depth in low risk gynecological surgery patients: a randomized controlled trial. BMC Anesthesiol. 2022;22:57.
21. Ehrenfeld JM, Rehman MA. Anesthesia information management systems: a review of functionality and installation considerations. J Clin Monit Comput. 2011;25(1):71-9.

CHAPTER 25

End of Life: Laws and Policies

Anjali Gera, Bimla Sharma

"Death is inevitable, but bad death is not."

ABSTRACT

End-of-life (EOL) care is a multidisciplinary approach to providing complete supportive care to patients with life-limiting terminal illnesses. It includes initiating palliative care after counseling the patients and their families. Countries with a good Quality of Death (QOD) index have palliative care integrated into their health services like the UK and Australia. Unfortunately, there is no legislation regarding EOL care in our country, and doctors often practice defensive treatment. The Supreme Court gave guidelines to execute advance directives (AD) in 2018, but the procedure needed to be more straightforward and practical. The apex court simplified the process in 2023, and these guidelines are valid until the parliament passes legislation. EOL laws are required so doctors can practice EOL care and make decisions ethically and honestly. This will help achieve the goal of dignified death for all.

Keywords: Euthanasia; Advance directives; Legal; End-of-life care

KEY POINTS

- End-of-life (EOL) decisions are based on the patient's autonomy.
- Patients who are terminally ill and lack decision-making ability usually end up dying in intensive care units (ICUs) because of a lack of EOL care policies.
- Aruna Shanbaugh judgment in 2012 legalized passive euthanasia and opened up debates on EOL care.
- Advance directives (AD) or Living Will was legalized in Common Cause judgment.
- The Supreme Court simplified the procedure for withdrawing/withholding treatment in the absence of AD in a recent judgment in 2023.

INTRODUCTION

End-of-life care is a multidisciplinary approach to providing physical, emotional, social, and spiritual support to patients suffering from incurable and life-limiting illnesses. The aim is to reduce suffering and give comfort to the patient. The process of care also extends to the family and caregivers. It can be initiated as soon as the competent patient can decide and the doctor has shared the decision that the curative treatment will be futile.

World Health Organization (WHO) explicitly recognized palliative care as a fundamental human right.[1] Unfortunately, <1% of the population in India has access to palliative care and pain relief.[2] The need for palliative and EOL care will grow as the aging population increases as well as the incidence of communicable and noncommunicable diseases.

There are several things that could be improved regarding EOL care, not only among the public at large but also among physicians. We will answer the following EOL care uncertainties in this chapter.

- Why do we need EOL policies?
- Is the right to death our fundamental right?
- Is withdrawal/withholding of treatment the same as physician-assisted death (PAD)?
- Who can decide on EOL initiation?
- Can the doctor or family go ahead with EOL decisions for incompetent patients in the absence of documented wishes of the patient?

NEED FOR END-OF-LIFE LAWS AND POLICIES

People suffering from incurable diseases or life-threatening illnesses like AIDS, malignancies, or neurodegenerative disorders may not have any hope of recovery. These patients usually end up dying in the ICU surrounded by tubings, machines, and ventilators that sustain life and its agony but result in lonely and undignified death. This causes mental trauma to the family and results in excessive financial burden on the aggrieved family. In our country, the penetration of healthcare insurance is scanty, and most of the healthcare expenses are borne by individual patients. These futile treatments drain the family's resources.

Without EOL policies, doctors continue practicing "defensive treatment" even when they know the treatment is not in the patient's best interest and will not cure the disease. It usually results in ordering multiple laboratory investigations and avoidance of discussions about poor outcomes of the disease with patients and their family members. It is imperative to have an EOL law so that doctors can fearlessly initiate EOL care for the patient when the treating doctors have taken the decision ethically. It will reduce the family's financial burden and facilitate the equitable distribution of resources in society. In our country, 78% of patients leave hospitals against medical advice (LAMA) because of a lack of EOL policies.[3] The patient's family usually decides on LAMA due to excessive financial burden, resulting in a harrowing death. Moreover, if the EOL policies are in place, a person can exercise autonomy until the end and have a dignified death.

The basic ethical reasoning behind EOL decisions is based on four principles given by Beauchamp and Childress—(1) autonomy, (2) beneficence, (3) nonmaleficence, and (4) social justice.[4]

Autonomy is an individual's right to self-determination, and respecting autonomy is the cornerstone of EOL decisions. The physician must disclose all relevant information to the patient and family members so that the patient can make an autonomous decision. AD or living will is an instrument for expressing autonomy in anticipation of loss of competence. A person's wishes expressed in AD should be included in EOL decisions. Mental Health Act 2017[5] also supports the use of AD. If the patient is not competent to make a decision and AD is also not there, then the patient's family or close friend who understands the patient's best interest can make a surrogate decision. The surrogate can be a spouse, children, siblings, parents, next of kin, or trusted friends.[6]

When discussing laws on EOL issues, it is essential to understand the terminologies such as euthanasia, assisted suicide, and withholding or withdrawing treatment. In legal literature, much debate is centered on euthanasia, the right to life, and the right to death.

■ EUTHANASIA

Euthanasia means good death, derived from the Greek word euthanatos (eu means good, and thanatos means death). House of Lords Select Committee on Medical Ethics has defined euthanasia as "a deliberate intervention undertaken with the express intention of ending a life, to relieve intractable suffering".[7] It has been classified based on consent as follows:

Voluntary Euthanasia

In voluntary euthanasia, a competent person makes voluntary and enduring requests for life-terminating measures, most likely due to terminal illness or intractable suffering. The person requests independently and is not imposed by any rule or person.

Involuntary Euthanasia

In this life-terminating decisions are taken without the person's or surrogate's consent, either as the paternalistic decision to end the victim's suffering or for political reasons. It is illegal all over the world.

Nonvoluntary Euthanasia

Here, life-terminating decisions are taken by a surrogate or proxy for the patients who are mentally incompetent to make decisions. Generally, the decision to end life is taken by family members of accident victims in the absence of AD.

Based on the nature of the act, euthanasia has been classified as active and passive.

Active Euthanasia

Active euthanasia is a merciful act in which a physician administers a lethal injection to end suffering and meaningless existence. This includes voluntary active euthanasia (VAE) and PAD. In VAE, a physician administers a lethal injection to the patient at his explicit request. In PAD, a physician prescribes or provides medication with a clear understanding that it will be used to end life at the patient's explicit request.

Passive Euthanasia

Passive euthanasia involves intentionally ending someone's life motivated solely by the person's best interest by withholding life-preserving treatment or withdrawing treatment necessary for sustaining life.

In active euthanasia, physicians are actively doing something to end someone's life; in passive, physicians are not doing something that would preserve someone's life. In both situations, explicit consent is required.

The term euthanasia has historical significance only and is not used by medical professionals. The terms being debated for legal support are withdrawal of treatment, withholding of life support treatment, foregoing life support treatment, and PAD. Instead of intent to hasten or achieve death, EOL care is about making life as comfortable and pain-free as possible when suffering from an incurable illness.

■ END-OF-LIFE LAWS IN OTHER COUNTRIES

Different countries have different laws for EOL according to cultural and religious differences.

The House of Lords in Airedale NHS vs. Bland permitted withdrawal of life-sustaining treatment (LST) in patients with a permanent vegetative state (PVS).[8] Tony Bland was in PVS with no hope of recovery and had been on artificial feed and other supportive measures to sustain life. The House of Lords observed that medical professionals are under no duty to continue treatment as, in their opinion, it is in the best interest of such patients.

The UK topped the survey, which ranked Quality of Death (QOD) according to the healthier environment, home resources, community engagement affordability, and quality.[9] Palliative care in the UK is provided through hospitals, community, and inpatient hospice centers and directly at home. 75% of people in England and Wales benefit from palliative care services during the end of life.[10] The UK's Health and Care Act 2022 includes a legal foundation for integrated care boards, including palliative and EOL care.[11]

In the United States, refusing medical treatment other than Jehovah's Witness started with the Re Quinlan case in 1976.[12] A 21-year-old Karen Ann Quinlan lapsed unconscious after intoxication with alcohol and drug and suffered a hypoxic brain injury. She was in PVS, requiring artificial ventilation and feeds to support life. The Supreme Court granted the request by the parents to remove LST. The court held that the "right to privacy" includes refusing medical treatment and extends to incompetent patients. The court imposed a condition that in such cases physician's diagnosis must be confirmed by the hospital's ethics committee.

In 1990 in the Cruzan case, the United States Supreme Court affirmed that artificial nutrition and hydration are medical interventions and can be withheld or withdrawn under the guidelines that apply to other medical interventions.[13]

A traditional Confucian country like South Korea, where policymaking is influenced by familial relations and social harmony rather than individual autonomy, passed the "Well Dying Act" in 2018.[14] The act legalized the autonomous decision of terminally ill patients to refuse resuscitation and LST. A study done by Lee and colleagues compared the quality of dying and death (QODD) as measured by the QODD questionnaire in years before the act and after the passage of the act. The authors found fewer patients admitted to the ICU for resuscitation and less time for "do not resuscitate" (DNR) to death after the act.[15] The QOD improved, and the patients had time to say goodbye to loved ones and had access to spiritual services.

Another law is France's Leonette's Law 2005, which helped improve interprofessional communication about withdrawing and withholding LST. After the law's passage, EOL decision-making has become transparent, and healthcare professionals can communicate openly with patients.[16]

■ THE LEGAL FRAMEWORK IN INDIA

In our country, there are no legislations regarding EOL that can guide and support the ethical decisions taken by medical professionals regarding EOL care of their patients. The current position includes certain judicial pronouncements, constitutional rights, the human organ transplantation act, and guidelines by the Indian Council of Medical Research (ICMR).[17,18] Indian Penal Code (IPC), Medical Council of India (MCI) Act (Professional Conduct, Etiquette, and Ethics), and Mental Healthcare Act also have some relevance.[5,19,20]

Section 6.7 of the MCI code of conduct states that practicing euthanasia is unethical.[20] However, a team of doctors will decide to withdraw life support systems for sustaining cardiopulmonary function even after brain death. This team shall consist of a doctor in charge of the patient, a chief medical officer (CMO)/medical officer in charge of the hospital, and a doctor nominated by the in-charge of the hospital by the provisions of the Transplantation of Human Organs and Tissues Act (THOTA) 1994.[17] The THOTA Act (amended in 2014) addresses the issue of organ retrieval from living and deceased donors. The act defines brain death as a stage at which all brain stem functions have permanently and irreversibly ceased. The ventilator can be disconnected once brain death is documented with appropriate safeguards.

These principles guide clinicians in making decisions in EOL situations. However, a dilemma remains because of multiple factors like medicolegal issues, advancing medical technology, and the need for more awareness among people. For example, suppose a clinician wishes to inform a competent patient with an advanced incurable disease about EOL care. The family, however, insists that the patient should not be told about the condition and that definitive treatment may be given. The clinician understands that the advanced treatment will not cure the illness, and a competent adult patient cannot make autonomous decisions.[21]

■ LEGAL EVOLUTION OF LAWS ON END OF LIFE

The right to life is a fundamental right enshrined under Article 21 of the Constitution of India.[22] It states that no person shall be deprived of his/her life or personal liberty. Courts have interpreted it very liberally and have included many rights under its ambit, like rights to education, shelter, livelihood, etc., so that people can have a dignified life. But whether the right to death comes under this or not has been a question of debate for a long time.

This issue arose in our courts for the first time in 1950 in the *State of Maharashtra vs. Maruti Sripati Dubal*.[23] The court held that the right to life also includes the right to death, and the Bombay High Court struck down Section 309 of IPC, which attempts to commit suicide as a criminal offense. A division bench of the *Supreme Court in P Ratiram vs. UOI* also held that the right to life includes the right to death and considered Section 309 unconstitutional.[24] Suicide and euthanasia are two different things, and the court in *Naresh Moratrao Sakhre vs. UOI* stated that suicide is an act of self-killing, an act of terminating one's own life, and without the aid or assistance of a human agency. Euthanasia or mercy killing, on the other hand, implies the interaction of other human agencies to end life. Mercy killing is thus not suicide, and the provision of Section 309 does not cover an attempt at mercy killing.[25]

In a landmark judgment in *Gian Kaur vs. the State of Punjab*, the court held that the right to death is not included with the right to life.[26] The court explicitly stated that the constitutional right to life and personal liberty, by no stretch of the imagination, can include the extinction of life. The Supreme Court upheld the validity of Sections 306 and 309 of IPC. It discussed assisted suicide, euthanasia, and withdrawal of life support and opined that assisted suicide can be legalized only by legislation. The court differentiated between the "right to die" and "right to die with dignity", and reference was made to Airedale NHS vs. Bland.[8]

In the case of euthanasia, there is an intention to kill the patient, even if it is in the patient's best interest. This comes under clause 1 of Section 300 of IPC.[27] In the case of voluntary euthanasia, there is the valid explicit consent of the act to attract exception 5 of Section 300 of IPC. Doctor will be held under Section 304 (culpable homicide not amounting to murder). Suicide is illegal in our country and is punishable under Section 305 (abetment of suicide of child/insane person), Section 306 (abetment of suicide), and Section 309 (attempt to commit suicide) of IPC.[19]

Aruna Shanbaug case was a historic case in the Indian legal system where the court dealt with the issue of permitting mercy killing for the first time. Aruna Shanbaug was a young nurse at KEM Hospital, Mumbai, who was sexually assaulted by one of the hospital staff. She survived the assault but developed irreversible brain damage secondary to hypoxia due to strangulation. She remained in a persistent vegetative state for 42 years till her natural death. Following a writ petition by a social activist seeking mercy killing for Aruna, the Supreme Court appointed a team of three medical experts for their opinion. The court analyzed the medical experts' report and the hospital staff and doctor's opinion and concluded that Aruna Shanbaug is in PVS but not brain dead. The court further said that taking her life was unjustified as she was in stable condition and the hospital staff was taking good care of her. Moreover, the right to decide on her behalf rested with the hospital's management, not some "friend".[28]

The bench, in this case, referred to overseas cases and discussed euthanasia at length. It was stated that the "general legal position all over the world seems to be that while active euthanasia is illegal unless legislation permits it, passive euthanasia is legal even without legislation provided certain conditions and safeguards are maintained".[28] The court ruled that active euthanasia is a criminal offense punishable under Sections 302 and 304 of the IPC, and PAD executed by a doctor is punishable under Section 306 of the IPC. The court gave certain safeguards—to discontinue life support, a decision must be taken by the parents, spouse, or other close relatives. In the absence of any of them, such a decision can be taken by a person acting as a close friend or by the doctors attending the patient. However, in all the above situations, approval of the concerned High Court is mandatory. It held that the High Court is parens patriae (parent of the nation) and has the power to decide what is best for the patient and extended the power under Article 226.

The supreme court gave another landmark judgment on March 19, 2018 in *Common Cause vs. UOI*.[29] Five judges' constitutional bench delivered the judgment in response to a writ petition filed by a registered society called Common Cause. The society prayed for declaring the "right to die with dignity" a fundamental right under Article 21 of the Indian Constitution. The society also prayed that people with terminal illnesses or deteriorating health might be allowed to execute "living wills authorized by attorney" and to legalize it so that it can be presented to the hospital authority for action in case they are admitted. As the opinions in Aruna Shanbaug and Gian Kaur cases had been inconsistent, a three-judge bench referred the matter to five-judge bench in 2014 to settle the issue. The constitution bench transferred the burden on parliament to draft a law on EOL care. As a response, the Health Ministry proposed the Medical Treatment of Terminally Ill Patients (Protection of Patients and Medical Practitioners) Bill 2016.[30] This was proposed by the Law Commission of India in its 241st report in 2012.[31]

The apex court said that the right to privacy is an essential right to human dignity, and both dignity and privacy are intimately related and are natural conditions for life through death. The court also took note of the case "Re Quinlan", which suggested that the right to privacy includes the right to refuse medical care.[12] It also relied upon the judgment in a European Court of Human Rights in the case of "Pretty vs. the UK".[32] In this case, it was concluded that a person has a choice to avoid what they consider an undignified and distressing end to their life, and such a choice would be guaranteed under the right to respect for private life under Article 8(1) of the European Convention on Human Rights.[33]

The Supreme Court, in this case, held that the right to die with dignity is a fundamental right under Article 21 and legalized passive euthanasia, and allowed to withdraw or withhold the life support system of terminally ill patients. AD was validated, and a person's autonomy and right to refuse treatment was safeguarded. The court laid down the procedure for altering AD and gave guidelines for cases without AD. The guidelines provided by the court regarding the execution of living wills and their authentication by the magistrate were very complicated and time-consuming. The treating physician of a terminally ill patient will refer the matter to a medical board consisting of the head of the treating department and at least three experts from general medicine: cardiology, neurology, psychiatry, or oncology with experience in critical care. The decision of the medical board will be communicated to the jurisdictional collector, who shall then constitute a board comprising the CMO of the concerned district as chairman and three medical experts in the same field, as mentioned earlier. The chairman of the medical board shall then authorize the implementation of the board's decision.

This process of execution of AD had been made to avoid its misuse, but it needed to be more practical to implement and create confusion around EOL care. A survey was conducted across seven cities on 2,400 urban Indians 1 year after this judgment. It found that 88% of respondents wanted to decide about the line of management during the end of life, only 27% were aware of AD, and only 6% had created an AD. This survey was guided by ELICIT (End of Life Care in India Taskforce), a group of senior specialists from three associations, namely, Indian Association of Palliative Care (IAPC), the Indian Society of Critical Care Medicine (ISCCM), and the Indian Academy of Neurology (IAN).[34]

Medical bodies like ISCCM and IAPC have laid down guidelines, and so also the All India Institute of Medical Sciences (AIIMS) and the Manipal Hospital. In 2012 and 2014, ISCCM gave a consensus ethical position statement on EOL guidelines in ICU.[35,36] ICMR guidelines published in 2018 enunciated the terminologies and issues clinicians face in EOL care. It has defined terms like futile treatment and inappropriate treatment.[18] The ICMR has also given guidelines for DNR.[37]

Manipal Hospital guidelines on the limitation of LST called Blue Maple were published by Salins et al.[38] Recently, AIIMS has developed a document for recognizing medical futility, palliative care initialization, family consensus and withholding LST allowing a natural death and audit by EOL care advisory committee.[39] None of these guidelines mention AD. These guidelines have discussed withholding the LST but have not mentioned the withdrawal of LST. This may be because of avoidance of conflict with the precedent for withdrawal laid down by the common cause verdict. However, medical ethicists and medicolegal experts have confirmed that withholding and withdrawing are ethically and legally the same.[40]

The government's involvement is necessary to enable, mandate, and support EOL care through legislative and executive action. Opioids have a "double effect" in patients with terminal illnesses but are the mainstay of EOL and palliative care treatment. Getting opioids was tough before 2014 because of stringent requirements under the Narcotic Drugs and Psychotropic Substances (NDPS) Act. The amendment of the act in 2014 was a huge step forward in EOL and palliative care.[41] The registered hospitals can procure opioids with just one license from the state drug controller rather than five.

World Health Organization recommends that palliative care be integrated with healthcare services and can be effective only if initiated early in a terminal illness.[1] WHO also recommends access to palliative care for children (in collaboration with UNICEF). World Health Association (WHA) insists that its member states should improve palliative care as a core component of health systems with an emphasis on primary health care and community/home-based care.

LAW COMMISSION OF INDIA REPORT

The 42nd Law Commission Report recommended that Section 309 be repealed, and an amendment bill was introduced in the Lok Sabha in 1978.[42] This bill could not be passed as the Lok Sabha was dissolved. In 2006, the Law Commission, in its 196th report, recommended the legalization of passive euthanasia.[43] It suggested having a law to protect terminally ill patients who refuse medical treatment, artificial nutrition, or hydration from Section 309C of the IPC and to protect doctors from Section 306 IPC. It suggested the law be termed "the Medical Treatment of Terminally Ill Patients (Protection of Patients and Terminally Ill Patients) Act". The report clearly defined competent patient, informed consent, and best interests. It recommended that treating doctors must only withdraw or withhold treatment if the opinion of three medical practitioners has been obtained.

In 2016 the "Medical Treatment of Terminally Ill Patients" bill was introduced in the Lok Sabha but is yet to be passed as legislation.[30] The bill must be relooked completely before being represented to the parliament.

RECENT JUDGMENT

The common cause verdict 2018 has given a process of execution of AD, which is very time-consuming and impractical. A constitutional bench of the Supreme Court issued guidelines in January, 2023 to simplify the execution of a living will.[44] Instead of attestation by a judicial magistrate, the AD can be signed by the executor in the presence of two independent witnesses and attested by a notary or a gazette officer. The executor may incorporate this AD as a part of digital health records, if any. The process of withholding the treatment has been made two-tier instead of three-tier. The hospital will constitute a primary medical board consisting primary physician and at least two physicians with at least 5-year experience who will visit the patient in the presence of their relatives and form an opinion within 48 hours regarding withholding of treatment. The hospital will then notify a secondary board comprising one medical practitioner nominated by the district's CMO and at least two subject experts with at least 5 years of experience in the specialty who were not part of the primary board. The secondary board shall have to give an opinion in 48 hours. The hospital must inform the first-class judicial magistrate in contrast to previous guidelines where authorization by the magistrate was necessary **(Flowchart 1)**.

The Supreme Court reiterated that these guidelines are valid until the parliament passes legislation.

Flowchart 1: Supreme Court's legal guidelines for a decision to withdraw or withhold treatment.

```
┌─────────────────────────────────────────────────────────────┐
│ Patients with terminal illness who are not competent to take│
│ decision and treatment is not going to improve the outcome  │
└─────────────────────────────────────────────────────────────┘
                              ↓
┌─────────────────────────────────────────────────────────────┐
│ Treating team decides that further life-sustaining treatment│
│ (LST) would not be beneficial to the patient                │
└─────────────────────────────────────────────────────────────┘
                              ↓
┌─────────────────────────────────────────────────────────────┐
│ Primary Medical Board (PMB):                                │
│ • Treating physician and two subject experts (≥5 years'     │
│   experience)                                               │
│ • Visit patient and family/surrogate                        │
│ • Certify to withdraw/withhold treatment (within 48 hours)  │
└─────────────────────────────────────────────────────────────┘
         Yes                              No
          ↓                                ↓
┌──────────────────────────────┐  ┌──────────────────────────┐
│ Secondary Medical Board (SMB)│  │ If PMB/SMB does NOT      │
│ • One district chief medical │  │ concur with treating     │
│   officer                    │  │ team, the aggrieved      │
│ • Two subject experts (≥5    │  │ family or the treating   │
│   years' experience) not part│——│ team or the hospital     │
│   of the PMB            No   │  │ may approach the         │
│ Certify to withdraw/withhold │  │ High Court               │
│ treatment (within 48 hours)  │  │                          │
└──────────────────────────────┘  └──────────────────────────┘
         Yes
          ↓
┌──────────────────────────────┐
│ Hospital shall record and    │
│ intimate the Judicial        │
│ Magistrate, AND treating     │
│ team shall implement the     │
│ decision to withdraw/withhold│
│ LST                          │
└──────────────────────────────┘
```

■ CONCLUSION

A comprehensible legal framework for EOL should be there in the country for all ethical decision-making and strict adherence. Guidelines for the hierarchy of surrogates must be established. Healthcare professionals must be well versed in EOL decision-making and empowered with good communication skills. Society must be aware of AD, and each institute or hospital must have EOL committees. EOL and palliative care must be covered under health insurance schemes.

■ REFERENCES

1. World Health Organization. (2020). Palliative care. [online] Available from: https://www.who.int/news-room/fact-sheets/detail/palliative-care [Last accessed September, 2023].
2. Bag S, Mohanty S, Deep N, Salins N, Bag S. Palliative and end of life care in India - Current scenario and the way forward. J Assoc Physicians India. 2020;68:61-5.
3. Mani RK. Limitation of life support in the ICU: Ethical issues relating to end of life care. Indian J Crit Care Med. 2003;7.

4. Beauchamp TL, Childress JF. Principles of Biomedical Ethics, 7th edition. Oxford: Oxford University Press; 2013. pp. 63-335.
5. Mishra A, Galhotra A. Mental Healthcare Act 2017: Need to wait and watch. Int J Appl Basic Med Res. 2018;8:67-70.
6. Gera A, Sharma B, Sood J. Legal issues in end-of-life care: Current status in India and the road ahead. Curr Med Res Pract. 2023;13:32-9.
7. UK Parliament. (1994). Medical Ethics: Select Committee Report. [online] Available from: https://api.parliament.uk/historic-hansard/lords/1994/may/09/medical-ethics-select-committee-report [Last accessed September, 2023].
8. Great Britain House of Lords. Airedale NHS Trust vs. Bland. All Engl Law Rep. 1993;1:821-96.
9. Economist Intelligence Unit. The 2015 Quality of Death Index: Ranking palliative care across the world. [online] Available from: https://impact.economist.com/perspectives/sites/default/files/2015%20EIU%20Quality%20of%20Death%20Index%20Oct%2029%20FINAL.pdf [Last accessed September, 2023].
10. Sleeman KE, Timms A, Gillam J, Anderson JE, Harding R, Sampson EL, et al. Priorities and opportunities for palliative and end of life care in United Kingdom Health Policies: A national documentary analysis. BMC Palliat Care. 2021;20:108.
11. Legislation.gov.uk. Health and Care Act 2022. [online] Available from: https://www.legislation.gov.uk/ukpga/2022/31/contents/enacted [Last accessed September, 2023].
12. Kennedy IM. The Karen Quinlan case: problems and proposals. J Med Ethics. 1976;2:3-7.
13. JUSTIA US Supreme Court. Cruzan v. Director, Missouri Dep't of Health, 497 U.S. 261 (1990). [online] Available from: https://supreme.justia.com/cases/federal/us/497/261/ [Last accessed September, 2023].
14. Dzeng E, Bein T, Curtis JR. The role of policy and law in shaping the ethics and quality of end-of-life care in intensive care. Intensive Care Med. 2022;48:352-4.
15. Lee YJ, Ahn S, Cho JY, Park TY, Yun SY, Kim J, et al. Change in perception of the quality of death in the intensive care unit by healthcare workers associated with the implementation of the "well-dying law". Intensive Care Med. 2022;48:281-9.
16. Blythe JA, Kentish-Barnes N, Debue AS, Dohan D, Azoulay E, Covinsky K, et al. An interprofessional process for the limitation of life-sustaining treatments at the end of life in France. J Pain Symptom Manage. 2022;63:160-70.
17. Ministry of Health and Family Welfare, Government of India. (2014). Transplantation of Human Organs Acts and Rules. [online] Available from: https://main.mohfw.gov.in/sites/default/files/THOA-amendment-2011%20%281%29.pdf [Last accessed September, 2023].
18. Salins N, Gursahani R, Mathur R, Iyer S, Macaden S, Simha N, et al. Definition of terms used in limitation of treatment and providing palliative care at the end of life: The Indian Council of medical research commission report. Indian J Crit Care Med. 2018;22:249-62.
19. Indian Kanoon. Indian Penal Code; Section 309; 1860. [online] Available from: https://indiankanoon.org/doc/1501595/#:~:text=309.,fine%2C%20or%20with%20both%5D [Last accessed September, 2023].
20. National Institute of Health and Family Welfare. The Indian Medical Council Act, 1956 (Professional Conduct & Ethics) Regulations, 2002. [online] Available from: http://www.nihfw.org/Legislations/THEINDIANMEDICALCOUNCILACT_1956.html [Last accessed September, 2023].

21. Herring J. Medical Law and Ethics, 4th edition. United Kingdom: Oxford University Press; 2012
22. Legislative Department, Ministry of Law and Justice, Government of India. The Constitution of India. 2020. [online] Available from: https://legislative.gov.in/constitution-of-india/ [Last accessed September, 2023].
23. Indian Kanoon. Maruti Shripati Dubal vs. State of Maharashtra; 1987.BomCR499; 1986,88.BOMLR589. [online]. Available from: https://indiankanoon.org/doc/490515/ [Last accessed September, 2023].
24. Indian Kanoon. P. Rathinam vs Union Of India on 26 April, 1994; 1994 AIR 1844, 1994 SCC (3) 394. [online] Available from: https://indiankanoon.org/doc/542988/ [Last accessed September, 2023].
25. Indian Kanoon. Naresh Marotrao Sakhre And ... vs Union Of India And Others on 17 August, 1994: 1996 (1) BomCR 92, 1995 CriLJ 96, 1994 (2) MhLj 1850. [online] Available from: https://indiankanoon.org/doc/1453319/ [Last accessed September, 2023].
26. Indian Kanoon. Smt. Gian Kaur vs The State Of Punjab. 1996 AIR 946, 1996 SCC(2) 648. [online] Available from: https://indiankanoon.org/doc/217501/ [Last accessed September, 2023].
27. Indian Kanoon. Section 300 in The Indian Penal Code. [online] Available from: https://indiankanoon.org/doc/626019/ [Last accessed on September, 2023].
28. Aruna Ramakrishna Shanbaugh vs. The Union of India and Ors; 2011 4 SCC 454 & 524. Also: AIR 2011 SC 1290. [online] Available from: https://indiankanoon.org/doc/235821/ [Last accessed September, 2023].
29. Indian Kanoon. Common Cause (A Regd. Society) vs. Union of India & Ors.,(2008)5 SCC 511. [online] Available from: https://indiankanoon.org/doc/184449972 [Last accessed September, 2023].
30. The Treatment of Terminally-Ill Patients Bill, 2016. [online] Available from: http://164.100.47.4/billstexts/lsbilltexts/asintroduced/2656.pdf [Last accessed September, 2023].
31. Indian Kanoon. (2012). 241st report on passive euthanasia—a relook. [online] Available from: https://indiankanoon.org/docfragment/133438875/?big=3&formInput=law%20commission [Last accessed September, 2023].
32. HUDOC. Pretty v. the United Kingdom - 2346/02. Judgment 29.4.2002 [Section IV]. Article 2. [online] Available from: https://hudoc.echr.coe.int/fre#{%22itemid%22:[%22002-5380%22]} [Last accessed September, 2023].
33. European Convention on Human Rights - European Court of Human Rights. [online] Available from: https://www.echr.coe.int/documents/d/echr/Convention_ENG [Last accessed September, 2023].
34. Vidhi Centre for Legal Policy. (2021). End of Life Care in India. Available from: https://vidhilegalpolicy.in/wp-content/uploads/2021/02/Model-End-of-Life-Care-Bill_Version-2.0.pdf [Last accessed September, 2023].
35. Mani RK, Amin P, Chawla R, Divatia JV, Kapadia F, Khilnani P, et al. Guidelines for end-of-life and palliative care in Indian intensive care units: ISCCM consensus ethical position statement. Indian J Crit Care Med. 2012;16:166-81.
36. Myatra SN, Salins N, Iyer S, Macaden SC, Divatia JV, Muckaden M, et al. End-of-life care policy: An integrated care plan for the dying: A Joint Position Statement of the Indian Society of Critical Care Medicine (ISCCM) and the Indian Association of Palliative Care (IAPC). Indian J Crit Care. Med. 2014; 18:615-35.

37. Mathur R. ICMR Consensus Guidelines on 'Do Not Attempt Resuscitation'. Indian J Med Res. 2020;151:303-10.
38. Pallium India. BLUE MAPLE End of Life Care 2021. [online] Available from: htttps://palliumindia.org/wp-content/uploads/2021/10/BLUE-MAPLE-End-of-Life-Care-Manipal.pdf [Last accessed September, 2023].
39. Guidelines for End of Life Care, AIIMS - All India Institute of Medical Science. [online] Available from: https://www.aiims.edu/images/pdf/notice/irch-9-3-20.pdf. [Last accessed September, 2023].
40. End of Life Care - The legal Framework. In: Nandimath OV, Thomas A, Arptha HC,1st ed. Health Law and Ethics: Critical Reflections. Gurgaon: Thomson Reuters South Asia Pvt. Ltd.; 2022:293.
41. The Narcotic Drugs and Psychotropic Substances Act, 1985 arrangement. [online] Available from: https://www.narcoticsindia.nic.in/legislation/ndpsact.pdf [Last accessed September, 2023].
42. Criminal Law Reforms. (1971). 42nd Report on Indian Penal Code. [online] Available from: https://cdnbbsr.s3waas.gov.in/s3ca0daec69b5adc880fb464895726dbdf/uploads/2022/08/2022082456.pdf [Last accessed September, 2023].
43. Medical Treatment of Terminally Ill Patients (For the Protection of Patients and Medical Practitioners) 196th Report of Law Commission of India; 2006. [online] Available from: http://www.commonlii.org/in/other/lawreform/INLC/2006/2.html [Last accessed September, 2023].
44. Mani RK, Simha S, Gursahani R. Simplified Legal Procedure for End-of-life Decisions in India: A New Dawn in the Care of the Dying? Indian J Crit Care Med. 2023;27:374-6.

Index

Page numbers followed by *b* refer to box, *f* refer to figure, *fc* refer to flowchart, and *t* refer to table

A

Aberrant stress response 321
Accidental dural puncture 67
Acetylcholine 321
Actinomycin 355
Activated clotting time 275
Activated partial thromboplastin time 275
Acute coronary syndrome 23, 81, 255, 268, 302
Acute kidney disease 241
    outcomes of 254
Acute kidney injury 83, 86, 241-243, 250
    outcomes of 254
    pathophysiology of 244
    risk factors for 86*t*
    staging of 243*t*
Acute liver disease 219
Acute liver failure 216, 221*t*
    management of 220
    pathophysiology of 220
    prognosis of 219
Acute lung injury 22
Acute Physiologic and Chronic Health Evaluation Score 279
Acute respiratory distress syndrome 298, 303
Adequate alpha-receptor blockade 136
Adjuvant therapy 366
Adult respiratory distress syndrome 24
Advanced cardiac life support 113
Aerospace medicine 177
Airway 200
    assessment 1
        ultrasound for 1
    equipment 106
    management 1, 174*t*
    problems 111
    ultrasound assessment 1
Alanine transaminase 224
Alcohol 263
    hepatitis 222
    withdrawal 327
Alfentanil 407
Alkaline phosphatase 224
Alpha glycoprotein inhibitors 355
Alpha-blockers 134

Alzheimer's disease 77
American Society of Anesthesiologists 71, 86, 384
    classification system 75*t*
American Society of Regional Anesthesia and Pain Medicine 267, 275
Aminoglycosides 246
Amitriptyline 138
Amlodipine 134
Amphetamine 138
Anaesthetist's non-technical skills framework 388, 394*t*
    elements of 391*f*
Analgesia 30
    labor 68, 68*t*
    nociception index monitoring 337
    postoperative 52
Analgesics 406*f*
    dose of 331
Anesthesia 68*t*, 130, 175*t*, 200, 216, 241, 388
    epidural 57
    field of 151
    general 57, 88, 104*f*, 137, 173-175
    hypotensive 105*f*
    induction 140
    intravenous 118
    low-flow 400
    machine 400
    management 71, 137, 200, 210
    monitoring, depth of 108
    neuraxial 267
    pediatric 183
    peripheral regional 270
    regional 30, 88, 175, 267, 268
    spinal 57, 59*f*, 83*fc*
    surgical 68
    techniques 57
    total intravenous 117, 124*f*, 127, 162, 174
    workstations 400, 401
Anesthesiology 390
    minimal monitoring standards for 155
Anesthetic
    agents, pharmacology of 157
    considerations 77*b*, 101
    drugs 104, 232
        reduced consumption of 405

Index

equipment 106
  management 231
  techniques 109
Anesthetist non-technical skills system 390*f*
Angiotensin-receptor blocker 247
Anterior superior iliac spine 102*f*
Anticholinergic drugs 320
Anticoagulation 267, 268, 308*t*
  management of 307
  monitoring of 307
Anti-factor Xa agents 272
Antifibrinolytic agents 110
Antiplatelet therapy 81
Antisialagogue administration 183
Antithrombotic drug withdrawal 271
Antithrombotic therapy, management of 274
Anxiolysis 183
Apixaban 272
Aprotinin 110
Arrhythmias, management of 142
Arterial blood gas analysis 26
Arterial oxygen, partial pressure of 289, 298, 303
Artificial intelligence 178, 331, 339
  based closed-loop systems 404
Artificial lung 299
Artificial manual breathing unit bag 107
Arytenoid cartilages 6*f*
Aspartate transaminase 224
Aspiration 22
Atelectasis 213
Atenolol 134
Atracurium 138, 264
Atrial fibrillation 268
Autologous donation, preoperative 109
Automated gas control 403
Autonomic nervous system 333, 337

B

Baker classification 402, 402*t*
Barbiturates 355
Basic vital parameters 331
Benzodiazepine 158, 233, 320
  antidote 157
Beta-adrenergic blockade 134
Beta-blockers 134
  nonspecific 227
Biochemical investigations 132
Biochemical tests 132
Biomarkers 247
Bispectral index 108
Bleeding 82
  blocks, high-risk 275*t*
  complications, severe 270

Blood 366
  brain barrier 321
  clots, embolisms of 112
  conservation strategies 97, 109
  loss 105*f*
  pressure 136
    control, pharmacological preparation for 133
    systolic 289
  tests 26
  transfusion 241, 320
Body mass index 86, 227, 407
Bone demineralization 165
Brachial plexus 101*f*, 112
Bristol model 123
Bristol regimen 117
Bronchospasm 213
B-type natriuretic peptide 71
Budd-Chiari syndrome 220, 222, 225
Bupivacaine 68

C

Calcium channel blockers 133-135
Cancer 366, 367
  care 370, 373
    intention-action gap in 371*f*
  recurrence 372, 373
  surgery 370
  therapy options 368
  treatment 366-368
    goals of 368
Cannabis 261
Cannulation
  challenges of 310
  potential complications of 310
Capnography 151
Carbamazepine 355
Carbon dioxide 298
  absorption 207
  partial pressure of 300
  production 299
Cardiac catheterization 301
Cardiac complications 79
Cardiac index 101
Cardiac myocytes 26
Cardiomyopathy, types of 135
Cardiovascular collapse 172
Cardiovascular system 205
Catecholamine
  release 138
  secreting neuroendocrine tumors 131
  synthesis inhibitor 134

Catheter
  breakage of 66
  kinking of 66
  over-the-needle set 62, 63, 63*f*
Cauda equina syndrome 60, 65, 66, 68
Cell division, errors of 368
Central nervous system 206, 320, 333
Cerebral edema 221
Cerebral vascular accident 75
Cerebrospinal fluid 321
Chemoradiotherapy 384
Chemotherapy 366
  neoadjuvant 384
Chest
  compression techniques 176
  X-ray 25, 25*f*
Child-Turcotte-Pugh score 228
Chloral hydrate 190
  use of 118
Chlorpromazine 138, 355
Cholecystectomy 45
Chromaffin tissue 130
Chronic kidney disease 76*b*
Chronic liver disease 216, 217, 222, 224, 227, 231
  clinical manifestations of 223
  etiology of 222*t*
  laboratory tests of 224*b*
  signs of 224*b*
  symptoms of 224*b*
Chronic obstructive pulmonary disease 77, 86
Chronic vasoconstriction, catecholamine induced 139
Ciprofloxacin 355
Circulatory failure 301
Cirrhosis 216, 222, 228
  uncompensated 217
Clavicle, nerve supply of 38*f*
Clavipectoral fascial plane block 37, 38*f*, 39*f*
Clinical decision support system 392
Clinical frailty scale 74*t*
Clinically significant portal hypertension, diagnosis of 226
Clonidine 183, 186
Clopidogrel 81
Closed-loop system 117
Coagulation 227
  cascade, multiple therapeutic targets of 80*fc*
Cobb angle 114
Cocaine 138
Cognitive impairment 77, 320
Colorectal liver metastases 366

Commercial spaceflight operations 177
Communication 392
Compartment syndrome 175, 213
Computerized tomography scan 25
Concentration 121*f*
Conox monitoring 333, 337
Consciousness, disturbance of 322
Continuous positive airway pressure 16
Continuous spinal anesthesia 57, 65*b*, 67
  advantages of 60*b*
  clinical indications of 67*t*
  complications of 57
  technique of 64
Coronavirus disease 2019 (COVID-19) 298
  infection 78
Corticosteroids 320
C-reactive protein, peripheral 321
Creatinine clearance 275
Cricoid cartilage 7*f*
Cricothyroid membrane 1, 2, 7*f*
Cricothyrotomy, evaluation for 11
Crystalloids, large volumes of 105*f*
Cyclooxygenase 194

D

Da Vinci surgical robot 202*f*
Damage control philosophy 167
Death index, quality of 413
Decompression surgeries 100
Deep learning 341
Deep posterior gluteal compartment block 51, 53*f*
Deep venous thrombosis 80
Dehydroepiandrosterone 166
Delirium 318, 327
  diagnosis of 323*t*
  features of 322
  hyperactive 318
  pathophysiology of 320
  postoperative 87, 87*t*
  prevention, nonpharmacological methods of 326*t*
Dementia 77
Desflurane 138, 407
Dexmedetomidine 183, 187
Diabetes mellitus 75
Dialysis 76
  general guidelines for 77
Diamorphine 183, 189
Diarrhea, *Clostridium difficile*-associated 312
Diazepam 139

Difficult airway
  assessment of 8
  evaluation 9
Digital health technologies,
    integration of 408
Diisopropylphenol 119
Diltiazem 134
Direct oral anticoagulation therapy 83fc, 272
Direct thrombin inhibitor 275
Disease-specific scoring systems 290
Disseminated intravascular coagulation 75
Disuse atrophy 166
Dopamine-2 antagonists 138
Double tract sign 10f
Doxarubecin 355
Doxazosin 133, 134, 138
Dräger Smartpilot view 405
Dräger workstation 406f
Droperidol 138
Drug
  addiction 260
  affecting renal function 245
  delivery
    innovations 404
    systems 404
  infusion rate of 124
  metabolism of 232
Duloxetine 138

E

Echocardiography
  findings 25
  role of 306t
E-cigarette 260
Edema
  cardiogenic pulmonary 22
  neurogenic pulmonary 22
  noncardiogenic 16
  nondependent 25f
  postextubation 16
  postobstructive pulmonary 17
  pulmonary 16
Edoxaban 272
Ejection fraction 75
Electroencephalogram-derived
    parameters 405
Electromyographic waves 333
Embolism 112
  pulmonary 268
Emphysema 264
  subcutaneous 213
Encephalopathy 216
Endobronchial intubation 213

End-of-life
  care 413, 414
  decisions 413
Endotracheal intubation 162, 173, 175f
  confirmation of 9
Endotracheal tube 2, 20, 98, 102, 103f, 107f
End-stage liver disease 216, 280
  score, model for 228, 280
End-stage renal disease 75
End-tidal carbon dioxide monitoring 154f
Enhanced gas delivery systems 401
Enhanced recovery after surgery 104f, 371f
  protocols 366
Entropy 108
  monitoring 333
Ephedrine 138
Epidural catheters 57
Epiglottis 5f
Epinephrine 143
Epsilon aminocaproic acid 110
Esmolol 143
Esophagus 10f
Estimated glomerular filtration rate 243
European Society of Anaesthesiology and
    Intensive Care 275
European Society of Regional
    Anaesthesia 275
Euthanasia 169, 413, 415, 416, 419
Excessive sedation, periods of 353
External iliac artery 49f
External oblique intercostal plane
    block 45, 46f
  sonographic image for 47f
Extracorporeal cardiopulmonary
    resuscitation 301, 302
Extracorporeal membrane oxygenation
    296-298, 301, 303
  associated bleeding 310
  components 305f
  configuration, basic 304f
  progress of 297
  support in intensive care 296
  use of 296
Extravascular compartment 16
Extubation 110

F

Facemasks 107
Facial
  anatomy 103f
  transversalis 271
Fatty liver disease, nonalcoholic 217
Federal aviation administration 177

Femoral artery 49f
Femoral neck 73, 73f
   fractures 73
Femoral vein 49f
Fentanyl 158, 190, 353, 407
Fiberoptic bronchoscopes 107
Finger with single-use sensor 344f
Fluconazole 355
Fluid
   intravenous 172
   overload 23
   redistribution 165
Flumazenil 157
Fluoxetine 355
Fluvoxamine 355
Fondaparinux 80, 272
Forearm block
   lateral cutaneous nerve of 40f, 41, 42, 42f
   medial cutaneous nerve of 39, 41f
Fractures
   extracapsular 73, 73f
   intracapsular 73, 73f
   repair 71
   types of 72
Frailty 71, 73
Fresh gas flow 402
   Baker classification of 402t
Functional residual capacity 101
Fundoplication 45
Fungal infections 222

G

Gamma-aminobutyric acid type A 194
Gamma-glutamyl transferase 224
Gas
   embolism 213
   exchange 299, 300
Gastrectomy 45
Gastric cancer 366
Gastroesophageal reflux 162, 173
Gastrointestinal system 206
Gastroparesis 173
Gel head ring 103f
General anesthesia 57, 88, 104f, 137, 173-175
   fundamental part of 331
Genetic polymorphisms 246
Geniohyoid muscle 4f
Genitofemoral nerve
   block 47
   course of 48f
Genome-wide association 246
Glasgow coma scale 174, 280, 289
Glomerular filtration rate 86

Glucagon 138
Glucocorticoids 355
Glycemic control 253

H

H1N1 298
Halogenated inhalational agents 105
Haloperidol 138, 318, 355
Halothane 138
Harlequin syndrome 306
Headache, postdural puncture 57, 67
Healthcare interventions, sedation for 151
Heart
   disease, ischemic 353
   failure
      congestive 79
      preoperative 79
   rate 289
Hematoma 66
Hemodilution, acute normovolemic 109
Hemodynamic monitoring 305
Hemorrhage 170
   cavitary 171
   intracerebral 75
   intrathecal 66
Heparin 270
   clearance of 81t
Hepatic circulations 232
Hepatic cytochrome p450 system, enzyme reactions of 232
Hepatic dysfunction 264
Hepatic lobule 218f
Hepatic resection 45
Hepatitis C virus 216
Hepatobiliary disease 216, 229
Hepatopulmonary syndrome 225
Hepatorenal syndrome 223
Hip
   fracture 71, 81, 86, 87t
      anticoagulant use in 82
      repair 83fc
      surgery 87t
   joint 53f
   surgery 52
Holmes-Adie syndromes 337
Horner's syndrome 36, 337
Hydromorphone 353
Hyoid bone 4f
Hyomental distance 4f
Hyperalgesia, opioids induced 333
Hypercarbia 213
Hyperkalemia 172

Index

Hypertension 75, 131
    management of 142
    portal 216, 225, 227
    pulmonary 302
Hypnosis, depth of 333
Hypnotics 406f, 407
Hypotension 88, 89, 89t, 213
    management of 143
Hypothermia, severe 302
Hypoxia 213

I

Ibuprofen 185
Ideal scoring system, desired
    characteristics of 290
Immune deficits 166
Infections 66, 78, 311
    bacterial 222
    viral 78, 222
Inflammatory response 245
Inhalational agents 138, 140
Injury, neurological 111
Inspired oxygen, fraction of 289, 303
Integrated decision support systems 408
Integrated Dräger Smartpilot view 406f
Intensive care 318
    delirium screening checklist 318
    unit 280, 283, 296, 318, 320, 413
    length of 279
Intention-action gap, concept of 370f
Interfascial plane blocks 30
Interleukin-18 250
Intermittent positive pressure
    ventilation 101
Intra-abdominal pressure 205
Intracranial pressure 165f
Intraoperative analgesic therapy,
    backbone of 333
Intraoperative bronchospasm,
    high risk of 260
Intraoperative cell salvage 109
Intraoperative hemodynamic
    control 143t
    disturbances 333
    response 142
Intrathecal catheter 57
Intravascular volume optimization 136
Intravenous fluids 172
    transfusion of 172
Intubation, difficult 1
Involuntary euthanasia 415
Isoflurane 407
Isolation 167

J

Joint capsule 73f

K

Kataria model 117
Ketamine 138, 183, 188
Kidney Disease Improving Global
    Outcomes
    bundle 253
    group 242
Kidney
    disease 76
        acute 241
        chronic 76b
    failure 355
    injury 83, 86, 241-243, 250
    normal physiology of 244
Kupffer cells 218

L

Labetalol 143
Laparoscopic retroperitoneoscopic
    approach 137f
Laparoscopic surgery 200, 201b, 204
Laparoscopic transabdominal
    approach 136f
Laryngeal edema assessment 10
Laryngeal mask airway 107f, 174
Laryngoscopy, difficult 1
Laryngospasm 16
Levopromazine 355
Lewy bodies 321
Limbic-hypothalamic-pituitary-adrenal
    axis 321
Liver
    cirrhosis 216
    disease 219, 223, 233
        acute 219
        chronic 216, 217, 222, 224, 227, 231
        end-stage 216, 280
    failure 355
        acute 216, 221t
        acute-on-chronic 217, 221, 222t
    function, rapid deterioration of 216
    sinusoidal endothelial cells 218
    transplantation 216
Logistic organ dysfunction
    score 280, 288, 289
Long-acting oral benzodiazepines 139
Lorazepam 139
Low-molecular-weight heparin 81, 275

Index

Lumbar
  plexus 271
  sympathectomy 271
Lung
  injury, acute 22
  point-of-care ultrasound of 24
  transplant 303
Lymph systems 366

M

Machine learning 331, 340
Macrolides 355
Magnesium sulfate 143
Marsh model 117, 123
Massive pulmonary embolism 302
Mean arterial pressure 111, 113, 289
Meconium aspiration syndrome 297
Melatonin 191
Membrane
  lung 299
  oxygenator 299, 305f
Mental health 167
  Act 415
Metabolic fresh gas flow 401
Metabolism 307
Methadone 352, 355t
  advantages 360
  history of 354
  interesting alternative 354
  major concerns 357
  pharmacokinetic properties of 355t
  pharmacology of 354
Metoclopramide 138
Metoprolol 134
Metyrosine 134
Microcatheters 57
Microcirculatory dysfunction 245
Microgravity, anesthesia in 162
Microporous hollow fibers 299
Microvascular thrombi, formation of 245
Midazolam 157, 183, 186
Minimally invasive surgery 169, 200, 366
Minto model 117, 124
Mivacurium 407
Modern anesthesia workstation, advanced features in 400
Monoamine oxidase inhibitors 138
Morphine 138, 188, 353
  pharmacokinetic properties of 355t
Mortality
  causes of 78
  long-term causes of 79
  prediction model 284
  probability model 280, 285
    score 279
  rates 74t
Motor-evoked potential 106, 106f
Multicomponent interventions 318
Multifaceted complex syndrome 255
Multiple logistic regression 285, 289
Multiple organ dysfunction
    score 280, 287, 289
Muscle
  atrophy of 172
  relaxant 173, 407
Myelopathy 100
Mylohyoid 4f
Myocardial function
  assessment of 135
  optimization of 135
Myocardial infarction 75, 301
Myocarditis 302

N

Naloxone infusion 352
Narcotic abstinence syndrome 260, 262
National Aeronautics and Space Administration 162
National Transport and Safety Board 177
Near-infrared spectroscopy 108
Negative pressure pulmonary
  edema 16, 19
    causes of 20t
  hemorrhage 19
Neoadjuvant therapy 366
Nephropathy, contrast-induced 246
Nephrotoxins 241
Nerve
  blocks 200
  pressure injury of 200
Neural integrity monitor 101f
Neural network 341
Neuraxial block 162, 175
Neuroinflammation 320
Neurologic damage 269
Neurological deficits 111
Neuromuscular agents 264
Neuromuscular blockers 138
  agents 141, 162, 172
Neuromuscular junctions 172
Neurotransmitter abnormalities 321
Neurovascular bundle 50f
Neutrophil gelatinase-associated lipocalin 250
Nicardipine 134
Nicotine 260, 264

Nifedipine 134
Nitroglycerin 143
Nitrous oxide 105
N-methyl-D-aspartate 194
  antagonist 352
Nociception level index 333
  monitor 342, 344f
Nociceptive flexor reflex 333, 339
Nonoperating room
  anesthesia 162
  sedation 152b
Nonopioid techniques 105f
Nonpharmacological prevention 318, 325
Nonsteroidal anti-inflammatory drugs 353
  inhibit cyclooxygenase enzymes 246
Nontechnical skills
  evaluation for 394
  performance of 394
Nonvoluntary euthanasia 416
Norepinephrine 143
Normal gas exchange physiology 298
North-south syndrome 306
Nursing
  activity score 280, 290
  manpower use score, nine equivalents of 280, 289

O

Objective pain monitoring 331, 333, 334t
Obstructive sleep apnea 16, 17
Olanzapine 138
Oliguria 353
Oncologic therapy 366, 368
Ophthalmic system 207
Opioids 105f, 106, 320
  analgesics 138
  shorter-acting 353
  use disorders 262
Oral space domain 9
Organ dysfunction scores 286
  comparison of 289t
Outcome prediction scores 281
Oxygen
  blender 305f
  carrying capacity 299
  consumption per minute, amount of 298
  delivery devices 154f

P

Paddles, anterior-posterior placement of 114
Pain 52, 332
  acute postoperative 333
  chronic postoperative 333

postoperative 200
  management of 212
Pancuronium 138, 407
Paracetamol 185, 264, 353
Paraneoplastic syndromes 325
Parasternal intercostal block 42, 43f-45f
Parkinson's disease 320, 321
Paroxetine 355
Passive euthanasia 416
Peak airway pressure 200
Pelvic fracture repair 51
Peptide hormones 138
Percutaneous tracheostomy,
  evaluation for 11
Perfusion pressure 105f
Perianal surgeries 51
Pericapsular nerve group 271
Perioperative pain, methadone for 352
Peripheral nerve blocks 270, 353
Peripheral nervous system injury 112
Peripheral oxygen saturation 156
Periprocedural support 301
Persistent ventricular arrhythmia storm 302
Pethidine 138
Pharmacokinetic 121, 122
Pharmacological preoperative blockade
  against 133
Pharmacological sedative agents 151
Pharmacology 157
Phenelzine 138
Phenoxybenzamine 134, 138
  efficacy of 133
Phentermine 138
Phentolamine 143
Phenylephrine 143
Phenytoin 355
Pheochromocytoma 130, 131, 138t, 144
  contemporary perioperative
    management of 130
  diagnosis of 132
  incidental 145
  preoperative preparation of 134t
  principles of 130
Plasma 123
  binding 355
  concentration 124
Plasminogen activation 83
Platelet membrane phospholipid 80
Plethysmography-based monitoring 338
Pneumomediastinum 213
Pneumonia, ventilator-associated 312
Pneumopericardium 213
Pneumoperitoneum 200, 204, 211
  physiological effects of 205

Pneumothorax 170, 213
Point-of-care ultrasound approach 12
Polypharmacy 247
Polyvinyl chloride 304
Portal hypertension 216, 225, 227
    causes of 225
    classification of 225
    management of 226
    pathophysiology of 226
Positive end-expiratory pressure 19
    use of 101
Postcardiac transplant 302
Posterior hip after surgery 52
Postextubation emergency 21
Prazosin 133, 134
Pregnancy 144
Preinduction 138
Pressure
    injury 204
    ulcer-associated infections 312
Prophylaxis 268
Propofol 106, 121f, 407
    infusion syndrome 120, 125
Propranolol 134
Prothrombin
    complex concentrate 82
    time 224
Proto-oncogenes 367
Pseudomonas aeruginosa 312
Psoas compartment 271
Pudendal nerve block 49, 50f
Pulmonary edema 16
    pathophysiology of 19fc
Pulmonary function test 99
Pupillary diseases 337
Pupillometry 333, 337

Q

qNOX Index 337
QT prolongation 352, 353, 358
Quadratus lumborum 271

R

Radiation, higher doses of 166
Radiculopathy 100
Radiotherapy 366
Rapid sequence intubation 174
Red blood cells 165f
Regional anesthesia 30, 88, 175, 267, 268
    advances in 30
    hazards 162
    techniques 30

Remifentanil 117, 407
    pharmacokinetics of 233
Remimazolam 158
Renal complications 85
Renal disease, end-stage 75
Renal function, intraoperative
        maintenance of 251
Renal hypoperfusion 244
Renal involvement 310
Renal perfusion, intraoperative
        maintenance of 251
Renal replacement therapy 254
    modality of 254
Renal resistive index 86, 87t
Renal system 206
Respiratory depression 352, 357
    apprehension of 352
    postoperative 333
Respiratory distress syndrome 206
Respiratory failure 301
Respiratory system 205
Response entropy index 333
Resuscitation,
        cardiopulmonary 162, 176, 303
Return to intended oncologic therapy 366,
    371, 373, 374t
Ribonucleic acid 250
Right ventricle 298
Rivaroxaban 272
Robotic interventions 178
Robotic laparoscopic surgery 200, 212, 213t
Robotic procedures, prerequisites for 208
Robotic surgery 200, 208
Robotic system 202, 203f
    concerns of 203
Rocuronium 407

S

Sacral multifidus plane block 51, 52f
Sacral plexus 271
Sacral spine surgery 51
Schneider model 124
Scoliosis 100, 101f
    anesthesia for 97
    correction 99
Scoring systems 227, 279-281
Seamless surgical experience 400
Sedation 151
    outside operating room 152
Sedative agents, pharmacology of 157
Selective trunk block 36
Sepsis 78, 83, 311

Sequential organ
    dysfunction score 289
    failure assessment score 279, 280
Serotonin
    reuptake inhibitors 138
    syndrome 353, 358
Sertraline 355
Serum creatinine concentration,
        elevation of 242
Severe acute respiratory distress
        syndrome 298
Severe clinical syndrome 217, 221
Sevoflurane 407
Shock
    cardiogenic 302
    postcardiotomy 302
    septic 78
Sibutramine 138
Simplified acute physiology score 279, 280,
        283, 285
Single-shot spinal anesthesia 57
Sinusoidal channels direct blood flow 218
Sinusoidal obstruction syndrome 222
Skin conductance 333, 338
Small bowel resection 45
Society for Intravenous Anaesthesia 117
Sodium nitroprusside 143
Somatosensory evoked potential 106f
Sonography 9
Sphenopalatine ganglion block 31, 32f, 33f
Spinal anesthesia 57, 59f, 83fc
Spinal catheter 57
Spinal reflex-based monitoring 333, 339
Spine
    specific assessment 99
    surgery 97, 101, 107f, 109
        anesthesia for 97
Splanchnic circulations 232
Stacked Venn diagram 164f
Standard epidural macrocatheters
        sets 62, 62f
State entropy index 333
Stomach neoplasms 366
Strap muscle 5f, 6f
Stressors 164
Substance abuse 260
    chronic 260
    prevalence of 260, 261
    screening for 262
Succinylcholine 138, 172
Sufentanil 353, 407
Superior trunk block 33
Supraclavicular fossa 36f
Supraclavicular nerves 35f

Surgery 372
    nonhepatic 229
    superficial 39, 41
Surgical oncology 366
Surgical pleth index 333, 338
Surgical site infections 384
Surrogate's consent 415
Sympathetic crashing acute pulmonary
        edema 23
Systemic inflammatory response
        syndrome 290

T

Takotsubo cardiomyopathy 17
Takotsubo syndrome 23
Target plasma concentration 124
Target-controlled infusion 117, 118, 124f, 125
Telemedicine technology 176
Terazosin 133, 134
Therapeutic intervention scoring
        system 280, 288
Thienopyridine 274
Thiopental 233, 355
Thoracic cage 114
Thoracic spine 100
    surgeries, anterior approach for 110
Thoracoscopic surgery, video-assisted 100
Thoracotomy 100
Thorax 271
Three-compartment model 117, 122f
Thrombin time 275
Thyroid cartilage 6f, 7f
Ticagrelor 81
Tissue
    factor 80
    pressure injury of 200
Total intravenous anesthesia 117, 124f, 127,
        162, 174
    benefits of 119
    disadvantages of 120
    fifteen rules for 125
    outside operating room 127
Touchscreen interfaces 410
Trachea 10f
Tracheal cartilage 7f
Tracheal intubation 140
Tranexamic acid 67, 71, 83, 110
Transducer, position of 43f
Transesophageal echocardiography 140
Transient ischemic attack 75
Transjugular intrahepatic portosystemic
        shunt 227
Transplantation of Human Organs and
        Tissues Act 418

Transverse foramen 35*f*
Transversus thoracic plane block 42
Traumatic spine fractures, surgeries for 100
Tricyclic antidepressants 78, 138
Tumor necrosis factor-alpha 320
Tumor suppressor genes 367
Typical total intravenous anesthesia set connector 126*f*

U

Ulnar nerve 112
Ultrashort-acting barbiturate 233
Ultrasonography 53*f*
Unfractionated heparin 271, 275
Upper abdominal surgeries 45
Upper airway
  obstruction 16, 19
  ultrasound anatomy of 3
Upper limb 271
Upper respiratory tract infection 165*f*
Urinary retention 353
  postoperative 333
Urogenital procedures 51

V

Vanlafaxine 355
Vascular complications 80
Vasoconstrictors 143
Vasodilators 143
Vasopressin 143
Vecuronium 407

Venoarterial extracorporeal membrane oxygenation 300
Venous air embolism 112
Venous thromboembolism 80, 275
  treatment for 268
Venovenous extracorporeal membrane oxygenation 300
Ventilation
  perfusion mismatch 19
  strategies 211
Verapamil 134
Vertebral canal hematoma 267, 269*t*
  risk of 82, 267
Videolaryngoscopes 107, 107*f*
Vinblastine 355
Visual loss, postoperative 105*f*
Vital organ 216
Vitamin K antagonist 81, 82, 273, 275
Vocal cord 6*f*
VOCAL-Penn model 228
Volatile agents 407
Volatile anesthetic vaporizers 172
Voluntary euthanasia 415

W

Wernicke's encephalopathy 263
White blood cell 289

Z

Zuckerkandl organ 131